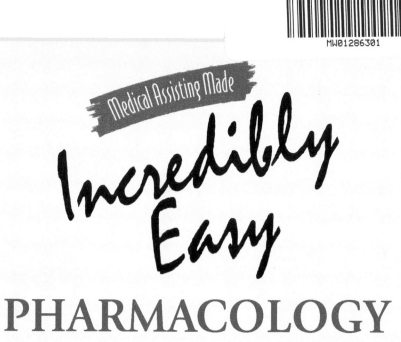

Medical Assisting Made

*Incredibly Easy*

# PHARMACOLOGY

## Joanna Holly, MSHSA, RN, CMA

Midstate College
Peoria, Illinois

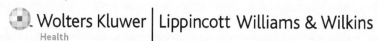
Wolters Kluwer | Lippincott Williams & Wilkins
Health

Philadelphia · Baltimore · New York · London
Buenos Aires · Hong Kong · Sydney · Tokyo

*Executive Editor:* John Goucher
*Managing Editor:* Renee Thomas
*Senior Marketing Manager:* Zhan Caplan
*Production Editor:* John Larkin
*Illustrator:* Bot Roda
*Designer:* Joan Wendt
*Compositor:* Circle Graphics

351 West Camden Street        530 Walnut Street
Baltimore, MD 21201           Philadelphia, PA 19106

Printed in Strategic Content Imaging

9  8  7  6  5  4  3

**Library of Congress Cataloging-in-Publication Data**

Holly, Joanna.
Pharmacology / Joanna Holly.
  p. ; cm.—(Medical assisting made incredibly easy)
ISBN 978-0-7817-7509-0
  1. Pharmacology—Textbooks. 2. Pharmaceutical arithmetic—Textbooks. 3. Medical assistants—Textbooks. I. Title. II. Series.
  [DNLM: 1. Pharmacology—methods—Handbooks. 2. Allied Health Personnel—Handbooks. 3. Drug Therapy—Handbooks. 4. Pharmacologic Actions—Handbooks. QV 39 H746p 2009]
  RM301.H58 2009
  615′.1—dc22

                    2008019829

## DISCLAIMER

# PREFACE

*Medical Assisting Made Incredibly Easy* is an exciting new series designed to make learning enjoyable for medical assisting students. Each book in the series uses a light-hearted, humorous approach to presenting information. Maria, a Certified Medical Assistant, guides students through the books, offering helpful tips and insight along the way.

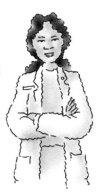

*Medical Assisting Made Incredibly Easy* takes a practical approach, providing students with the critical information that they need to know, including complete coverage of the core skills they must master in their studies. The series covers all competencies based on the standards and guidelines established for medical assisting by the Commission on Accreditation of Allied Health Educational Programs (CAAHEP) and the Accrediting Bureau of Health Education Schools (ABHES).

## About This Book

*Medical Assisting Made Incredibly Easy: Pharmacology* provides instruction in the CAAHEP and ABHES competencies that pertain to drug administration and preparation and other pharmacologic principles. These are among the skills that students must master to pass the test required to become either a Certified Medical Assistant or a Registered Medical Assistant.

## Special Features

*Medical Assisting Made Incredibly Easy: Therapeutic Communications* is designed to be enjoyable to read, as well as highly informative. Each chapter in this book includes special features designed to guide students in their study. These elements will help students identify the most important information in the chapter and to understand all of it.

- *Chapter Checklist* includes a list of skills and other important information that students will gain after reading the material.

- *Chapter Competencies* highlights the ABHES and CAAHEP competencies covered in each chapter.

- *Closer Look* explores chapter information in more detail in a list or summary form.

- *Running Smoothly* features situations that medical assistants may encounter in a medical office and shows how students can apply what they have learned to those situations.

- *Ask the Professional* offers expert advice on how to handle difficult situations that medical assistants may face in the workplace.

- *Secrets for Success* provides tips for studying, remembering important material, and success in a career as a medical assistant.

- *Legal Brief* provides important legal and ethical information.

- *Your Turn To Teach* provides students with valuable information regarding patient education.

- *Safety First* offers helpful tips and information pertaining to safety, an important issue for medical assistants.

- *You Try It* provides practice problems so students can strengthen their medical math skills.

- *Hands On* contains procedures for important skills and tasks.

- *Chapter Highlights* summarizes a chapter's key content.

In addition to the above features, this book also includes bolded key terms throughout each chapter and a Glossary in the back of the book, as well as many other boxed features and tables. In addition, special Drug Spotlight tables in chapter 5 give students an overview of different types and examples of common drugs found in various drug classifications.

## Additional Resources

In addition to the text, the following resources are available for students and instructors:

- *Study Guide for Medical Assisting Made Incredibly Easy: Pharmacology* includes learning activities and exercises, quizzes, puzzles, certification review questions, and competency evaluation forms so students can practice their skills and measure their success.

- An **Instructor's Resource CD-ROM** with test generator, PowerPoint slides, answers to study guide questions, and customizable competency evaluation forms helps instructors optimize their teaching. The Instructor's Resource CD-ROM also includes information on where in the book each ABHES and CAAHEP competency is covered.

- A complete set of **Lesson Plans** is also available to instructors.

*Medical Assisting Made Incredibly Easy: Pharmacology* is designed to make the study of medical assisting fun and effective. The purpose of this book, and the entire *Medical Assisting Made Incredibly Easy* series, is student success!

# USER'S GUIDE

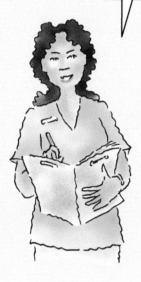

Hello, my name is Maria. I'm a Certified Medical Assistant and educator, as well as your guide through this textbook. There are a number of features in this **Medical Assisting Made Incredibly Easy** text to help you learn everything you need to become a successful medical assistant. Read through this User's Guide to orient yourself to everything the text has to offer. Good luck in your medical assisting studies!

## Chapter Checklist

- Explain how drugs are classified
- Identify the uses for antibiotics and discuss the therapeutic actions of these drugs
- Recognize the conditions topical drugs are commonly used to treat and explain how these medications are thought to work
- List the uses for anti-inflammatory drugs and describe how they work
- List the uses for analgesics and antipyretics and describe how these drugs work
- Explain why muscle relaxants may be prescribed and discuss the two ways these drugs work in the body
- Identify the various conditions cardiac drugs are used to treat and describe the different therapeutic actions of these drugs
- List the uses for respiratory medications and explain the various ways in which these medications work
- Recognize the indications for digestive drugs and discuss how these drugs work
- Explain why urinary drugs may be used and identify the therapeutic actions of these drugs
- Discuss the main use for diuretic drugs and how these drugs accomplish their purpose
- Identify the uses for nervous system medications and recognize where these drugs work in the body

**Chapter Checklists** orient you to the material that's covered in the current chapter.

## Chapter Competencies

- Perform within legal and ethical boundaries (CAAHEP Competency 3.c.2.b.)
- Demonstrate knowledge of federal and state health care legislation and regulations (CAAHEP Competency 3.c.2.e.)
- Monitor legislation related to current health care issues and practices (ABHES Competency 5.g.)
- Maintain medication and immunization records (CAAHEP Competency 3.b.4.h.; ABHES Competency 4.n.)
- Use methods of quality control (CAAHEP Competency 3.c.4.d.; ABHES Competency 4.i.)
- Perform risk management procedures (ABHES Competency 5.h.)
- Document appropriately (CAAHEP Competency 3.c.2.d.)
- Document accurately (ABHES Competency 5.b.)
- Determine needs for documentation and reporting (ABHES Competency 5.a.)

**Chapter Competencies** tell you which skills are covered in each chapter, as outlined by CAAHEP and ABHES.

## Running Smoothly

### KEEPING UP WITH THE DRUG ENFORCEMENT ADMINISTRATION

**Running Smoothly** boxes feature situations that you may encounter in a medical office. These boxes are designed to show you how to apply what you've learned to real-life situations.

*What if you're assigned the task of keeping up with the physician's DEA registration?*

A DEA number is valid for three years, after which the physician's registration must be renewed. The DEA does not send out reminders to renew soon-to-expire registrations. As a medical assistant, you may be responsible for maintaining registration or reminding the physician or practitioner about registering with the DEA. You can do this by tracking the physician's DEA registration and submitting a renewal application at the appropriate time. The DEA's Office of Diversion Control handles renewal applications. These applications can now be completed online by visiting the Office of Diversion Control's Web site at www.deadiversion.usdoj.gov.

## Ask the Professional

### ISN'T THERE A UNIT SYSTEM OF MEASUREMENT, TOO?

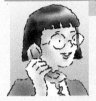

**Q:** My sister has type 1 diabetes and gives herself insulin injections. I noticed that her insulin bottles are labeled *100 units/mL*. What are units?

**A:** You get an A+ for being observant! The strength of the active ingredient in some drugs is measured simply in units. How much of the actual unit depends on the kind of drug. Units are unique to each kind.

Insulin is one of the drugs measured this way. The injectable form of penicillin is another. The label *100 units/mL* means that 100 units of your sister's insulin are in each milliliter of liquid.

You'll usually find units labeled in one of two ways:

- USP, for United States Pharmacopoeia
- IU, for International Units

Handle units like any other measurement you encounter.

**Ask the Professional** boxes offer expert advice on how to handle difficult situations that you may face in the workplace.

**Secrets for Success** boxes provide tips for studying, for remembering important material, and for success in your career as a medical assistant.

## Secrets for Success — FINDING COMMON GROUND

Another way to find a common denominator is to list the multiples of each denominator. Compare them until you get the first match. The number that you find this way is the **lowest common denominator**.

For example, look at the fractions 1/4, 1/6, and 1/8

...inators are 4, 6, and 8.

...les of 4 are 4, 8, 12, 16, 20, 24 . . .

...les of 6 are 6, 12, 18, 24 . . .

...les of 8 are 8, 16, 24 . . .

...atch is 24.

...common denominator of these fractions is 24.

## Legal Brief — MISLEADING CLAIMS FOR OXYCONTIN BRING FINES

In May 2007, Purdue Pharma was fined $600 million for giving false or misleading information about oxycodone (OxyContin) to physicians and the public.

The drug manufacturer asserted that OxyContin users were less likely to abuse the drug or become addicted to it than to fast-acting narcotic painkillers such as oxycodone with acetaminophen (Percocet). OxyContin's time-release formula was the reason.

However, according to evidence given in federal court, the product did not live up to these claims. Recreational users soon discovered that they could get an immediate heroin-like high from O... break the tablets open a... the drug. Inside was pure, p...

**Legal Briefs** provide important legal and ethical information.

## Your Turn to Teach — VITAMIN C AND THE COMMON COLD

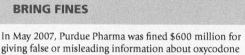

Many patients that you see have probably heard that vitamin C can cure the common cold and respiratory infections. However, large clinical trials have shown that taking vitamin C doesn't reduce the risk of getting a cold. It also doesn't have any effect on the severity of the cold. For a small number of people, it reduces the length of a cold. So, what should you say to a patient who asks if it will help to start taking vitamin C after the cold starts? Break ...tly: the studies say no. Although it won't hurt ... drink some extra orange juice, it's not likely ...ffect on the patient's cold.

**Your Turn To Teach** boxes provide helpful information about patient education.

## Safety First — ADVERSE REACTIONS TO NONPRESCRIPTION DRUGS

Although nonprescription drugs may be easily available, they still carry some risk. For example, some people react poorly to acetylsalicylic acid, commonly known as aspirin. In some patients, taking aspirin can cause gastrointestinal bleeding, or bleeding in the stomach and intestines. Medical practitioners often recommend that such patients take products that contain acetaminophen instead. Acetaminophen is sold under a variety of brand names, including Tylenol.

Often, over-the-counter medications may have additional ingredients. For example, Excedrin contains aspirin and caffeine, and Tylenol PM has acetaminophen and diphenhydramine, which is an antihistamine originally sold as Benadryl. Patients should be aware of these ingredients and not mix medications because they can cause unpleasant or dangerous adverse reactions.

Some drugs may be released as over-the-counter medications at a lower strength, whereas a higher dosage of these drugs, such as cimetidine (Tagamet) and famotidine (Pepcid), requires a prescription. This can be confusing for patients, so you need to stay up to date on the latest information about drug releases.

**Safety First** boxes offer tips and information about lab safety, an important issue for medical assistants.

## FIGURING OUT FRACTIONS

Find the lowest common denominator.

1. $\frac{1}{5}$ and $\frac{2}{3}$

2. $\frac{5}{8}$ and $\frac{3}{16}$

3. $\frac{1}{5}$ and $\frac{1}{7}$

4. $\frac{1}{16}$ and $\frac{3}{4}$

5. $\frac{2}{3}$ and $\frac{1}{2}$

Reduce to the lowest term

**You Try It** provides practice problems to help you strengthen your medical math skills.

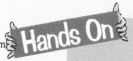

## HANDS ON PROCEDURE 8-1: ADMINISTERING ORAL MEDICATIONS

This procedure should take five minutes.

1. Wash your hands and gather your supplies, including the physician's order, the correct oral medication, a disposable calibrated cup, a glass of water, and the patient's medical record.

2. Check the medication label and compare it to the physician's order. Note the expiration date. Remember to check the medication label three times—when taking the medication from the shelf, when measuring, and when returning it to the shelf.

3. If necessary, calculate the correct dose.

4. For a multidose container, remove the cap from the container. Touch only the outside of the lid to avoid contaminating the inside. Single, or unit-dose, medications come individually wrapped. Packages may be opened by pushing the medication through the foil backing or by peeling back a tab on one corner.

5. Remove the correct dose of medication according to your calculations and the label.

A. For solid medications:
   • Pour the correct dose into the bottle cap to pre-

**Hands On** boxes contain step-by-step, easy-to-follow procedures for important skills and tasks.

### Chapter Highlights

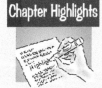

• Fat-soluble vitamins are stored inta fatty tissues for up to six months. The body does not break them down into other substances. Vitamins A, D, E, and K are the fat-soluble vitamins.

• Water-soluble vitamins pass through the bloodstream and leave the body through the kidneys. Vitamin $B_1$, $B_2$, $B_3$, $B_6$, $B_9$, $B_{12}$, and C are the water-soluble vitamins.

• Vitamins help maintain normal body functions such as formation of bone and tissue, production of white and red blood cells, and cell repair. Lack of vitamins can cause disease, poor eyesight, and other problems.

• Dietary minerals in different quantities are among the building blocks of bone, teeth, soft tissue, muscles, blood, and nerve cells. The body also uses minerals to make hormones and regulate the heartbeat.

• Multivitamins usually contain small amounts of minerals.

**Chapter Highlights** summarizes a chapter's key content.

# REVIEWERS

**Nina Beaman**
Bryant and Stratton College
Richmond, Virginia

**Robyn Gohsman, AAS**
Medical Careers Institute
Newport News, Virginia

**Elizabeth Hoffman**
Baker College
Clinton Township, Michigan

**Helen Houser**
Phoenix College
Phoenix, Arizona

**Maureen Messier**
Bradford Hall Career Institute
Southington, Connecticut

**Linda Romines**
Ivy Tech Community College
Fort Wayne, Indiana

**Amy Semenchuk**
Rockford Business College
Rockford, Illinois

**Paula Silver**
Medical Careers Institute
Newport News, Virginia

# TABLE OF CONTENTS

# EXPANDED TABLE OF CONTENTS

# DRUG FUNDAMENTALS

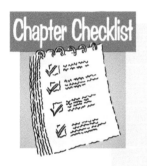

- Explain the differences between the generic, trade, and chemical names of drugs.

- Identify the five major drug laws and explain why they are important.

- Describe the Food and Drug Administration's role in the development of new medications.

- Compare and contrast over-the-counter (OTC), prescription, and controlled substances.

- Name the four sources from which we get drugs.

- List the advantages of synthetic medications.

- Explain the differences between parenteral and enteral medications.

- Identify two written resources for drug information.

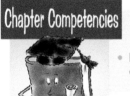

- Demonstrate knowledge of federal and state health care legislation and regulations (CAAHEP Competency 3.c.2.e.)
- Determine needs for documentation and reporting (ABHES Competency 5.a.)

Welcome to the exciting career of medical assisting! This career will allow you to do many things that help people maintain their good health, live more comfortably, and recover from illness. This text includes a personal hostess, Maria. Like many medical assistants, she is eager to begin working with live patients. However, you and she will find that there is a lot of important textbook information that medical assistants must know in order to help ensure patients' safety.

As a clinical medical assistant, you may be responsible for handling medications under the supervision of a physician or other health care professional. Therefore, there are a number of important things that you need to know about medications, which are covered throughout this book.

This chapter focuses on the following topics:

- Naming drugs
- Major drug laws
- How drugs are developed
- Major drug categories
- Drug sources
- Drug forms

## What's in a Name?

Medications are available in many forms and are administered in various ways to produce therapeutic, or medically helpful, effects. The names of drugs can give you important information about them.

Drugs often have three names:

- the chemical name
- the generic name
- the trade name

A patient may refer to a drug by one name, whereas a health care professional may use a different name for the same medication. It's important to be familiar with the various names and how they are used.

### CHEMICAL NAME

A medication's chemical name identifies the exact chemical make-up of the drug, including the placement of the atoms or the molecular structure. The chemical name of one common medication found in many first-aid kits is acetylsalicylic acid. This drug is also known as:

$$C_9 H_8 O_4$$

Its name tells us that there are nine atoms of carbon, eight atoms of hydrogen, and four atoms of oxygen in each molecule of this drug.

You may notice that the name does not begin with a capital letter. That's not a mistake! Chemical names are not capitalized.

> Ummm, acetyl-sali-what? That's a mouthful! But do not worry—the chemical name is mainly used by medical researchers, not in the medical office.

## GENERIC NAME

The generic name is the name given to a drug during the research and development stage. It becomes the official name of the drug.

The generic name refers to the chemical ingredients in the drug. Like the chemical name, the generic name is also not capitalized. For example, aspirin is the generic name of the common medication with the chemical name you just read. You'll need to be familiar with generic names because medical professionals often use the generic name of drugs in the medical office.

## TRADE NAME

A drug's trade name is also called its brand name. This is the name that the manufacturer gives the drug when it's distributed commercially. Before putting the drug on the market, the manufacturer registers the drug's trade name and chemical formulation with the U.S. Patent Office. You can recognize a trade name because the first letter of the name is capitalized. The trade name also may be followed by the trademark (™) or registered trademark (®) symbol.

You may find aspirin in a drug store under names such as Bayer Aspirin and St. Joseph's Aspirin. Only the manufacturer can use the trade name. However, after the patent on a medication expires, other companies may manufacture generic versions of the drug and supply their own trade names.

The table on page 4 shows the chemical, generic, and trade names for some different medications.

## Major Drug Laws

Medications can have such powerful effects on the human body that the U.S. government enforces a wide variety of laws to protect consumers from unsafe and harmful drugs. There are

## Examples of Drug Names

| Chemical Name | Generic Name | Trade Name(s) |
| --- | --- | --- |
| Ethyl4-(8-chloro-5,6-dihydro-11H-benzo[5,6]cyclohepta[1,2-b]-pyridin-11-ylidene)-1-piperidinecarboxylate | loratadine | Alavert, Claritin, Claritin Reditabs, Claritin Syrup, Tavist ND Allergy |
| 7-Chloro-1,3-dihydro-1-methyl-5-phenyl-2H-1,4-benzodiazepin-2-one | diazepam | Diastat, Diazepam Intensol, Valium |
| DL-Threo-2-(methylamino)-1-phenylpropan-1-ol | pseudoephedrine | Dimetapp, PediaCare Infants' Decongestant Drops, Sudafed, Triaminic |
| 4'-Hydroxyacetanilide | acetaminophen | Tylenol |
| 4-[4-(p-Chlorophenyl)-4-hydroxypiperidino]-4'-fluorobutyrophenone | haloperidol | Haldol |

Every drug has three different names.

two main government agencies that are involved in controlling drugs and their uses.

- The United States **Food and Drug Administration (FDA)** is the federal agency responsible for approving and monitoring the sale of drugs and food products. It ensures that drugs are safe to use and that drug labels are accurate and easy to understand.

- The **Drug Enforcement Administration (DEA)** monitors the use of **controlled substances**, or those drugs that may result in dependency or abuse.

> The DEA has created the Schedule of Controlled Substances, which organizes certain drugs according to their tendencies to cause dependence and abuse. You'll learn more about this drug classification system later in the chapter.

## THE PURE FOOD AND DRUG ACT

The FDA was first established by the **Pure Food and Drug Act of 1906**. The government passed the Pure Food and Drug Act of 1906 to regulate questionable practices within the food and drug industries. The drug-related provisions of this law banned false and misleading product labeling.

In addition, the Pure Food and Drug Act forced manufacturers to list on the label the presence and amount of 11 dangerous ingredients. These substances included alcohol, heroin, and cocaine, which were common ingredients in medicines at that time. In the late 1800s, the Sears Roebuck & Co. Catalogue sold a morphine-laced tonic that was to be "slipped into the coffee of a wayward husband to keep him home."

## Legal Brief | PROTECTING THE PUBLIC

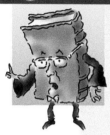

**The Federal Food, Drug, and Cosmetic Act of 1938** was passed to protect consumers from harmful health and beauty aids already on the market. There were specific products that prompted the new legislation. These products showed the need for product testing before products reached consumers. The following were included among the products:

- *Lash Lure*, an eyelash dye that caused blisters, blindness, tissue necrosis, and death in many women

- *Elixir Sulfanilamide*, an untested liquid version of a drug commonly used to treat streptococcal infections. The liquid used to dissolve powdered sulfanilamide was diethylene glycol, a substance used in antifreeze. The product was tested for taste, appearance, and fragrance, but not toxicity, or harmfulness. More than 100 people in 15 states died from taking Elixir Sulfanilamide.

- *Radithor*, a popular tonic that was advertised to "speed up healing," contained the highly toxic element radium. Using Radithor caused a slow and painful death.

## FEDERAL FOOD, DRUG, AND COSMETIC ACT OF 1938

In 1938, Congress strengthened the Pure Food and Drug Act. The new regulations required that a drug's safety be proved before it can be dispensed to the public. As a result of this legislation, manufacturers had to prove that their products were safe before selling them to consumers.

## THE DURHAM-HUMPHREY AMENDMENT

In 1951, the Durham-Humphrey Amendment banned many drugs from being dispensed without a prescription. For the first time, the law drew a clear distinction between two categories of drugs:

- **nonprescription drugs**, which patients can purchase on their own for their own use
- **prescription drugs**, which must be taken under a medical practitioner's supervision

However, already approved, non-habit-forming drugs that were on the market did not have to be reclassified.

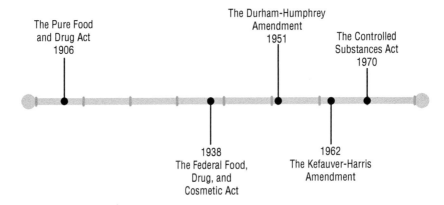

The Pure Food
and Drug Act
1906

The Durham-Humphrey
Amendment
1951

The Controlled
Substances Act
1970

1938
The Federal Food,
Drug, and
Cosmetic Act

1962
The Kefauver-Harris
Amendment

## THE KEFAUVER-HARRIS AMENDMENT

The Kefauver-Harris Amendment of 1962 was passed after many people suffered from severe **adverse reactions** (side effects) to the sedative thalidomide, which caused birth defects. The act:

- required reporting of adverse reactions to the FDA
- required drug manufacturers to disclose the risks and benefits of a drug
- reformulated the FDA's new drug applications

## THE CONTROLLED SUBSTANCES ACT OF 1970

The **Controlled Substances Act of 1970** was passed to regulate the manufacture and distribution of dangerous drugs. This act required that anyone who manufactures, prescribes, adminis-

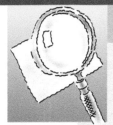

## Closer Look    WHAT'S THE DIFFERENCE BETWEEN SIDE EFFECTS AND ADVERSE REACTIONS?

Adverse reactions are undesirable drug effects. Some texts use both the terms *side effect* and *adverse reaction*. Often, *side effects* refer to mild, common, and nontoxic reactions, whereas *adverse reactions* refer to more severe or life-threatening reactions. In this text, only the term *adverse reaction* is used, referring to reactions that may be mild, severe, or life-threatening. (You'll learn more about adverse reactions in Chapter 4.)

ters, or dispenses controlled substances must register with the U.S. government. All these controlled items are substances that have a potential for dependency or abuse. You'll read more about controlled substances later in this chapter.

## Drug Development

As a medical assistant, you'll see and hear the names of many medications during your workday. It's useful for you to know what researchers and drug manufacturers must do to bring a drug to market in the United States. However, keep in mind that this process differs in other countries. Some drugs from other countries might not be safe to use.

> Drug companies often test a medicine for 7 to 12 years before they submit it to the FDA for approval, which can take another 2 years.

### TIME FRAME

It takes the drug companies many years and tens of millions of dollars to bring a drug to market. The process, from preclinical research through clinical studies and final review by the FDA, can take from 7 to 12 years, and sometimes even longer.

### STAGES OF TESTING

Testing occurs in two main stages:

- the pre-FDA stage
- the FDA stage

Many research projects undertaken in drug company labs are dead ends that do not lead to new products. However, as investigations continue, some projects may start to show interesting results. Some even have the potential to become new and breakthrough treatments for a medical condition. The company then selects these projects for further study and funding.

The company may spend millions of dollars on research and testing before a medication ever reaches a physician's office. These promising projects enter what is formally called the pre-FDA stage of testing.

### The Pre-FDA Stage

In the pre-FDA stage, the researchers first test the drug under laboratory conditions, using animal and human cells. They then test the drug on living animals. If the results still look promising, the company applies for *investigational new drug (IND)* status.

IND status allows the company to begin formal clinical testing of the new but still unapproved drug. Clinical testing means trying out the new drug on human subjects. There are three phases of clinical testing. Researchers carefully record the drug's effects during each phase.

### Phase I

Phase I generally lasts 4 to 6 weeks. The clinical trial team, made up of physicians, nurses, and other health care professionals, administers the drug to 20 to 80 healthy volunteers. The team is studying how the drug is metabolized and excreted from the body, and learning about any potential adverse reactions that the drug may cause.

### Phase II

If the results of phase I are positive, the test moves on to phases II and III. In each new phase, the drug is given to a larger number of volunteers. About 100 to 300 volunteers are needed for phase II. These volunteers include individuals who suffer from the disease or condition that the drug is intended to treat. The clinical trial team gathers safety data and early data about the drug's effectiveness.

### Phase III and Beyond

If phase II shows that the adverse reactions and other risks are acceptable and the beneficial effects of the drug are significant, testing will move on to phase III. The participants in phase III may number from 1,000 to 3,000, all of whom have the condition the drug is intended to treat. Phase III studies also provide researchers with information about infrequent or rare adverse reactions.

All three phases last anywhere from 2 to 10 years, with an average of 5 years. After the three phases of testing, the manufacturer is confident that the drug is safe and effective. The manufacturer then submits the drug to the FDA for approval. However, sometimes the monitoring may continue with a voluntary phase IV. This phase involves postmarket research of the drug's therapeutic effects. Physicians provide the pharmaceutical companies with reports on any adverse reactions to the drug, as well as results for the drug's effectiveness for different populations, such as children.

## The FDA Stage

When the drug company is ready to submit a medication for approval, there are certain steps that must be followed.

1. First, the company submits an *NDA*, or *new drug application*. Along with the application, the company submits all the data it collected during the clinical trials.

## Closer Look     IDENTIFYING PROBLEM DRUGS

The three phases of pre-FDA testing allow time for any problematic or dangerous drugs to be identified. If a problem is found with a drug, the drug should be dropped from study. Drugs may be dropped if they:

- fail to work at all
- fail to work in humans
- are less effective than expected
- are **toxic**, or harmful
- cause unacceptable adverse reactions
- are not as effective as drugs already on the market

2. A panel of experts reviews the application, examines the data, and submits a recommendation to the FDA. Panelists include pharmacologists, or drug experts, chemists, physicians, and other professionals. Their decision tells the FDA whether to approve or disapprove the drug for use.

3. The FDA stage of the review process lasts about 2 years.

Even after the drug is released to the market, its effectiveness continues to be monitored. Health care professionals are encouraged to help with this monitoring by reporting adverse reactions to drugs to the FDA.

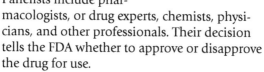

Even after a drug has been released to the market, it must be monitored. The FDA won't allow a drug to get away with too many adverse reactions!

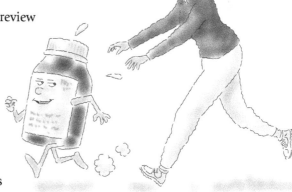

### THE FDA ACCELERATED PROGRAM

It takes close to 12 years for most drugs to get FDA approval. However, the FDA has special programs, such as the accelerated program, to meet special needs.

## Legal Brief — MEDWATCH

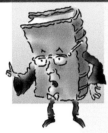

As a medical assistant, you might be asked to process paperwork for the FDA's MedWatch reporting program (www.fda.gov/medwatch) or other similar reporting programs. Health care professionals who notice serious adverse reactions to a drug are encouraged to report their findings to the FDA. The FDA wants to know about any drug reactions that result in the following:

- death
- life-threatening illness
- hospitalization
- disability

The FDA protects the identities of participants.

The FDA also wants to know about any reactions that may require medical or surgical intervention. A special MedWatch reporting form is used for this purpose. This form is also used to report problems caused by medical products, such as latex gloves, pacemakers, infusion pumps, and other such items.

---

The FDA is sometimes willing to grant accelerated, or faster, approval to a drug early in its development process, even during phase I and phase II clinical trials. This is done primarily for drugs and treatments for life-threatening illnesses that pose a significant health risk to the public.

### THE FDA COMPASSIONATE ACCESS PROGRAM

The compassionate access program is another program that allows patients to receive drugs that the FDA has not formally approved. This program provides experimental drugs to patients in a compassionate, or sympathetic, attempt to relieve their suffering if no alternative therapy exists. In all likelihood, these patients will die before the drug is approved for general use. They may also be too sick to take part in controlled clinical studies.

To participate in the compassionate access program, the drug company must follow these steps:

1. The drug company first approaches the FDA with a proposal to target this group of patients for special consideration.

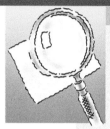

## Closer Look

### THE FDA ACCELERATED PROGRAM AT WORK

One example of a disease that poses a significant health risk to the public is **acquired immunodeficiency syndrome (AIDS)**. This disease remains a worldwide threat. Untreated, AIDS can be devastating to the men and women afflicted with it. Because it's easily spread, AIDS also poses a major health threat to the general public. The FDA and the drug companies are working together to speed up the IND approval process so that AIDS drugs that promise positive results can be administered to the people who could benefit from them. This approval is *provisional*, or temporary. With provisional approval comes a written commitment from the drug company to complete a product's clinical studies and to show the drug's expected benefits formally.

AIDS patients are not the only ones to benefit. Accelerated programs have also placed new treatments for cancer, childhood leukemia, and other diseases at the physician's disposal.

2. All participants must grant their full informed consent in writing.

3. The company then provides the medication for free to these patients and collects data about how they respond to it.

4. The drug company analyzes the data and presents its findings to the FDA.

The compassionate access program offers benefits but also problems.

- The patients who receive the drug may be sicker than those who would normally receive the treatment in its final form. Thus, patients may be at greater risk for adverse reactions.

- Supplies of the drug may be limited.

- The number of patents in the program may also be limited or selected too much at random.

- The data this test provides may be faulty or inaccurate, thus giving the drug a bad reputation before its full program has been completed.

The FDA accelerated program and compassionate access program can help patients receive the treatments they need ahead of the standard drug-approval time frame.

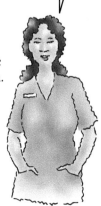

## *Drug Categories*

After approving a drug, the FDA assigns it to a specific category. As a medical assistant, you need to become familiar with the differences among the three main categories of drugs:

- nonprescription drugs
- prescription drugs
- controlled substances

### NONPRESCRIPTION DRUGS

Nonprescription drugs are drugs that the FDA classifies as safe if they are taken as directed. These drugs are available without prescriptions. Consumers may purchase them without any restrictions in many different places, including pharmacies, drug stores, supermarkets, and convenience stores. Another name

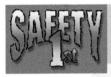

### ADVERSE REACTIONS TO NONPRESCRIPTION DRUGS

Although nonprescription drugs may be easily available, they still carry some risk. For example, some people react poorly to acetylsalicylic acid, commonly known as aspirin. In some patients, taking aspirin can cause gastrointestinal bleeding, or bleeding in the stomach and intestines. Medical practitioners often recommend that such patients take products that contain acetaminophen instead. Acetaminophen is sold under a variety of brand names, including Tylenol.

Often, over-the-counter medications may have additional ingredients. For example, Excedrin contains aspirin and caffeine, and Tylenol PM has acetaminophen and diphenhydramine, which is an antihistamine originally sold as Benadryl. Patients should be aware of these ingredients and not mix medications because they can cause unpleasant or dangerous adverse reactions.

Some drugs may be released as over-the-counter medications at a lower strength, whereas a higher dosage of these drugs, such as cimetidine (Tagamet) and famotidine (Pepcid), requires a prescription. This can be confusing for patients, so you need to stay up-to-date on the latest information about drug releases.

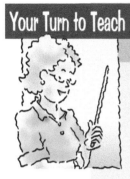

## DISCUSSING NONPRESCRIPTION DRUGS WITH PATIENTS

Many patients take nonprescription drugs regularly because they are convenient and easily available. However, it's important to caution patients about self-diagnosing or taking medications for conditions without checking with the physician. Here are some things to keep in mind when discussing nonprescription medications with patients.

- Explain to the patient that OTC medications are convenient, but they might not offer the same benefits as prescription drugs when treating the same condition.

- Remind the patient that it's fine to take OTC medications occasionally. However, if a condition persists, the patient should contact the physician immediately. Some OTC medications can cover up symptoms. Others can be harmful when taken with certain medications.

- Urge the patient to tell the physician about any OTC medications that they take on a regular basis or even just occasionally.

- Advise the patient to read the drug label carefully on all medications, including nonprescription drugs. It's essential that the patient understands how to take the medicine as well as how to store it safely. The patient should also be aware of when the medicine expires.

for this category is over-the-counter drugs (OTC). People commonly use OTC drugs to treat:
- headaches
- muscle aches
- symptoms of the common cold
- constipation
- diarrhea
- upset stomach
- skin disorders

## PRESCRIPTION DRUGS

Prescription drugs are drugs that need to be taken under the supervision of a licensed health care provider, such as a physician, physician's assistant, nurse practitioner, or dentist. A **prescription**

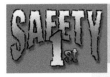

## ADVERSE REACTIONS TO PRESCRIPTION DRUGS

Even though prescription drugs have been tested for safety and have FDA approval for general use, they may cause adverse reactions in some individuals. (Keep in mind that an adverse reaction isn't a drug allergy, but a drug allergy is a type of adverse reaction.) For example, patients may report that certain antibiotics such as penicillin or amoxicillin cause upset stomach or nausea. Any adverse reactions should be noted in a patient's medical record.

is a written order to the pharmacist. The health care provider must sign the prescription form, or the prescription can't be filled. (You'll learn more about prescriptions in Chapter 3.)

Prescription drugs are also called *legend drugs* because by law their labels must carry the legend, or statement, "Caution: Federal law prohibits dispensing without prescription."

### Prescription Drugs and Pregnancy

Medical assistants often work in offices that serve women who are or may become pregnant. Accordingly, you should be aware of the effects of prescription drugs on an unborn baby (fetus). Drugs that a woman takes in the first trimester (3 months) of pregnancy may cause birth defects. Drugs taken during the later stages of pregnancy may also cause problems. Therefore, many common drugs are not recommended during pregnancy or breast-feeding. The physician may make an exception if the potential benefit of taking the drug outweighs the risks to the fetus or infant.

### The Pregnancy Categories of Drugs

To prevent birth defects and other problems, the FDA has set up five pregnancy categories for drugs. Information about the pregnancy category of a specific drug may be found in drug reference books and in the paper inserts that manufacturer's package with the drugs.

Regardless of the pregnancy category or the likely safety of the drug, no drug should be given during pregnancy unless it's clearly needed. The potential benefits must outweigh the potential risks to the fetus.

The table on page 15 shows the pregnancy categories for various drugs.

## Pregnancy Categories

| Pregnancy Category | Potential Risks |
|---|---|
| Pregnancy Category A | Controlled studies show that there is no danger to the fetus. Adequate well-controlled studies in pregnant women have not demonstrated risk to the fetus. |
| Pregnancy Category B | There is no evidence of risk in humans. Animal studies show risk, but studies in humans do not. If no adequate human studies have been done, then animal studies are negative. |
| Pregnancy Category C | Risk can't be ruled out. Human studies are lacking. Animal studies are either lacking or show possible risk to the fetus. The drug may be used during pregnancy if the potential benefits of the drug outweigh the potential risks. |
| Pregnancy Category D | There is positive evidence of risk to a human fetus both before and after the drug was approved for use. However, potential benefits may outweigh the risk to the fetus. If the situation is life-threatening or if the mother suffers from a serious disease, the drug may be used if safer drugs can't be found. |
| Pregnancy Category X | The drugs should not be used during pregnancy. Studies in humans and animals show risk to the fetus that clearly outweighs any benefits. |

## CONTROLLED SUBSTANCES

The FDA lists certain drugs as **controlled substances** because using them often leads to abuse or dependency. The Controlled Substances Act of 1970 puts strict controls on who may make these drugs and how they are handled in the medical office. It also puts strict controls on how they can be administered and prescribed.

The DEA is the government agency that is responsible for enforcing the Controlled Substances Act. It's a branch of the Department of Justice. The DEA's mission is to control the use of all drugs listed as controlled substances by the Bureau of Narcotics and Dangerous Drugs (BNDD).

Controlled substances are grouped into five categories, based on their potential for abuse. A label on the drug's container indicates the schedule, or category, of drugs that have the same restrictions and controls.

The table on page 16 shows the Schedule of Controlled Substances.

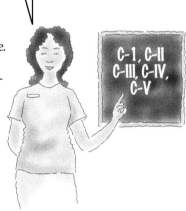

Look for one of these symbols on a bottle or package that contains a controlled substance. These symbols tell which schedule a substance belongs to.

C-1, C-II
C-III, C-IV,
C-V

## Schedule of Controlled Substances

| Schedule | Potential for Abuse | Examples |
|---|---|---|
| Schedule I (C-I) | High potential for abuse<br>No acceptable medical use in the United States | heroin<br>marijuana<br>LSD (lysergic acid diethylamide)<br>peyote |
| Schedule II (C-II) | Potential for high abuse with severe physical or psychological dependence | narcotics such as meperidine, methadone, morphine, and oxycodone<br>amphetamines<br>barbiturates |
| Schedule III (C-III) | Less potential for abuse than Schedule II drugs<br>Potential for moderate physical or psychological dependence | nonbarbiturate sedatives<br>nonamphetamine stimulants<br>limited amounts of certain narcotics<br>aspirin, butalbital, caffeine, and codeine (Fiorinal with Codeine)<br>paregoric (Camphorated Tincture of Opium) |
| Schedule IV (C-IV) | Less potential for abuse than Schedule III drugs<br>Limited potential for dependence | some sedatives and anxiety medications<br>nonnarcotic analgesics (painkillers)<br>valium (Diastat, Diazepam Intensol, Valium)<br>midazolam (Versed, Versed Syrup)<br>zolpidem (Ambien, Ambien CR) |
| Schedule V (C-V) | Limited potential for abuse | small amounts of narcotics (codeine) used to control coughing (antitussives) or diarrhea (antidiarrheals) |

## Drug Sources

Companies make drugs from a variety of natural sources, including plants, minerals, and animals. Some drugs are **synthetics**; that is, they're made in the laboratory. The table on page 17 includes some examples of drugs from a variety of sources.

Scientists can create and build synthetic drugs to do specific things, such as act as analgesics (painkillers). In fact, many of the most common painkillers are synthetics. These include such common medications as:

- acetaminophen (Tylenol)
- ibuprofen (Advil, Motrin, and Nuprin)
- naproxen sodium (Aleve)
- ketoprofen (Orudis KT)

Synthetic drugs offer some advantages. They are more readily available, and they are less expensive to make than drugs from other sources. Unfortunately, many illegal drugs are also laboratory-made synthetics. These include "club drugs" such as ecstasy, methamphetamines, and other recreational drugs that can be harmful.

## Common Drugs and Their Sources

| Source | Drug | Use |
| --- | --- | --- |
| **Plants** | | |
| Cinchona bark | quinidine (Quinaglute Dura-Tabs, Quinidex Extentabs) | antiarrhythmic (affects the rhythm of the heartbeat) |
| Purple foxglove | digoxin (Digitek, Digoxin, Lanoxin, Lanoxicaps) | cardiotonic (stimulates the heart) |
| Opium poppy | paregoric (Camphorated Tincture of Opium) | antidiarrheal |
| | morphine (Avinza, DepoDur, Infumorph, MS Contin, RMS Uniserts, Roxanol) | analgesic (painkiller) |
| | codeine | antitussive (cough suppressant), analgesic |
| Leaves and beans of coffee plant, Guarana berries, kola nut | caffeine | stimulant |
| **Minerals** | | |
| Magnesium | magnesium hydroxide (Milk of Magnesia, Milk of Magnesia-Concentrated, Phillips' Milk of Magnesia) | antacid, laxative |
| Silver | silver nitrate | placed in eyes of newborns to kill *Neisseria gonorrhoeae,* a bacteria that causes gonorrhea |
| Gold | aurothioglucose (Solganal) | arthritis treatment |
| **Chemical** | | |
| Bismuth | bismuth subsalicylate (Bismatrol, Bismatrol Extra Strength, Children's Kaopectate, Extra Strength Kaopectate, Kaopectate, Pepto-Bismol, Pepto-Bismol Maximum Strength Liquid, Pink Bismuth) | treats upset stomach and indigestion |
| **Animal proteins** | | |
| Pork, beef pancreas | insulin (Novolin R, Humulin R) | antidiabetic hormone |
| Animal thyroid glands | thyroid, dessicated (Armour Thyroid) | hypothyroidism |
| **Synthetics** | | |
| | meperidine hydrochloride (Demerol) | analgesic |
| | diphenoxylate hydrochloride and atropine sulfate (Logen, Lomanate, Lomotil, Lonox) | antidiarrheal |
| | sulfisoxazole acetyl (Gantrisin) | sulfonamide (used to treat bacterial diseases) |
| **Semisynthetics** | | |
| *Escherichia coli* bacteria, altered DNA molecules | humulin | antidiabetic hormone |

## *Drug Forms*

Medicines do not do the patient much good if they aren't taken correctly. A physician or other health care professional often chooses one medication rather than another for a patient because of how the drug enters the bloodstream. Cost, safety, and the speed at which the drug can be absorbed are important considerations.

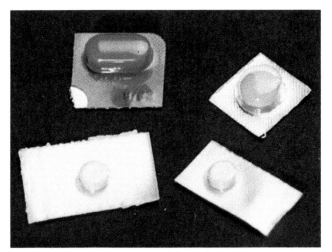

Many oral medications are packaged in unit doses. A unit dose
contains the amount of the drug for one dose.

Physicians choose from two main groupings of medications.

- enteral medications
- parenteral medications

## ENTERAL MEDICATIONS

> Enteral medications enter the body through the gastrointestinal tract.

**Enteral medicines** enter the body through the stomach
and intestines—the gastrointestinal tract. Most patients prefer
to take drugs by mouth, which is the easiest way to get a drug
into the body. Most medicines of this kind come in a form that
a patient can swallow, such as:

- tablets
- capsules
- liquids

### Solid Forms of Oral Medications

As a medical assistant, you may encounter a variety of solid
forms of oral medications.

#### Capsules

A **capsule** provides medicine in powdered or granulated form
that's packaged inside a gelatin casing. A capsule is designed to
dissolve in stomach acids or in the small intestine.

Not all capsules are designed the same way.

- A **gelcap** is a soft gelatin capsule with an oil-based drug
  inside.

- A **time-release capsule,** also called a *spansule,* is a gelatin capsule that will release the medicine inside over time rather than all at once. You should not open a time-release capsule unless the manufacturer recommends it.

### Tablets

**Tablets** are shaped and colored for easy identification. They usually dissolve in the gastrointestinal tract. You may break them in half only if they are scored, or have a shallow ridge cut into them, for this purpose. Some tablets are scored rectangles so they can be divided into thirds.

**Buffered caplets** have an ingredient that prevents stomach irritation. **Enteric coated tablets** have dry, compressed medication inside a coating that can resist stomach acids. You should not break or crush these tablets. The coating on these tablets resists stomach acid and in turn allows the medication to dissolve in the intestines. Without the coating, these medications might be harmful to the stomach (e.g., aspirin).

### Powders

A **powder** is a finely ground form of a medication. Some patients may find a powder hard to swallow, so most powders are stirred into a liquid. For example, many people use psyllium (Fiberall Tropical Fruit Flavor, Genfiber, Hydrocil Instant, Konsyl, Metamucil, Serutan) as a bulk laxative and follow directions to stir an amount of the powder into an 8-ounce glass of water for ingestion.

### Lozenges or Troches

A **lozenge** or **troche** is a small, flavored tablet that is often used to release medication into the mouth or throat. The simplest and most common form is a cough drop. Lozenges should be allowed to dissolve slowly. You should tell patients to avoid drinking fluids after using lozenges.

## Liquid Forms of Oral Medications

Oral medications are also available in a variety of liquid forms, such as syrups, elixirs, emulsions, suspensions, extracts, and gels.

**Syrups** are very sweet, flavored forms of a medication that are high in sugar. They are often given to children. Be aware that the sugar in syrups makes them a poor choice for diabetic patients.

An **elixir** is dissolved in alcohol and flavored. Given mainly to adults, an elixir is less sweet than a syrup. You shouldn't give elixirs to alcoholic or diabetic patients because these medications contain alcohol and sugar.

An **emulsion** is a medication that is combined with water and oil. It must be thoroughly shaken before it's taken so that the medication is evenly dispersed.

**Suspensions** are particles of medication that are dissolved in liquid. Like emulsions, suspensions must be shaken well before they can be effectively used.

An **extract** is a highly concentrated form of a medication. It may be given as drops. It's typically given in a liquid to hide its strong taste.

A **gel** is a medication that is suspended in a thin gelatin or paste.

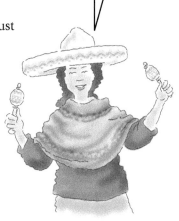

When it comes to using emulsions and suspensions, remember to shake things up!

## Advantages of Oral Medications

Oral medications have a number of important advantages. They are:

- easiest to administer
- available in a variety of forms
- preferred by most patients
- often available in unit dose packages for ease of administration in the medical office
- administered with a high degree of safety

## Disadvantages of Oral Medications

Oral medications also have some important disadvantages. These medications:

- have variable speeds at which they take effect
- can't be given to someone who is unconscious
- can't be given to someone who is experiencing nausea or vomiting
- may be difficult for a patient to swallow (in the case of tablets, pills, or capsules)
- can't be given to someone who has been ordered to take nothing by mouth
- may have a taste that patients dislike
- are less predictable in their effects on the body than when given by injection

The speed at which certain oral medications take effect depends on how they are administered. For example, when medication is given sublingually (under the tongue), it enters the bloodstream and takes effect rapidly. But when oral medications are swallowed, the onset of action is very slow.

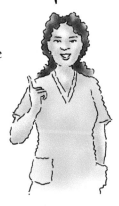

## PARENTERAL MEDICATIONS

Some medicines can't be given by mouth, or the body can't absorb the drug fast enough if it's taken that way. Sometimes, a patient is unconscious or not physically able to swallow a tablet or a liquid. Thus, there is another category of medications to fit these circumstances. These medications are called parenteral medications. They do *not* go through the gastrointestinal tract.

Here are some of the most common ways to administer parenteral medications:

- by needle through the skin
- in mist and spray form for inhalation
- in drop form, such as eye drops
- by patches placed on the skin
- in tablets under the tongue
- in suppositories placed in the rectum or vagina
- in tablets placed between the cheek and gum (buccal)

Parenteral medications can be grouped by their delivery method.

## Injectables

Injectables can be broken down into three categories.

- *Subcutaneous (SubQ) medications* are injected under the skin. Some examples are insulin used to treat diabetes, morphine to control pain, and epinephrine for serious allergic reactions.
- *Intramuscular (IM) medications* are injected directly into the muscle. Many vaccines and antibiotics are administered this way.
- *Intravenous (IV) medications* are injected directly into the vein. IV medication has the quickest action because it enters the bloodstream immediately.

## Inhalants

**Inhalants** are medications that are absorbed directly into the lungs by breathing, or *inspiration*. Inhalants are absorbed quickly into the capillaries, making them a popular choice for patients with chronic pulmonary (breathing) disorders.

Patients who suffer from asthma or other breathing disorders may self-administer medications through a handheld **nebulizer** or inhaler. These nebulizers produce a fine spray of medication that is inhaled directly into the lungs. Albuterol inhalers are commonly used for asthma relief.

Health care professionals may administer inhalants in a medical facility. Anesthetics such as nitrous oxide can be inhaled directly into the lungs before surgical treatments.

## Transcutaneous or Transdermal Medications

**Transcutaneous medications**, also known as **transdermal medications**, are absorbed directly through the skin. Dermal medications, which are applied to the skin, include the following:

- topical creams
- lotions
- ointments
- transdermal patches

Most topical medications, such as creams and sprays, produce only local effects, meaning they affect only one area or part of the body. These medications are commonly used for treatments of skin conditions such as rashes or acne. Eye drops are another common topical medication. However, some medications in a topical form may cause systemic effects; that is, they affect the entire body. For example, nitroglycerin (Nitro-Bid, Nitro-Dur, Nitrostat, Transderm-Nitro) can be delivered by pill, patch, cream, or spray to relieve chest pain. The topical forms of this medication cause systemic effects.

Transdermal patches also produce systemic effects. A transdermal patch is placed directly on the skin, usually on the chest, back, upper arm, buttocks, or sometimes behind the ear. Delivery is slow and maintains a steady, stable level of absorption. This means that you should never cut a transdermal patch because that can change the rate of absorption. Two popular examples include the nicotine patch to stop smoking and the birth control patch.

## Sublingual Medications

**Sublingual medications** are placed under the patient's tongue. The drug should not be swallowed; instead it's left under the tongue to dissolve by saliva. As the drug is dissolved, it's

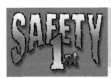

### PLAYING IT SAFE WITH NITROGLYCERIN PATCHES

Remind patients who are using topical or transdermal nitroglycerin to dispose of any unused medication properly. Careful disposal of the patch or cream-coated paper must be done to avoid others coming into contact with the medication. Individuals who empty wastebaskets, small children, and pets need protection from unwelcome systemic effects such as vasodilatation (an increase in blood vessel size) and severe headaches.

absorbed directly into the bloodstream. Patients should not eat or drink anything until the medication has completely dissolved. Some common examples of drugs that can be administered sublingually include the following:

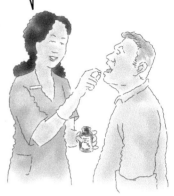

Some solid medications are used sublingually because they dissolve quickly and pass into tiny capillaries under the tongue.

- lorazepam (Ativan, Lorazepam Intensol), a sedative
- nitroglycerin, which is used in the treatment of heart attacks
- cyanocobalamin (vitamin $B_{12}$)
- nifedipine (Adalat, Adalat CC, Nifedical XL, Procardia, Procardia XL)

## Rectal and Vaginal Drug Administration

Some medications may be inserted directly into a patient's rectum or vagina. Rectal medications can provide a local effect, or they may be absorbed into the body for a systemic effect. Rectal medications may be used to treat patients who can't take anything by mouth or those who are experiencing nausea or vomiting.

The most common form of rectal medications is a **suppository** that is inserted directly into the rectum. A suppository is made partly of glycerin and cocoa butter and melts at body temperature. You usually store them in a refrigerator until they are needed. Patients typically insert rectal suppositories at home. However, sometimes, as a medical assistant, you may need to teach patients the proper technique for inserting them.

Vaginal medications are used to treat local effects such as infections. Vaginal medications include suppositories, tablets, hormonal creams, antibiotics, antifungal preparations, and solutions for douches. Many vaginal medications come with special applicators and instructions for administration. These instructions are to be followed carefully. Patients should be educated about the proper way to use these medications.

## Advantages of Parenteral Medications

Parenteral medications have a number of important advantages.

- They are released into the body very quickly and can start to act fast.
- Their dosage can be tailored to the patient's exact needs.
- They can be concentrated in the specific body area, such as a joint, where they are needed.

- They are ideal for patients who can't take medication by mouth because of an illness.
- They are ideal for patients whose stomach acids would destroy the medication.
- Transcutaneous delivery can maintain a slow, steady, stable level of medication.

### Disadvantages of Parenteral Medications

Parenteral medications also have some important disadvantages.

- Once given to a patient, an injected medication can't be taken back.
- The needles used to inject them can injure bone, soft tissue, nerves, or blood vessels.
- Infections can develop if sterile technique procedures are not followed.
- Needles can break in soft tissue.
- The medication can be accidentally injected into the vein instead of the soft tissue.
- Disease conditions may make it difficult to determine how well an inhaled medication is absorbed.
- The patient may experience discomfort upon insertion of the needle and burning with some parenteral medications.

## Resources for Drug Information

Physicians and other health professionals often consult the following three important sources of information about drugs:

- *Physician's Desk Reference*
- *United States Pharmacopeia and National Formulary*
- *United States Pharmacopeia Dispensing Information*

Medication packaging inserts are also frequently used in the medical office for information about drugs.

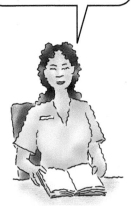

Use available resources to find out more about the drugs the physician prescribes.

### THE *PHYSICIAN'S DESK REFERENCE*

Most medical offices have a copy of the *Physician's Desk Reference* (PDR) on hand. This widely used reference is intended for physicians. However, as a medical assistant, you'll also find it a very useful reference to learn about

## Closer Look    THE PDR: NOT JUST A PICTURE BOOK

The photographs in the PDR are not just for decoration. You may find them useful to help family members identify an unknown pill or capsule that a child found and swallowed by accident. The PDR is also helpful when patients can't remember the name of a medication they have been taking but say something such as, "It's the little pink blood pressure pill."

the drugs the physician prescribes. The PDR includes the following information about drugs:

- the chemical names, the brand names they are sold under, and their generic names
- the properties of each drug, including indications (a listing of the diseases or conditions the drug is intended to treat), dosage information, and adverse reactions
- photographs of various medications

### THE *NATIONAL FORMULARY*

Each year the United States Pharmacopeial Convention publishes the *United States Pharmacopeia and National Formulary* (USP-NF). The book is in two parts: the USP and the NF. The Federal Food, Drug, and Cosmetic Act designates the USP-NF as the official source of information for drugs marketed in the United States. Drug products sold in the United States must conform to USP-NF standards.

The USP-NF contains valuable information that can help you as a medical assistant. This information includes the following:

- information about specific drugs, including their ingredients and dosage forms
- FDA-enforceable standards for medicines, dosage forms, drug substances, and other ingredients in drugs, medical devices, and dietary supplements
- requirements for packaging, storing, and labeling each drug product
- standards and procedures for medical tests

## UNITED STATES PHARMACOPEIA DISPENSING INFORMATION

The two-volume *United States Pharmacopeia Dispensing Information* (USPDI) also provides drug information to health care professionals. The USPDI:

- defines a drug's sources and chemical make-up
- gives the physical properties of the drug and lists tests for identification
- provides information about proper dosage and storage

Unlike the PDR, the USPDI does not contain photographs.

---

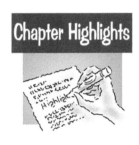

### Chapter Highlights

- Drugs are given three names. The chemical name gives the drug's chemical make-up, the generic name is the official name of the drug, and the trade name is registered by the manufacturer.
- Major drug laws include the Pure Food and Drug Act; the Federal Food, Drug, and Cosmetic Act; the Durham-Humphrey Amendment; the Kefauver-Harris Amendment; and the Controlled Substances Act. These laws are in place to protect consumers from unsafe or harmful drugs.
- The FDA must approve new medications before they can be made available to the public. The FDA also monitors new medications for adverse reactions by using reporting programs such as MedWatch.
- OTC drugs can be purchased without a prescription. Prescription drugs and controlled substances, however, may be obtained only through a licensed health care provider with prescribing privileges.
- Medications made from synthetic sources have several advantages. They are more readily available, and they are less expensive to make than drugs from other sources.
- Medications can be administered in many different forms. Enteral medications are designed to enter the body through the gastrointestinal tract. Parenteral medications, on the other hand, enter the body in other ways, such as by injection or direct application to the skin.
- The *Physician's Desk Reference, The United States Pharmacopeia and National Formulary,* and the *United States Pharmacopeia Dispensing Information* are excellent resources for drug information.

## Chapter 2

# MATH OF MEDICATIONS AND CALCULATING DOSAGES

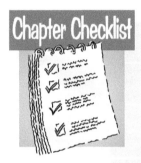

## Chapter Checklist

- Explain the steps necessary to add fractions and reduce them to lowest terms.

- Explain the steps necessary to multiply and divide fractions and decimals.

- Describe the place value of decimals.

- Correctly use a calculator to add, subtract, multiply, and divide.

- Calculate the percentage of any given number.

- Explain how to convert percentages into fractions and fractions into percentages.

- Describe the relationships between ratios, fractions, and proportions.

- Use dimensional analysis to convert between the metric, apothecary, and household systems of measurement.

- Calculate adult medication doses using the formula $W/H \times V$.

- Apply Clark's Law to calculate pediatric doses.

- Use the formula *dosage/kg of body weight* to calculate dosages for individuals of unique size.

As a medical assistant, one of your jobs may be to assist the physician with administering medications. When a pharmacy dispenses a medication to you personally, the dosage is already measured for you. However, when you're working with patients, the measuring may be your job. The information in this chapter will help you brush up on the math skills you'll need to accurately measure medication dosages in the office.

A whole number can also be written as a fraction.

$1 = \frac{3}{3}$

## Fractions

The numbers you'll be working with are whole numbers and fractions.

- **Whole numbers** are the counting numbers 1, 2, 3, 4, 5, and so on.
- **Fractions** are parts of a whole number, such as 1/3, 2/3, 1/8, and 7/8. You read these fractions in words as "one-third," "two-thirds," "one-eighth," and "seven-eighths."

When it comes to fractions, there are a few terms you'll need to know. For example, the number on top is called the **numerator**, and the number on the bottom is called the **denominator**. The denominator tells you the total number of equal parts in the whole. The numerator tells you how many parts of the whole are being considered; for example, a fraction such as 1/2 means the same as one part of two parts total, or 1 divided by 2, 1 ÷ 2, and 1:2.

### FINDING COMMON DENOMINATORS

When you work with fractions that have different denominators, it's hard to tell which fractions are bigger or smaller. That's why you have to find a denominator that's the same for all of the fractions: a **common denominator**.

One way to find a common denominator for a set of fractions is to multiply all the denominators. For example, to find a common denominator for the fractions 2/5 and 7/9, multiply the denominators 5 and 9 to get the multiplied common denominator 45.

$$\frac{2}{5} \quad \frac{7}{9}$$
$$\downarrow \quad \downarrow$$
$$5 \times 9 = 45$$

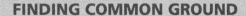

**Secrets for Success**    **FINDING COMMON GROUND**

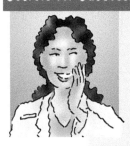

Another way to find a common denominator is to list the multiples of each denominator. Compare them until you get the first match. The number that you find this way is the **lowest common denominator**.

For example, look at the fractions 1/4, 1/6, and 1/8 again.

- The denominators are 4, 6, and 8.
- The multiples of 4 are 4, 8, 12, 16, 20, 24 . . .
- The multiples of 6 are 6, 12, 18, 24 . . .
- The multiples of 8 are 8, 16, 24 . . .
- The first match is 24.
- The lowest common denominator of these fractions is 24.

This method also works to find the common denominator for three or more fractions. For example, to figure out the common denominator for the fractions 1/4, 1/6, and 1/8, simply multiply all of the denominators. The common denominator is 192.

$$4 \times 6 \times 8 = 192$$

## REDUCING FRACTIONS TO THE LOWEST TERMS

When you find a common denominator, the number can be very large. For simplicity, you should usually reduce fractions to their lowest terms. This means that you find the smallest numbers possible in the numerator and the denominator. To simplify fractions, follow these steps:

1. Find the largest number that you can divide equally into the numerator and the denominator. You should have nothing left over when you divide.
2. Divide that number into the numerator and the denominator to reduce the fraction to its lowest terms.

### How Low Can You Go?

To reduce or simplify the fraction 8/10 to its lowest terms:

1. Find the largest number you can divide into both 8 and 10. That number is 2.

2. Divide the numerator and the denominator by 2 to reduce the fraction to its lowest terms, or 4/5.

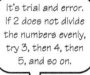

It's trial and error. If 2 does not divide the numbers evenly, try 3, then 4, then 5, and so on.

$$\frac{8}{10} \text{ is } \frac{8 \div 2}{10 \div 2} \text{ is } \frac{4}{5}$$

### Trimming Down the Numbers

To reduce the fraction 7/14 to its lowest terms:

1. Find the largest number you can divide into both 7 and 14. That number is 7.

2. Divide the numerator and the denominator by 7 to reduce the fraction to its lowest terms, or 1/2. This fraction can't be reduced further.

$$\frac{7}{14} \text{ is } \frac{7 \div 7}{14 \div 7} \text{ is } \frac{1}{2}$$

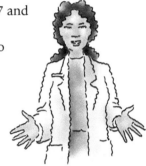

### Third Time's a Charm

To reduce the fraction 3/9 to its lowest terms:

1. Find the largest number you can divide into both 3 and 9. That number is 3.

2. Divide the numerator and the denominator by 3 to reduce the fraction to its lowest terms, or 1/3.

$$\frac{3}{9} \text{ is } \frac{3 \div 3}{9 \div 3} \text{ is } \frac{1}{3}$$

## ADDING FRACTIONS

To add fractions when the denominators are the same, just add the numerators.

$$\frac{1}{3} + \frac{1}{3} = \frac{2}{3}$$

But what if the denominators aren't the same? Then you need to rewrite them as fractions with the same denominator. For example, here's how to add the fractions 1/7 and 1/3:

1. Find the lowest common denominator.
   - The multiples of 7 are 7, 14, 21 . . .
   - The multiples of 3 are 3, 6, 9, 12, 15, 18, 21 . . .
   - The first match is 21.
   - The lowest common denominator of these fractions is 21.

2. Rewrite each fraction so that it has a denominator of 21. To do this, multiply the bottom number by a number that

will make it 21. Multiply the top number by the same number.

$$\frac{1}{7} = \frac{1 \times 3}{7 \times 3} = \frac{3}{21} \qquad \frac{1}{3} = \frac{1 \times 7}{3 \times 7} = \frac{7}{21}$$

3. Now add the fractions. To do this, add the numerators. Put them over the common denominator. This fraction is your answer.

$$\frac{3}{21} + \frac{7}{21} = \frac{3+7}{21} = \frac{10}{21}$$

> When adding or subtracting fractions, remember to convert them to fractions with common denominators. That way, you'll be comparing apples to apples.

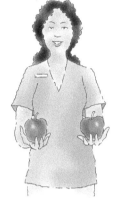

## SUBTRACTING FRACTIONS

Now, suppose you want to subtract these two fractions:

$$\frac{5}{12} - \frac{1}{6} = \underline{\hspace{1cm}}$$

Follow these steps:

1. Find the lowest common denominator. In this example, the lowest match when you compare the multiples of 6 and 12 is 12. So, the lowest common denominator is 12.

2. Rewrite the second fraction so that both fractions have a denominator of 12.

$$\frac{1}{6} = \frac{1 \times 2}{6 \times 2} = \frac{2}{12}$$

> The number you get when you multiply other numbers is called the *product*. Here, 25 is the product.

3. Now subtract the fractions. To do this, subtract the numerators and place them over the common denominator.

$$\frac{5}{12} - \frac{2}{12} = \frac{5-2}{12} = \frac{3}{12}$$

4. Reduce this fraction to its lowest terms, 1/4.

$$\frac{3}{12} = \frac{1}{4}$$

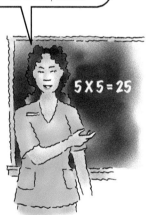

5 X 5 = 25

## MULTIPLYING FRACTIONS

Multiplying fractions is simple: All you have to do is multiply the numerators and then the denominators.

## Multiplying Two Fractions

Suppose you wanted to multiply 4/7 by 5/8. Here's what to do:

1. Set up the problem.

$$\frac{4}{7} \times \frac{5}{8} = \underline{\quad\quad}$$

2. Multiply the numerators. Then multiply the denominators.

$$\frac{4 \times 5}{7 \times 8} = \frac{20}{56}$$

3. Reduce the answer to its lowest terms.

$$\frac{20}{56} = \frac{10}{28} = \frac{5}{14}$$

## Multiplying a Fraction and a Whole Number

Suppose you wanted to multiply 1/9 by 4. Notice that 4 is a whole number, not a fraction. Follow these steps.

1. Set up the problem.

$$\frac{1}{9} \times 4 = \underline{\quad\quad}$$

2. Write the whole number, 4, as a fraction (i.e., the whole number over 1). Put this fraction in the problem instead of the whole number.

$$4 = \frac{4}{1} \qquad \rightarrow \qquad \frac{1}{9} \times \frac{4}{1} = \underline{\quad\quad}$$

3. Multiply the numerators and the denominators.

$$\frac{1}{9} \times \frac{4}{1} = \frac{1 \times 4}{9 \times 1} = \frac{4}{9}$$

## DIVIDING FRACTIONS

When you write an equation for dividing fractions, you usually use the division symbol ÷, which means "divided by." You're dividing the second fraction into the first fraction.

Here's how you read the equation below: "Five-sevenths divided by two-thirds equals how much?"

$$\frac{5}{7} \div \frac{2}{3} = \underline{\quad\quad}$$

See *Know the Lingo* for a quick review of the terms **divisor**, **dividend**, and **quotient**.

# Closer Look    KNOW THE LINGO

Before you can divide numbers, it's helpful to know what each part of a division problem is called. In the examples below, you can see that a division problem can be written in two different ways, although the terms remain the same.

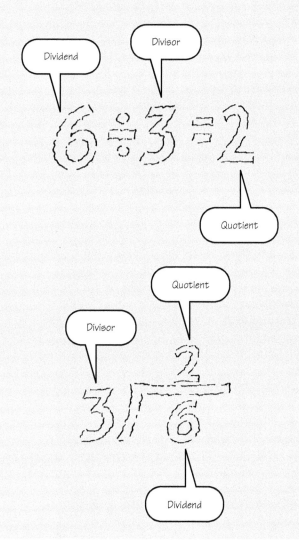

Dividend

Divisor

6 ÷ 3 = 2

Quotient

Quotient

Divisor

$3\overline{)6}^{\,2}$

Dividend

### Dividing a Fraction by a Fraction

Three simple steps are all it takes to divide fractions. Just remember this important part of the process: turn the second fraction upside down and then multiply. For example, to divide 1/2 by 1/4:

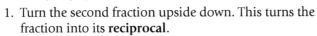

To multiply fractions, you multiply the two top numbers and the two bottom numbers.

1. Turn the second fraction upside down. This turns the fraction into its **reciprocal**.

$$\frac{1}{4} \rightarrow \frac{4}{1}$$

2. Multiply the first fraction by the reciprocal of the second fraction.

$$\frac{1}{2} \div \frac{1}{4} = \frac{1}{2} \times \frac{4}{1} = \underline{\quad\quad}$$

$$\frac{1 \times 4}{2 \times 1} = \frac{4}{2}$$

3. Simplify the fraction.

$$\frac{4}{2} = 2$$

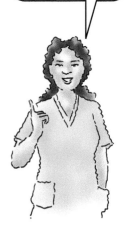

### Dividing a Fraction by a Whole Number

To divide a fraction by a whole number, you follow the same steps. To divide 3/5 by 2:

1. Turn the whole number into its reciprocal. To do this, you use the whole number as the bottom number of a fraction and 1 as the top number.

$$2 \rightarrow \frac{1}{2}$$

2. Multiply the first fraction by the reciprocal of the whole number.

$$\frac{3}{5} \div 2 = \frac{3}{5} \times \frac{1}{2} = \frac{3 \times 1}{5 \times 2} = \frac{3}{10}$$

3. Simplify the fraction (if needed). In this case, 3/10 can't be simplified any further.

## Decimals

As a medical assistant, you'll probably encounter decimals every day at work. This will happen most often if you're assisting with administering medications or collecting money. The metric

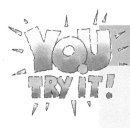

## FIGURING OUT FRACTIONS

Find the lowest common denominator.

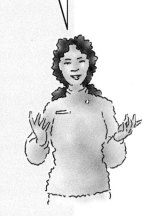

In the real world, you do not get three tries to get it right. So now is the time to practice, practice, practice!

1. $\frac{1}{5}$ and $\frac{2}{3}$

2. $\frac{5}{8}$ and $\frac{3}{16}$

3. $\frac{1}{5}$ and $\frac{1}{7}$

4. $\frac{1}{16}$ and $\frac{3}{4}$

5. $\frac{2}{3}$ and $\frac{1}{2}$

Reduce to the lowest terms.

6. $\frac{3}{12}$

7. $\frac{2}{4}$

8. $\frac{8}{64}$

9. $\frac{3}{9}$

10. $\frac{15}{45}$

Add. Reduce and convert to a mixed number if needed.

11. $\frac{1}{9} + \frac{3}{9}$

12. $\frac{1}{4} + \frac{3}{4}$

13. $\frac{2}{3} + \frac{2}{3}$

14. $\frac{1}{5} + \frac{1}{9}$

15. $1 + \frac{1}{2}$

Subtract. Reduce if needed.

16. $\dfrac{3}{5} - \dfrac{2}{5}$

17. $\dfrac{7}{8} - \dfrac{3}{8}$

18. $\dfrac{15}{16} - \dfrac{3}{16}$

19. $\dfrac{9}{16} - \dfrac{1}{8}$

20. $\dfrac{3}{4} - \dfrac{3}{8}$

Multiply. Reduce if needed.

21. $\dfrac{1}{4} \times \dfrac{1}{4}$

22. $\dfrac{2}{3} \times \dfrac{1}{3}$

23. $\dfrac{1}{2} \times \dfrac{4}{9}$

24. $\dfrac{3}{8} \times 3$

25. $\dfrac{1}{2} \times 4$

Divide. Reduce if needed.

26. $\dfrac{1}{3} \div \dfrac{1}{2}$

27. $\dfrac{5}{6} \div \dfrac{1}{3}$

28. $\dfrac{1}{9} \div \dfrac{1}{2}$

29. $\dfrac{1}{8} \div \dfrac{1}{3}$

30. $\dfrac{3}{4} \div \dfrac{1}{4}$

Solve.

31. Suppose you need to calculate a patient's fluid intake for the last 8 hours. The patient reports that he drank 1/2 cup broth, 2/3 cup ginger ale, and 3/4 cup water. How many cups of liquid did the patient drink?

> Hint: Add the fractions. Remember to use the lowest common denominator.

system is the most commonly used system for measuring medications, and it's based on decimal numbers.

## UNDERSTANDING PLACE VALUES

You already know something about place value from handling money. You know the following:

- $1.05 is less than $1.10.
- $1.15 is less than $1.25.
- $2.00 is more than any of the amounts listed above.

Counting with decimals is very similar to counting with dollars and cents. Dollars are whole dollars, and cents are parts of dollars. **Decimal numbers** have whole numbers to the left of the decimal point and parts of a whole number to the right of the decimal point. For example, in the number 2.25, the decimal point separates the whole number from the decimal fraction. A **decimal fraction** is a proper fraction (meaning the numerator is less than the denominator) in which the denominator is a power of 10, indicated by a decimal point placed at the left of the numerator. An example of a decimal fraction is 0.2, which is the same as 2/10.

### Reading Numbers with Decimals

When you talk about money, you usually say "and" where the decimal point is. You say $5.20 as "five dollars and twenty cents." When you say a decimal aloud, you use the word *point* to identify where the decimal point is. You say 5.2 as "five point two" and 0.25 as "zero point two five" or "point two five."

There are names for all of these places to the left and right of the decimal point. (See *Places, Everyone!*)

### What Zeros Tell You

Zeros are important. The more zeros there are to the left of the decimal point in a number, the larger the number is. The more zeros there are to the right of the decimal point, the smaller the number is. The following table provides some examples.

## Closer Look  PLACES, EVERYONE!

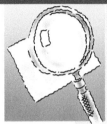

Based on its position in relation to the decimal point, each decimal place represents a power of 10, or a fraction with a denominator that's a power of 10, as shown below:

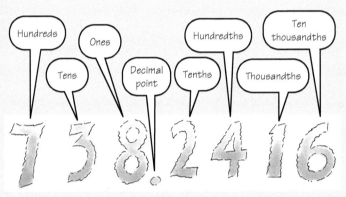

### How Big and How Small?

| Larger | Smaller |
| --- | --- |
| 1.0 | 0.1 |
| 10.0 | 0.01 |
| 100.0 | 0.001 |
| 1000.0 | 0.0001 |

## Secrets for Success  WHEN TO ADD AND DROP ZEROS

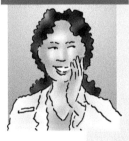

Use the letters *L* and *R* and the words *left* and *right* to remember what to do about zeros when you work with decimals.

- *Leave* a zero to the *left* of the decimal point if you need a placeholder to show a decimal quantity that is less than 1—for example, 0.5 mL.
- *Remove* any trailing zeros to the *right* of the decimal point if no other number follows and you do not need a placeholder to add or subtract. For example, 4.40 mg becomes 4.4 mg.

## ADDING AND SUBTRACTING DECIMALS

Before you add or subtract decimals, be sure to line up all the decimal points. This will help you keep track of the decimal positions. To maintain column alignment, add zeros as place-holders where you need them.

Suppose you need to add these three decimals: 2.61, 0.315, and 4.8.

1. Write the problem correctly. Line up the decimal points. Add any zeros you need.

2. Add the numbers.

$$
\begin{array}{r}
2.610 \\
0.315 \\
+\,4.800 \\
\hline
7.725
\end{array}
$$

### It All Adds Up

Here's another example of adding decimal fractions. Add 0.017, 4.8, and 1.22:

$$
\begin{array}{r}
0.017 \\
4.800 \\
+\,1.220 \\
\hline
6.037
\end{array}
$$

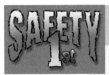

## DOUBLE-CHECK THOSE DECIMALS!

Decimal points and zeros are big deals on medication orders and administration records. When you read a drug order, study it closely. If a dose does not sound right, maybe a decimal point was left out or put in the wrong place.

For instance, an order that calls for ".5 mg lorazepam PO" may be misread as "5 mg of lorazepam PO." The correct way to write this order is to use a zero as a placeholder to the left of the decimal point. The order would then be written as "0.5 mg lorazepam PO."

## Secrets for Success    A HELPING HAND FROM CALCULATORS

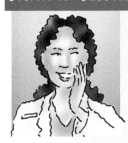

Here are some things to keep in mind when using a calculator.

- Every calculator has function keys (+, −, ×, and ÷).
- When you add or multiply, the order in which you enter the numbers does not matter. 5 + 4 is the same as 4 + 5 and 5 × 4 is the same as 4 × 5.
- When you subtract, however, you have to enter the numbers in the correct order. You often (but not always) subtract the smaller number from the larger number.
- Likewise, when you divide, the order in which you enter the numbers is important. Remember that ÷ means "divided by." To divide 5 into 14, you have to enter it as "14 divided by 5." For example:
  1. Enter the dividend, 14.
  2. Press ÷.
  3. Enter the divisor, 5.
  4. Press = to obtain the quotient, 2.8.

### Line 'Em up and Subtract

Use the same method to subtract decimal fractions. To subtract 0.05 from 4.726:

$$\begin{array}{r} 4.726 \\ -\,0.050 \\ \hline 4.676 \end{array}$$

## MULTIPLYING DECIMALS

You multiply decimals in the same way you multiply whole numbers. You do not have to align the numbers. But you have to do one more step: you have to decide where to place the decimal point.

1. Multiply the numbers. Write the product, or answer.
2. Count the number of decimal places in each of the numbers you're multiplying.
3. Then count out the same number of places in the answer, starting from the right. Put the decimal point after that number.

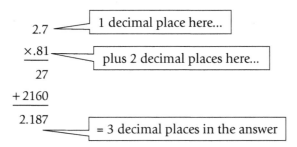

2.7 ← 1 decimal place here...

×.81 ← plus 2 decimal places here...
_____
27
+2160
_____
2.187 ← = 3 decimal places in the answer

Here's another example of multiplying decimal fractions. Notice how to determine where the decimal point in the answer goes. To multiply 1.423 and 8.59:

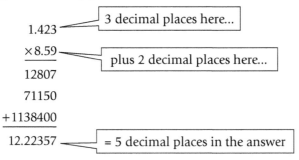

1.423 ← 3 decimal places here...

×8.59 ← plus 2 decimal places here...
_____
12807
71150
+1138400
_____
12.22357 ← = 5 decimal places in the answer

## DIVIDING DECIMALS

When dividing decimal fractions, align the decimal points.

The following example shows how to divide using a whole number divisor. Here's the easy way to know where to place the decimal point:

1. Divide the numbers. Remember to divide by the whole divisor each time.

2. Line up the decimal point in the quotient with the decimal point in the dividend.

$$12\overline{)1.464}$$
quotient: 0.122

Here's another example. Notice how to decide where the decimal point in the answer goes.

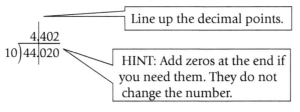

Line up the decimal points.

$$10\overline{)44.020}$$
quotient: 4.402

HINT: Add zeros at the end if you need them. They do not change the number.

Remember: The number to be divided is the dividend, the number that does the dividing is the divisor, and the answer is the quotient.

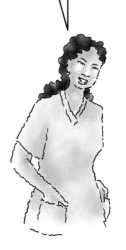

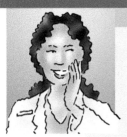

## Secrets for Success

### WORKING WITH DIVISORS THAT CONTAIN DECIMALS

When dividing one decimal fraction by another, move the divisor's decimal point all the way to the right to convert it to a whole number. Then, move the dividend's decimal point the same number of places to the right. After completing the division problem, place the quotient's decimal point directly above the new decimal point in the dividend. For example, to divide 10.45 by 2.6:

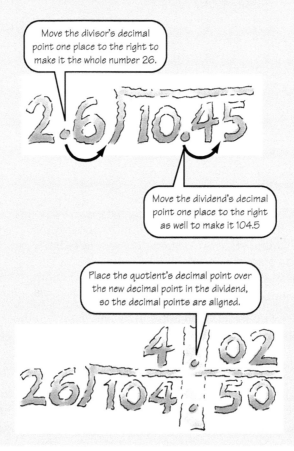

Move the divisor's decimal point one place to the right to make it the whole number 26.

Move the dividend's decimal point one place to the right as well to make it 104.5

Place the quotient's decimal point over the new decimal point in the dividend, so the decimal points are aligned.

## ROUNDING OFF DECIMALS

Most of the instruments and measuring devices you'll use as a medical assistant measure accurately only to a tenth or maybe a hundredth. You'll need to round off decimal fractions. That means converting long fractions to those with fewer decimal places.

Here's what to do. When you round off a decimal fraction, the magic number is 5. Check the number to the right of the decimal place that will be rounded off.

- If that number is greater than or equal to 5, add 1 to the number to the left of it.
- If that number is less than 5, do not add 1.

The following examples demonstrate rounding numbers to the nearest tenth (one decimal place).

| | | |
|---|---|---|
| 98.46 | → | 98.5 |
| 98.44 | → | 98.4 |
| 104.252 | → | 104.3 |
| 104.245 | → | 104.2 |

The next examples show rounding numbers to the nearest hundredth (two decimal places).

| | | |
|---|---|---|
| 72.345 | → | 72.35 |
| 72.343 | → | 72.34 |
| 25.1171 | → | 25.12 |
| 25.1101 | → | 25.11 |

# Percentages

Percentages are another way to express fractions and numerical relationships. The percent symbol may be used with a whole number such as 21%, a mixed number such as 34 1/2%, a decimal number such as 0.9%, or a fraction such as 1/8%. You should know how to convert easily from percentages to decimal fractions and common fractions, and vice versa.

## CONVERTING PERCENTAGES TO DECIMAL FRACTIONS

To change a percentage to a decimal fraction, remove the % sign and multiply the number in the percentage by 1/100, or 0.01. For example, you would convert 84% and 35% to decimal fractions in this way:

$$84 \times 0.01 = 0.84$$

$$35 \times 0.01 = 0.35$$

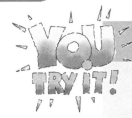

## DECIPHERING DECIMALS

Add. Round to the nearest tenth (one decimal point).
1. $4.218 + 5.03$
2. $0.277 + 4.33 + 7.8$
3. $1.2 + 2.1 + 3.77$
4. $90.75 + 3.45 + 2.23$
5. $2710 + .25 + .355$

Subtract. Round to the nearest hundredth (two decimal points).
6. $77.339 - 27.274$
7. $100.965 - 84.009$
8. $1791.791 - 1500.002$
9. $1.986 - 1.497$
10. $5.6995 - 4.0005$

Multiply and round to the nearest tenth (one decimal point).
11. $3.5 \times 0.05$
12. $55.2 \times 1.3$
13. $5.23 \times 18.98$
14. $45.1 \times 10.875$
15. $100 \times 0.0659$

Divide and round to the nearest hundredth (two decimal points).
16. $2\overline{)2.468}$
17. $4\overline{)16.084}$
18. $10\overline{)0.895}$
19. $25\overline{)25.625}$
20. $25\overline{)24.8}$

Solve.
21. During today's office visit, the physician changed Martin's dosage from 0.25 mg of atenolol daily to 0.75 mg daily. However, the patient just had his old

prescription for the lower dosage of the drug refilled. He has 88 tablets left in the bottle.

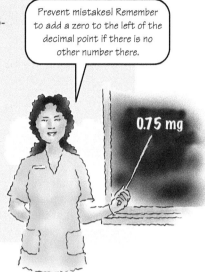

Prevent mistakes! Remember to add a zero to the left of the decimal point if there is no other number there.

0.75 mg

a. How many of the lower-strength tablets should Martin take each day to get the full new dose?

b. For how many days can he do this until he has to have the new prescription filled? The physician has warned him not to break tablets into pieces and not to take a partial dose.

Make sure that you shift the decimal point in the correct direction (to your left, when converting a percentage to the decimal); otherwise you could calculate a drug dose incorrectly.

## CONVERTING PERCENTAGES TO COMMON FRACTIONS

Suppose you want to convert 50% to a common fraction. To convert a percentage to a common fraction, follow these steps:

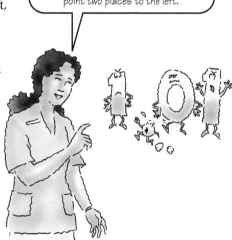

It's all about the decimal point! When converting a percentage to a fraction, remember to begin by moving the decimal point two places to the left.

1. Remove the percent sign and put a decimal point two places to the left, creating the decimal fraction 0.50.

   $$50\% = 0.50$$

2. Convert 0.50 to a common fraction with a denominator that's a factor of 10. The result is 50/100 because 0.50 has two decimal places.

   $$0.50 = \frac{50}{100}$$

3. Reduce the fraction to its lowest terms, which is 1/2.

   $$\frac{50}{100} = \frac{1}{2}$$

## CONVERTING COMMON FRACTIONS TO PERCENTAGES

Converting a common fraction to a percentage involves two simple steps. Suppose you want to convert 2/5 to a percentage. First, create a decimal fraction by dividing the numerator, 2, by the denominator, 5. You can do this by hand or with a calculator. The calculation looks like this:

$$\frac{2}{5} = 5\overline{\smash{)}\begin{array}{r} 0.4 \\ 2.0 \end{array}}$$

Next, convert the decimal fraction to a percentage by moving the decimal point two places to the right (you'll need to add a zero as a placeholder) and then adding the percentage sign. Here's what the calculation looks like:

$$0.40 = 40\%$$

## SOLVING PERCENTAGE PROBLEMS

Solving percentage problems involves three types of calculations. They are:

- finding a percentage of a number
- finding what percentage one number is of another
- finding a number when a percentage of it is known

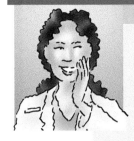

## Secrets for Success

### A WORD ABOUT PERCENTAGE PROBLEMS

When a percentage problem is worded this way: "What is 25% of 80?" mentally change the word *of* to a multiplication sign. Therefore, the problem becomes "What is 25% (or using a decimal fraction, 0.25) × 80?" Then continue with the calculation:

$$0.25 \times 80 = 20$$

If a problem is worded as "25 is what percentage of 80?" treat the word *what* as a division sign so the problem becomes 25/80. Then continue with the calculation:

$$25 \div 80 = 0.3125 = 31.25\%$$

## Finding a Percentage of a Number

The question "What is 40% of 200?" is an example of the first type of calculation. To solve it, change the word *of* to a multiplication sign. This gives you:

40% × 200 = ?

Next, convert 40% to a decimal fraction by removing the percent sign and moving the decimal point two places to the left. This gives you:

0.40 × 200 = ?

Then multiply the numbers to get the answer, 80:

0.40 × 200 = 80 —— | 40% of 200 is 80. |

## Finding What Percentage One Number Is of Another

The question "10 is what percentage of 200?" is an example of this type of calculation. To solve it, restate the question as a division problem, with the number 10 as the dividend and the number 200 as the divisor. Here's how the calculation looks so far:

$$\frac{0.05}{200 \overline{)10.00}}$$

Now, move the decimal point in the quotient two places to the right and add a percent sign.

0.05 = 5% —— | 10 is 5% of 200. |

## Finding a Number When You Know a Percentage of It

Finding a number when you know the percentage of it requires division. For example, consider the following question: "70% of what number is 7?" Here's how to do the calculation.

First, convert 70% into a decimal fraction by removing the percent sign and moving the decimal point two places to the left.

70% = 0.70

Next, divide 7 by 0.70. Move the decimal point two places to the right in both the divisor (to make it a whole number) and the dividend. The quotient is 10.

$$\frac{10.0}{0.70 \overline{)7.00\,0}}$$    | 70% of 10 is 7. |

## Closer Look    WHAT TO DO WITH THE REMAINDER

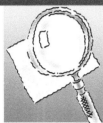

Sometimes, when determining what percentage one number is of another number, the divisor won't divide exactly into the dividend. In these cases, state the quotient as a mixed number by turning the remainder—the undivided part of the quotient—into a common fraction.

Here's how to do this using the problem, "3 is what percent of 11?"

First, restate the question as a division problem, making 11 the divisor and 3 the dividend. Work out the quotient to two decimal places; then take the remainder, 3, and make it the numerator of a fraction with the divisor, 11, as the denominator. Here's what the calculation looks like:

$$
\begin{array}{r}
0.27 \\
11\overline{)3.00} \\
2\,2 \phantom{0}\\
\hline
80 \\
77 \\
\hline
3
\end{array}
$$

The remainder as a common fraction is 3/11.

Next, move the decimal point in the quotient two places to the right and add a percent sign. (The remaining fraction, 3/11, is placed to the left of the percent sign.)

0.27 and 3/11 = 27 3/11%

When calculating dosages, you'll use ratios, fractions, and proportions frequently.

## Ratios, Fractions, and Proportions

Ratios, fractions, and proportions describe relationships between numbers. Ratios use a colon between the numbers in the relationship, as in 4:9. Fractions use a slash between numbers in the relationship, as in 4/9.

Proportions are statements of equality between two ratios. For example, to show that 4:9 is equal to 8:18, you would write:

4:9::8:18

or

$$\frac{4}{9} = \frac{8}{18}$$

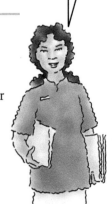

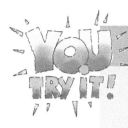

## PERCENTAGE PRACTICE

Convert the following percentages to common fractions. Reduce to lowest terms.

1. 81%

2. 32.7%

3. 20.05%

Convert the fractions below to percentages.

4. $\dfrac{1}{3}$

5. $\dfrac{3}{8}$

6. $\dfrac{7}{25}$

Find the percentage of the number.

7. What is 5% of 150?

8. What is 7% of 300?

9. What is 68% of 425?

Find what percentage one number is of another.

10. What percentage of 28 is 14?

11. What percentage of 30 is 6?

12. What percentage of 22 is 5?

Find the number when you know the percentage of it.

13. 30% of what number is 90?

14. 70% of what number is 28?

15. 28% of what number is 112?

Solve.

16. The physician prescribes amoxicillin (Amoxil) to treat a young patient's ear infection. The patient is to take one 400-mg chewable tablet twice a day. If the medication bottle originally contained 20 tablets, what percentage of these tablets will be left if the patient takes the medication as directed for four days?

Ratios and fractions are numerical ways to compare items. For example, if 100 syringes come in a box, then the number of syringes compared to the number of boxes is 100 to 1. This can be written as the ratio 100:1 or as the fraction 100/1. Conversely, the number of boxes to syringes would be 1:100 or the fraction 1/100, so pay attention to which item is mentioned first.

Here's another example. Suppose a vial has 8 mg of a drug in 1 mL of solution. By using a ratio, you can express this as 8 mg:1 mL. By using a fraction, you can describe it as 8 mg/1 mL.

## EXPRESSING PROPORTIONS WITH RATIOS

When using ratios in a proportion, separate them with double colons. Double colons represent equality between the two ratios.

For example, if the ratio of syringes to boxes is 100:1, then 200 syringes are provided in two boxes. This proportion can be written as:

100 syringes:1 box::200 syringes:2 boxes

or

100:1::200:2

meaning

100 is to 1 as 200 is to 2

Similarly, if you have a vial that contains 8 mg of a drug in 1 mL of a solution, you can state this as the ratio 8 mg:1 mL. This proportion equals 16 mg:2 mL and can be expressed with ratios as follows:

8 mg:1 mL::16 mg:2 mL

or

8:1::16:2

meaning

8 mg:1 mL = 16 mg:2 mL

## EXPRESSING PROPORTIONS WITH FRACTIONS

Any proportion that can be expressed with ratios can also be expressed with fractions. Also, any proportion that's expressed as two ratios can also be expressed as two fractions.

For example, if 100 syringes come in a box, this means that 200 syringes come in two boxes. Using fractions, you can write this proportion as:

$$\frac{100 \text{ syringes}}{1 \text{ box}} = \frac{200 \text{ syringes}}{2 \text{ boxes}}$$

or

$$\frac{100}{1} = \frac{200}{2}$$

Likewise, if there are 8 mg of a drug in 1 mL, this means there are 16 mg in 2 mL. This proportion can be expressed with fractions as:

$$\frac{8 \text{ mg}}{1 \text{ mL}} = \frac{16 \text{ mg}}{2 \text{ mL}}$$

or

$$\frac{8}{1} = \frac{16}{2}$$

## Units of Measurement

In the medical world, the three systems of measurement that are commonly used are the:

- metric system—used by medical staff and drug companies and in professional journals.
- apothecary system—an older system sometimes still used by pharmacists. Most pharmacists and physicians now use the metric system.
- household system—used by individuals at home when following recipes in a cookbook.

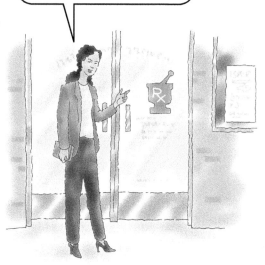

A pharmacist was once called an apothecary or a chemist. In the 19th and early 20th centuries, pharmacists made medicines from scratch.

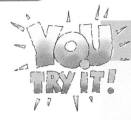

## RATIO REHEARSAL

Convert the following to ratios.

1. 50 capsules in each medication bottle
2. 40 mg of a drug in 5 mL of solution
3. 125 mg of a drug in 2 tablets

Use ratios to express the following proportions.

4. If the ratio of adhesive bandages to boxes is 25:1, then 50 bandages are provided in two boxes. What is the proportion?

5. If there are 5 mg of a drug in 2 mL of a solution, you can state this as the ratio 5:2. Based on this ratio, it follows that there are 20 mg of the drug in 8 mL of solution, or 20:8. Express these ratios as a proportion.

6. If there are 2.5 mg of a drug in each tablet, the ratio would be expressed as 2.5:1. Based on this ratio, you can determine that there are 7.5 mg of the drug in three tablets, or 7.5:3. What is the proportion?

Use fractions to express the following proportions.

7. 1:5::2:10
8. 27:2::81:6
9. 12:3900::3:975

Solve.

10. The physician prescribes 240 mg of acetaminophen (Tylenol) to relieve a 5-year-old patient's pain and fever and would like the first dose to be administered in the medical office. On hand is an oral suspension that contains 160 mg/5 mL. How many milliliters should be administered to the patient?

## THE METRIC SYSTEM

Scientists around the world use the metric system for volume, weight, length, and distance. Medical science does, too. If you're not familiar with the metric system from high school science class, you'd be wise to learn it now. You'll use it every day at work in the medical office.

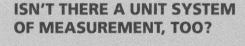

**ISN'T THERE A UNIT SYSTEM OF MEASUREMENT, TOO?**

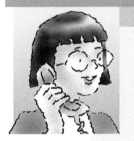

**Q:** My sister has type 1 diabetes and gives herself insulin injections. I noticed that her insulin bottles are labeled *100 units/mL*. What are units?

**A:** You get an A+ for being observant! The strength of the active ingredient in some drugs is measured simply in units. How much of the actual unit depends on the kind of drug. Units are unique to each kind.

Insulin is one of the drugs measured this way. The injectable form of penicillin is another. The label *100 units/mL* means that 100 units of your sister's insulin are in each milliliter of liquid.

You'll usually find units labeled in one of two ways:

• USP, for United States Pharmacopoeia

• IU, for International Units

Handle units like any other measurement you encounter.

---

Using the metric system makes it easier to calculate drug doses. You do not have to worry about fractions, using decimals instead. And like decimals, the metric system is based on the number 10 and multiples of 10 or parts of 10.

### Basic Metric Units

The following table describes the three basic units you need to know.

| Basic Metric Units | | |
| --- | --- | --- |
| **Unit** | **What It Measures** | **Abbreviation** |
| meter | length or distance | m |
| liter | volume | L |
| gram | weight | g |

### Making Prefixes Work for You

Different prefixes are used to indicate larger or smaller metric units. The prefix tells you the number by which to multiply the

## Prefixes for Metric Units

| Prefix | Multiply by | Example | Abbreviation |
|--------|-------------|---------|--------------|
| kilo- | 1,000 | kilometer | km |
| | | kiloliter | kL |
| | | kilogram | kg |
| deci- | 10 | deciliter | dL |
| centi- | 1/100 | centimeter | cm |
| | | cubic centimeter | cc or cm³ |
| | | centigram | cg |
| milli- | 1/1,000 | millimeter | mm |
| | | milliliter | mL |
| | | mg | mg |

basic unit. These prefixes are the ones you'll see and use most often in your work as a medical assistant.

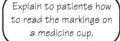

Explain to patients how to read the markings on a medicine cup.

### Metric System Do's and Do Not's

Remember these tips when you use the metric system.

- DO use the correct abbreviations. They always follow a number. For example, abbreviate five kilograms as *5 kg.*

- DO use decimals, not fractions. Always write *2.5 mg* instead of *2 ½ mg.*

- DO add a zero to the left of the decimal point if the amount is less than one. For example, write *0.5 mg* instead of *.5 mg.*

- DO NOT add extra zeros at the end of a decimal because they could be misunderstood. Write *5 mg* instead of *5.0 mg* and write *0.5 mL* instead of *0.500 mL.*

- DO remember that 5 mL = 1 teaspoon; this will allow you to find equivalents with any measurement in the household system.

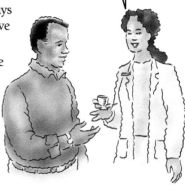

## THE APOTHECARY SYSTEM

Physicians and pharmacists used the apothecary system before the metric system was introduced. Even though the apothecary system is rarely used these days, you should be familiar with it.

### Basic Apothecary System Units

The following table lists the basic units you need to know. Some of the units are also common household measurements.

## Secrets for Success

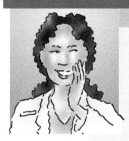

### USING PLACE VALUE TO CONVERT WITHIN THE METRIC SYSTEM

Sometimes, you'll get a medication order in a quantity that does not match what's on the bottle. To get it right, you'll need to convert between two sizes. It could be between liters and milliliters or between grams and milligrams.

Here's an easy way to do the conversion.

1. Write the problem. For example, 4750 mg = _____ g.

2. Identify each quantity (milligrams and grams) as smaller or larger than the other one.

3. Write the letter *L* (for "larger") or *S* (for "smaller") over each quantity.

4. Read the letters you wrote from left to right.
   - SL means *slide* the decimal point the appropriate number of places to the *left*. For example, 4750 mg = 4.75 g.
   - LS means move the decimal point the appropriate number of places to the right. Add extra zeros if necessary. For example, 3.5 L = 3500 mL.

## Apothecary System of Measurement

| Use | Unit | Abbreviation |
|-----|------|--------------|
| Measuring liquids (volume) | | |
| | minim | m |
| | fluid dram | fl dr |
| | fluid ounce | fluid oz |
| | pint | pt |
| | quart | qt |
| | gallon | gal |
| Measuring solids (weight) | | |
| | grain | gr |
| | dram | dr |
| | ounce | oz |
| | pound | lb |

One way to remember the smallest units is to picture the minim as about the size of a drop of water, which weighs about the same as a grain of wheat. For example:

1 drop = 1 minim = 1 grain

More about the grain:

- The grain is probably the most commonly used apothecary measurement; for example, aspirin is often measured in grains.
- The abbreviation for grain is *gr*, and the abbreviation for gram is *g*.
- When medicine is prescribed in grains, it's often ordered with the abbreviation *gr* followed by roman numerals—for example, *aspirin gr x*.
- Remember that 60 or 65 mg = 1 grain. (Use whichever is the easiest to calculate.)
- Use the idea of a clock when trying to figure out a fraction of a grain, for example, 0.5 gr = 30 mg; 1/3 gr = 20 mg; 0.75 gr = 45 mg.

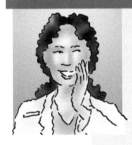

## Secrets for Success   CONVERTING BETWEEN UNITS

Just like you need to know how many pints are in a quart, you may sometimes need to know how many drams are in an ounce. Use the information in the following table to help you find this and other equivalents.

### Apothecary System Equivalents

Liquid Volume

| | | |
|---|---|---|
| 60 minim (m) | = | 1 fluid dram |
| 8 fluid drams | = | 1 fluid ounce (oz) |
| 16 fluid oz | = | 1 pint (pt) |
| 2 pt | = | 1 quart (qt) |
| 4 qt | = | 1 gallon (gal) |

Solid Weight

| | | |
|---|---|---|
| 60–65 grains (gr) | = | 1 dram |
| 8 drams | = | 1 oz |

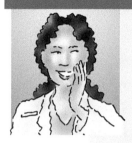

## Secrets for Success · THE ROAD TO ROMAN NUMERALS

Here's a handy review of Roman numerals.

| | | |
|---|---|---|
| 1 = I | 11 = XI | 40 = XL |
| 2 = II | 12 = XII | 50 = L |
| 3 = III | 13 = XIII | 60 = LX |
| 4 = IV | 14 = XIV | 70 = LXX |
| 5 = V | 15 = XV | 80 = LXXX |
| 6 = VI | 16 = XVI | 90 = XC |
| 7 = VII | 17 = XVII | 100 = C |
| 8 = VIII | 18 = XVIII | 200 = CC |
| 9 = IX | 19 = XIX | 500 = D |
| 10 = X | 20 = XX | 1,000 = M |
| | 30 = XXX | |

To help you remember Roman numerals in the correct order, recite this sentence: 1 Very Xtra Large Cow Drinks Milk.

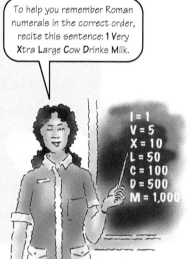

I = 1
V = 5
X = 10
L = 50
C = 100
D = 500
M = 1,000

### Roman Numerals

Some physicians and pharmacists use Arabic numerals (1, 2, 3, and so on) to express dosages in the apothecary system. When written, these look like any other dosage, for example, 5 drams, 20 fluid ounces.

However, you may also see dosages written in the more traditional form, using Roman numerals. Here's what you'll need to know about dosages written this way.

- The Roman numeral usually comes after the unit of measurement. For example, 5 grains is written *grains v.*
- The Roman numerals from I to X (1 to 10) are usually written in lowercase.
- All other fractions are written with Arabic numerals.

### Converting Between Arabic and Roman Numerals

To convert an Arabic numeral into a Roman numeral, follow these steps:

1. Break the Arabic numeral into its parts.

   125 = 100 + 20 + 5

2. Translate each part into Roman numerals.

$$125 = 100 + 20 + 5 = C + XX + V = CXXV$$

When determining the value of a Roman numeral, however, there are two rules to keep in mind:

- When a smaller numeral precedes a larger numeral, subtract the smaller numeral from the larger numeral. For example:

  $$IX = 10 - 1 = 9$$

- When a smaller numeral follows a larger numeral, add the numerals. For example:

  $$XI = 10 + 1 = 11$$

## THE HOUSEHOLD SYSTEM

When physicians prescribe liquid medications such as cough syrup and liquid antibiotics, they'll give the dosages in household measurements. Often, though, eardrops will come with a dropper marked with measurement. Also, some bottles of eye drops can be adjusted to dispense two drops at the same time. However, for those medications that are measured using the household system, most families have or can easily get the measuring tools they'll need:

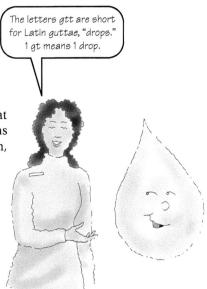

The letters gtt are short for Latin guttae, "drops." 1 gt means 1 drop.

- teaspoons
- tablespoons
- medication cups

Occasionally, you may have to convert between sizes in the household system. Use this chart of equivalents to help you.

## Household Measurement Equivalents

| | | |
|---|---|---|
| 60 drops (gtt) | = | 1 teaspoon (tsp) |
| 3 tsp | = | 1 tablespoon (tbs) |
| 2 tbs | = | 1 ounce (oz) |
| 8 oz | = | 1 cup |
| 16 oz (2 cups) | = | 1 pint (pt) |
| 2 pt | = | 1 quart (qt) |
| 4 qt | = | 1 gallon (gal) |

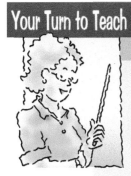

**Your Turn to Teach**

## TIPS FOR MEASURING MEDICATIONS AT HOME

Will the patient be taking medication at home? If so, show him how to use the devices below correctly.

### Medication Cup

A medication cup often has markings that use household, metric, and apothecary measurements.

- Help the patient find the right set of markings to use. If the prescription reads teaspoons, the patient should look for teaspoons on the cup.

- Tell the patient to set the cup on a counter or a flat surface. Then have the patient check at eye level to see how much liquid is inside.

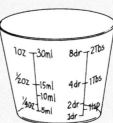

### Dropper

A dropper has markings that use household or metric measurements. It can also have special markings for medication strength or concentration.

- Help the patient find the right set of markings to use.

- Tell him to hold the dropper at eye level to check how much liquid is inside.

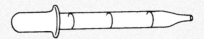

### Hollow-Handle Spoon

The markings on a hollow-handle spoon show teaspoons and tablespoons.

- Help the patient find the right set of markings to use.

- Teach the patient to check the dose after filling by holding the spoon upright at eye level.

• Show the patient how to take the medicine. First, tilt the spoon until the medication fills the bowl of the spoon. Then, tell the patient to place the spoon in his mouth and swallow the dose.

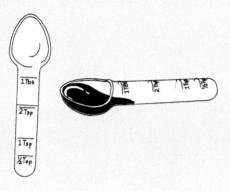

## Translating Tablespoons to Teaspoons

The physician tells a patient to take four tablespoons of milk of magnesia. How many teaspoons does this equal?

First, determine what you know. For example, there are three teaspoons of liquid in one tablespoon. To find out how many teaspoons are in four tablespoons, follow these steps:

1. Set up an equation. *X* is the unknown quantity.

$$\frac{3 \text{ tsp}}{1 \text{ tbs}} = \frac{X}{4 \text{ tbs}}$$

2. Solve for *X* by cross-multiplying the fractions, dividing each side of the equation by 1 tbs, and canceling the units of measurement that appear in both the numerator and the denominator.

$$\frac{X \times 1 \text{ tbs}}{1 \text{ tbs}} = \frac{3 \text{ tsp} \times 4 \text{ tbs}}{1 \text{ tbs}}$$

$$X = 12 \text{ tsp}$$

## A Drop in the Bucket

The physician has ordered 15 drops of a medication for a small infant. However, the drug label gives instructions in teaspoons.

How many teaspoons should be administered to the infant?

You know that there are 60 drops (gtt) of liquid in each teaspoon (tsp). So, to find out how many teaspoons are in 15 gtt, follow these steps:

1. Set up an equation, using $X$ as the unknown quantity.

$$\frac{60 \text{ gtt}}{1 \text{ tsp}} = \frac{15 \text{ gtt}}{X}$$

2. Cross-multiply the fractions.

$$X \times 60 \text{ gtt} = 1 \text{ tsp} \times 15 \text{ gtt}$$

3. Solve for $X$ by dividing each side of the equation by 60 gtt and canceling the units of measurement that are in both the numerator and the denominator.

$$\frac{X \times 60 \cancel{\text{ gtt}}}{60 \cancel{\text{ gtt}}} = \frac{1 \text{ tsp} \times 15 \cancel{\text{ gtt}}}{60 \cancel{\text{ gtt}}}$$

$$X = \frac{1 \text{ tsp} \times 15}{60}$$

$$X = 15/60 \text{ or } 1/4 \text{ tsp}$$

## *Dimensional Analysis*

Dimensional analysis gives you a basic and simple way to figure out drug dosages because you do not have to memorize any formulas. You need to solve only one equation to find your answer.

Dimensional analysis is a method of problem solving. You can use it whenever two quantities are directly proportional to each other. You use conversion factors, or common equivalents, to do the hard work.

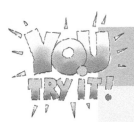

**HOUSEHOLD MEASUREMENT CONVERSIONS**

A patient is following a clear liquid diet. For lunch he drank six tablespoons of chicken broth. How many ounces of chicken broth did he have?

## CONVERSION FACTORS

A conversion factor tells you that two units equal the same thing. Here are five conversion factors you can use to figure out times.

- 1 year = 52 weeks
- 1 week = 7 days
- 1 day = 24 hours
- 1 hour = 60 minutes
- 1 minute = 60 seconds

Planning a vacation? You can use these conversion factors to figure out how many hours you have left in the 3 weeks before you leave. Just multiply the number of weeks by the number of days in a week by the number of hours a day. You can write this in an equation:

$$\frac{3 \text{ weeks}}{1} \times \frac{7 \text{ days}}{1 \text{ week}} \times \frac{24 \text{ hours}}{1 \text{ day}} = 504 \text{ hours}$$

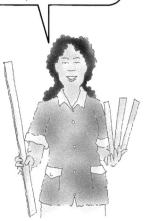

Remember, the equal sign means that the conversion works both ways. Three feet equals one yard and one yard equals three feet.

## USING CONVERSION FACTORS IN THE MEDICAL OFFICE

You can also use conversion factors to convert between metric, household, and apothecary systems. This may be necessary, for example, when the physician prescribes a dosage in milliliters and you need to convert the dosage to teaspoons or tablespoons for the patient.

The following table lists some of the most useful conversion factors. After you read the chart, you'll find out how to put these conversion factors to work for you.

### Common Conversion Factors

| Length | Weight | Volume |
|---|---|---|
| 1 m = 3.28 ft | 1 kg = 2.2 lb | 1 oz = 30 mL |
| 1 cm = 0.4 in. | 1 lb = 0.45 kg | 8 oz = 1 cup |
| 1 mm = 0.04 in. | 1 oz = 28.4 g | 1 tsp = 5 mL |
| 1 in. = 25.4 mm | 1 lb = 16 oz | 2 tbs = 1 oz |
| 1 in. = 2.54 cm | 1 grain = 60 or 65 mg | 1 tbs = 15 mL |
| 1 ft = 30.48 cm | | 1 pt = 480 mL |
| 1 yd = 0.914 m | | 1 qt = 960 mL |

## Ounce for Ounce

Suppose you're sending a shipment to a lab for testing. You know the package weighs 38 ounces but the shipping form asks for the weight in pounds. Here's how to calculate how many pounds the package weighs.

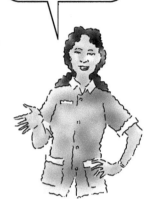

Notice how you turn the conversion factor into a fraction. It's the same as multiplying by 1 because $\frac{16\ oz}{16\ oz} = 1$.

1. Identify what you know.

   38 oz

2. Identify what you want to find out. Use $X$ to mean "unknown."

   $X$ pounds

3. Identify the conversion factor.

   1 lb = 16 oz

4. Set up the equation.

   $$\frac{38\ oz}{1} \times \frac{1\ lb}{16\ oz} = X$$

5. Cancel units that appear in both the numerator and the denominator.

   $$\frac{38\ \cancel{oz}}{1} \times \frac{1\ lb}{16\ \cancel{oz}} = X$$

6. Multiply the numerators and the denominators. Then divide the results to get your answer.

   $$\frac{38 \times 1\ lb}{1 \times 16} \times \frac{38\ lb}{16} = 2.375\ lb$$

   38 ounces equals 2.375 pounds.

## Going Metric

Now take this example a little further. If the package weighs 38 ounces, what does it weigh in kilograms? Follow the same steps.

1. Identify what you know.

   38 oz

2. Identify what you want to find out. Use $X$ to mean "unknown."

   $X$ kilograms

3. Identify the conversion factor(s). In this case, there are two.

1 lb = 16 oz

1 kg = 2.2 lb

> Here you're making two conversions—from ounces to pounds and from pounds to kilograms. That's because the conversion factor you're using, 1 kg = 2.2 pounds, is expressed in pounds.

4. Set up the equation.

$$\frac{38 \text{ oz}}{1} \times \frac{1 \text{ lb}}{16 \text{ oz}} \times \frac{1 \text{ kg}}{2.2 \text{ lb}} = X$$

5. Cancel units that appear in both the numerator and the denominator.

$$\frac{38 \ \cancel{oz}}{1} \times \frac{1 \ \cancel{lb}}{16 \ \cancel{oz}} \times \frac{1 \text{ kg}}{2.2 \ \cancel{lb}} = X$$

6. Multiply the numerators and the denominators. Then divide the results to get your answer.

$$\frac{38 \times 1 \text{ lb} \times 1 \text{ kg}}{1 \times 16 \times 2.2} \times \frac{38 \text{ kg}}{35.2} = 1.0795455 \text{ kg} = 1.08 \text{ kg}$$

38 ounces equals 1.08 kg.

## Cough Syrup Quandary

You've been ordered to give a patient at the clinic two ounces of cough syrup. The medicine cup you have is calibrated in milliliters. How many milliliters are in two ounces? Follow the same six steps you've learned.

1. Identify what you know.

2 oz

2. Identify what you want to find out. Use $X$ to mean "unknown."

$X$ mL

3. Identify the conversion factors.

1 tsp = 5 mL

2 tbs = 1 oz

3 tsp = 1 tbs

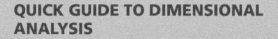

**Secrets for Success**

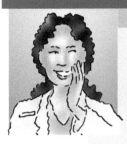

## QUICK GUIDE TO DIMENSIONAL ANALYSIS

Need to calculate a dosage? Do not panic. Just review this step-by-step guide to come up with the number you need quickly.

1. *Given*. What quantity is given in the problem?
2. *Wanted*. What quantity do you want to find out?
3. *Conversion factor*. What conversion factor do you need to change between systems of measuring?

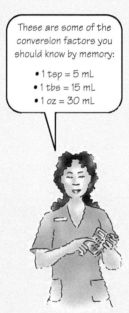

> These are some of the conversion factors you should know by memory:
> - 1 tsp = 5 mL
> - 1 tbs = 15 mL
> - 1 oz = 30 mL

1. *Set up the problem as an equation.* Set up the fractions so that the units you need to cancel are in the top and bottom parts of the fractions. You can't cancel units unless they appear in both the numerator and the denominator.
2. *Cancel unwanted units.* Isolate the unit you want to solve for. Cancel unwanted units in the top and bottom parts of the fractions.
3. *Multiply, multiply, and divide.* Here's where you use your math skills or a calculator to solve the problem. Multiply the numerators. Multiply the denominators. Then divide the bottom number into the top number.

4. Set up the equation.

$$\frac{2 \text{ oz}}{1} \times \frac{2 \text{ tbs}}{1 \text{ oz}} \times \frac{3 \text{ tsp}}{1 \text{ tbs}} \times \frac{5 \text{ mL}}{1 \text{ tsp}} = X$$

5. Cancel units that appear in both the numerator and the denominator.

$$\frac{2 \text{ o\hspace{-0.6em}/z}}{1} \times \frac{2 \text{ t\hspace{-0.6em}/bs}}{1 \text{ o\hspace{-0.6em}/z}} \times \frac{3 \text{ t\hspace{-0.6em}/sp}}{1 \text{ t\hspace{-0.6em}/bs}} \times \frac{5 \text{ mL}}{1 \text{ t\hspace{-0.6em}/sp}} = X$$

6. Multiply the numerators and the denominators. Then divide the results to get your answer.

$$\frac{2 \times 2 \times 3 \times 5 \text{ mL}}{1 \times 1 \times 1 \times 1} = \frac{60 \text{ mL}}{1} = 60 \text{ mL}$$

2 ounces equals 60 milliliters.

## Calculating Adult Dosages with the Formula W/H × V

A medicine's strength is usually based on its use in adults. A dose that is appropriate for the standard 150-pound adult could be lethal to a child.

When you're working with medications, the package label is very important to read. Most drugs come in a variety of strengths. Many times, the physician will prescribe one of those standard strengths.

However, sometimes, the needed dose might not be available for some reason. The supply on hand, for example, may all be at the lowest strength, and the patient needs a higher dose. So, the problem you have to solve is this: How can you make the dose more or less than what the package label tells you?

The answer is simple when you use the formula $W/H \times V$. Here's how it works. The letters stand for this:

$$\frac{\text{Want}}{\text{Have}} \times \text{Vehicle}$$

- *Want* means what the physician has ordered or wants given.
- *Have* means the strength of the drug you have on hand.
- *Vehicle* refers to how the drug is given. For drugs in tablet form, the vehicle is a single tablet. For an injectable drug, the vehicle is how much of the fluid you'll need to inject to give the amount of the drug you "have."

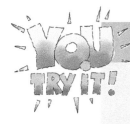

## ANOTHER DIMENSION

1. How many milligrams of phenobarbital does a 1/2-grain tablet contain?

2. A combination pain reliever contains 300 milligrams of acetaminophen in each tablet. How many grains of acetaminophen are in each tablet?

3. The package contains a roll of gauze that is 20 meters long. How many inches of gauze are there on the roll?

4. A new patient from South America has been losing weight rapidly. She told you that on the scale back home last summer, she weighed 73 kg. For your records, what was her weight in pounds?

5. How many 1-tsp doses of cough medicine are in a 375-mL bottle?

6. A patient is supposed to get an injection of 0.05 mg of levothyroxine sodium (Synthroid). The drug is available as 0.2 mg per 5 mL. How many milliliters should be prepared for the injection?

7. The physician prescribes 75 mg of a drug. The patient's pharmacy stocks a solution at a strength of 100 mg/mL. What dose, in milliliters, should the patient take?

8. The physician prescribes 250 mg of amoxicillin, which comes in a suspension of 25 mg/mL. You need to give the dose in teaspoons. How many teaspoons of the amoxicillin should you give?

For example, suppose a medication label reads *4 mg/2 mL*. That means you'd have to inject 2 mL of the liquid to give the patient a 4-mg dose of the drug.

The following examples demonstrate how to make the formula *W/H × V* work for you.

## HOW MANY TABLETS?

How many tablets do you give when the patient needs 0.125 mg of a medication and each tablet is 0.25 mg?

1. Identify what the physician has ordered or wants given.

Want = 0.125 mg

2. Determine the dosage you have available in a vehicle.

Have = 0.25 mg per tablet

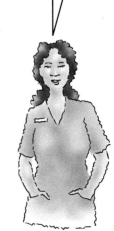

If one unit is different, convert it.

3. Make certain "Want" and "Have" are in same unit of measurement. In this case, both are in milligrams.

4. Do the math.

$$\frac{W}{H} \times V = \frac{0.125}{0.250} \times 1 \text{ tablet} = 0.5 \text{ or } \frac{1}{2} \text{ tablet}$$

## DOLING OUT DIAZEPAM

How much do you draw up in the syringe when the patient needs 4 mg of diazepam (Valium) and the label reads 10 mg/2 mL?

1. Identify what the physician has ordered or wants given.

Want = 4 mg

Yes! Both measurements are in milligrams. You can cancel units that are the same in both the numerator and the denominator of a fraction.

2. Determine the dosage you have available in a vehicle.

Have = 10 mg

3. Make certain "Want" and "Have" are in the same unit of measurement.

$$\frac{4 \text{ mg}}{10 \text{ mg}}$$

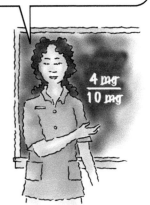

4. Do the math.

$$\frac{W}{H} \times V = \frac{4}{10} \times 2 \text{ mL} = \frac{8}{10} \text{ or } 0.8 \text{ mL}$$

# Clark's Law for Calculating Children's Dosages

The standard dose of a drug is based on the effect it has on a 150-pound adult. However, a dose that is appropriate for an adult could be an overdose for a child.

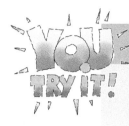

## USING THE FORMULA *W/H × V*

1. How many tablets of ezetimibe (Zetia) do you give when the patient needs 0.5 mg and each tablet is 0.25 mg?

2. How many tablets of pioglitazone hydrochloride (Actos) do you give when the patient needs 0.25 mg and each tablet is 0.5 mg?

3. How many tablets of aspirin do you give a patient if the physician orders 650 mg and the tablets in the bottle contain 325 mg?

4. How many milliliters do you draw up in the syringe when the patient needs 2700 units of penicillin and the label reads 900 units/mL?

5. How many milliliters of an oral suspension do you give the patient when the patient needs 150 mg of the medication and the label reads 50 mg/5 mL?

A formula called Clark's Law comes to the rescue. This formula helps you figure out a dose that's proportional to the child's weight.

$$\frac{\text{child's weight}}{150 \text{ lbs}} \times \text{adult dose} = \text{child's dose}$$

For example, Mindy weighs 30 pounds. If the adult dose of a drug is 600 mg, what dose should Mindy get?

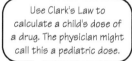

Use Clark's Law to calculate a child's dose of a drug. The physician might call this a pediatric dose.

1. Find out the child's weight in pounds. Put it in the equation.

$$\frac{30 \text{ lb}}{150 \text{ lb}} \times \text{adult dose} = \text{child's dose}$$

2. Fill in the adult dose.

$$\frac{30 \text{ lb}}{150 \text{ lb}} \times 600 \text{ mg} = \text{child's dose}$$

3. Do the math.

$$\frac{30 \text{ lb}}{150 \text{ lb}} \times 600 \text{ mg} = 120 \text{ mg}$$

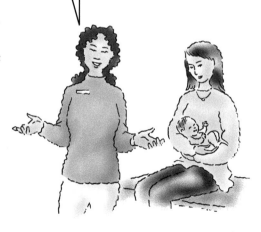

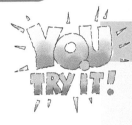

## USING CLARK'S LAW

1. Priya weighs 50 pounds. If the adult dose of a drug is 300 mg, what dose should Priya receive?
2. Jamal weighs 75 pounds. If the adult dose of a drug is 160 mg/mL, what dose should Jamal receive?
3. Eric weighs 100 pounds. If the adult dose of a drug is 300 mg, what dose should Eric receive?
4. Danisha weighs 80 pounds. If the adult dose of a drug is 1000 mg, what dose should Danisha receive?
5. José weighs 60 pounds. If the adult dose of a drug is 750 mg, what dose should José receive?

## Calculating Dosages for Persons of Unique Size

For patients of unique size, the physician may prescribe a certain number of milligrams of a medication per kilogram of body weight. When this occurs, use the following formula to calculate the correct dose:

$$\text{patient's weight in kg} \times \frac{\text{number of mg prescribed}}{\text{kg}}$$

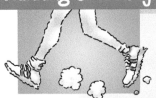

## Running Smoothly    WHEN ONE DOSE DOES NOT FIT ALL

*What if a patient weighs significantly more or less than the average adult weight of 150 pounds?*

A look around the waiting room of a medical office will soon convince you that patients come in all body sizes. Just like children need less of a medication to get the full benefit, other patients may need to take less or more than the standard adult dose, too. The physician has to decide how to adjust the dose to do the most good.

In cases like these, the physician may tell you, based on experience, how many milligrams of a drug per kilogram of body weight (mg/kg) a patient should get. You can calculate the exact dose by using this number. You multiply it by the patient's total body weight.

## MORE WEIGHT = LARGER DOSE

Homer weighs 440 pounds. The physician does not believe a standard dose of antibiotic will work. Dr. Lee wants Homer to receive 5 mg/kg of body weight.

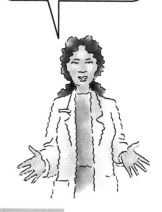

> Do not mix up measurement systems! If the dosage is in a metric measurement, then you'll have to convert the patient's weight to kilograms before making your calculations.

1. Convert the patient's weight from pounds to kilograms.

$$440 \text{ lb} \times \frac{1 \text{ kg}}{2.2 \text{ lb}} = 200 \text{ kg}$$

2. Multiply body weight by the dose.

$$200 \text{ kg} \times \frac{5 \text{ mg}}{\text{kg}} = 1,000 \text{ mg}$$

Homer needs 1000 mg of the antibiotic.

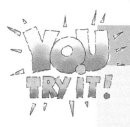

## CALCULATING UNIQUE DOSES

1. Jordan is a very muscular athlete who weighs 242 pounds. The physician wants to start him on a new antibiotic that might clear up a persistent infection. If the physician prescribes a dose that is 5 mg/kg of body weight, how much of the antibiotic should Jordan get?

2. 22-year-old Nicole has an eating disorder. Her present weight is 88 pounds. The physician wants to give her a prescription at a level of 2 mg per kilogram of body weight. How many milligrams should she receive per dose?

3. Gilberto weighs 100 pounds. The physician wants to give him an injection at a level of 10 mg per kilogram of body weight. What dose should Gilberto receive?

4. Ella weighs 220 pounds. The physician orders a sleep aid for her at a level of 0.25 mg per kilogram of body weight. How many milligrams of the medication should Ella get per dose?

5. Steve, a college athlete, weighs 198 pounds. The physician wants to give him an oral antibiotic at a level of 4 mg per kilogram of body weight. How much antibiotic should he receive per dose?

## LESS WEIGHT = SMALLER DOSE

Lexi is a 3-month-old baby. She weighs 11 pounds. She needs the same antibiotic as Homer and is to receive 5 mg/kg of body weight.

1.  Convert the patient's weight from pounds to kilograms.

$$11 \text{ lb} \times \frac{1 \text{ kg}}{2.2 \text{ lb}} = 5 \text{ kg}$$

2.  Multiply body weight by the dose.

$$5 \text{ kg} \times \frac{5 \text{ mg}}{\text{kg}} = 25 \text{ mg}$$

Lexi needs 25 mg of the antibiotic.

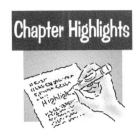

## Chapter Highlights

- When you reduce a fraction to its lowest terms, you find the largest possible number you can divide equally into the numerator and the denominator. For example, 3/9 = 1/3.
- To add fractions when the denominators are the same, just add the numerators. For example, 1/3 + 1/3 = 2/3.
- To add fractions with denominators that are not the same, rewrite them as fractions with the same denominator. For example, 1/7 + 1/3 = 3/21 + 7/21 = 10/21.
- To multiply fractions, multiply the numerators and then the denominators. Then reduce the answer to its lowest terms. For example, 4/7 × 5/8 = 20/56 = 5/14.
- To divide fractions, multiply the fraction by its reciprocal. (the reciprocal of 1/7 is 7/1). For example, 1/2 ÷ 1/4 = 1/2 × 4/1 = 4/2 = 2.
- Decimals have whole numbers to the left of the decimal point and parts of a whole number to the right of the decimal point. For example, one place to the right of the decimal point is a tenth, two places is a hundredth, three places is a thousandth, and so on.
- When you use a calculator, remember that you can add or multiply numbers in any order. When you divide or subtract, however, the order in which you enter the numbers is important. Remember that the ÷ function key means "divided by." To divide 5 into 14, enter it as "14 divided by 5."

- When solving percentage problems, remember to watch the wording. For example, "What is 25% of 80?" becomes "What is 25% × 80?" Similarly, if a problem is worded as "25 is what percentage of 80?" treat the word *what* as a division sign so the problem becomes 25/80.

- Ratios use a colon and fractions use a slash between the numbers in the relationship. Proportions are statements of equality between two ratios. When calculating dosages, you'll use ratios, fractions, and proportions frequently.

- In the medical world, the three systems of measurement that are commonly used are the metric system, the apothecary system, and the household system.

- Dimensional analysis is a method of problem solving. You can use it whenever two quantities are directly proportional to each other.

- Conversion factors, or common equivalents, let you convert between metric, household, and apothecary systems when you calculate dosages.

- If you need more or less of a drug, you can calculate adult dosages with the formula $W/H \times V$. In this formula, $W =$ "Want" (the dosage prescribed by the physician); $H =$ "Have" (the strength of the drug you have on hand); and $V =$ "Vehicle" (the quantity or strength in which the drug is given, e.g., 1 tablet, 10 mg/mL of solution).

- Using Clark's Law lets you calculate a dose of a drug that is appropriate for a child's weight. The formula is:

$$\frac{\text{child's weight}}{150 \text{ lbs}} \times \text{adult dose} = \text{child's dose}$$

- You can calculate dosages for persons of any weight if the physician tells how many milligrams of a drug per kilogram of body weight (mg/kg) a patient should get. You multiply the patient's weight (in kg) by the dose the physician orders.

## Chapter 3

# THE ROLE OF THE MEDICAL ASSISTANT

**Chapter Checklist**

- Name two legal issues concerning medical assistants administering medicine.

- Identify professional records regarding medication administration that must be properly maintained.

- State the six rights of safe medication administration.

- Describe ways to decrease the possibility of medication errors.

- Read and record medication orders.

- Read medication labels.

- Correctly document the administration of drugs.

**Chapter Competencies**

- Perform within legal and ethical boundaries (CAAHEP Competency 3.c.2.b.)
- Demonstrate knowledge of federal and state health care legislation and regulations (CAAHEP Competency 3.c.2.e.)
- Monitor legislation related to current health care issues and practices (ABHES Competency 5.g.)
- Maintain medication and immunization records (CAAHEP Competency 3.b.4.h.; ABHES Competency 4.n.)
- Use methods of quality control (CAAHEP Competency 3.c.4.d.; ABHES Competency 4.i.)
- Perform risk management procedures (ABHES Competency 5.h.)
- Document appropriately (CAAHEP Competency 3.c.2.d.)
- Document accurately (ABHES Competency 5.b.)
- Determine needs for documentation and reporting (ABHES Competency 5.a.)

Depending on the state in which you work, your lawful duties as a medical assistant with regard to medication administration will vary. However, you're always required to act under the direct supervision of a physician. In this chapter, you'll learn about handling medications, maintaining professional records, administering medications, and documenting information regarding medication administration. This chapter also explains the general rules for safely giving medications to patients.

## Handling Medications

One of your most important tasks in the medical office will be to assist with medication administration. Taken incorrectly, they can do much harm and even cause loss of life. No medication-related task should ever be taken lightly or done with anything less than your best effort.

### WORKING UNDER SUPERVISION

Handling medications is always done under the direction of a physician. Some of the tasks you may assist with include these:

- preparing medications to be given to patients in the medical office
- authorizing drug refills, as directed
- writing out prescriptions for the physician's signature
- phoning prescriptions to the pharmacy, as directed
- maintaining professional records

### STATE LAWS VARY

Medical assisting duties that can be performed legally differ from state to state. Some states have medical practice acts that clearly define what a medical assistant is allowed to do. For example, in California, the work of the medical assistant is clearly defined. Medical assistants in the state of California are permitted by law to inject, handle, and provide medications to patients, but only if a physician or podiatrist has verified the medications first.

Other states delegate specific skills to certain health professionals. Under those circumstances, the medical assistant performs skills not specifically designated to someone else. For example, if a state delegates intravenous (IV) and intramuscular (IM) injections only to the registered nurse, but does not specify subcutaneous (SubQ) or intradermal (ID) injections, it would be presumed that a patient, family member, or medical assistant would be allowed to give SubQ or ID injections.

Before acting on your own initiative, ask questions, and keep asking them until you fully understand what authority has been delegated to you by state law and the licensed professional in charge.

> Check with your state board of professional regulation to determine what tasks medical assistants are allowed to perform in your state.

## SUPPLYING PATIENTS WITH MEDICATIONS

As a medical assistant, you need to be aware of the three chief ways in which patients receive medications.

- Depending on state law, medications may be **administered** by medical assistants, nurses, physicians, and other qualified health care personnel. This means that the medications are given to the patient in the office. Medications given this way include flu shots, vaccinations for hepatitis and various childhood diseases, injections of penicillin and other antibiotics, and local anesthetics such as those given in a dentist's office before a procedure.

- Pharmacists may **dispense** medications to patients. The physician may also dispense a supply of medications for the patient's later use. Some of these may be samples that drug manufacturers give physicians for this purpose. Examples of medications given to patients for later use include antibiotics, pain medications, antidepressants, and other medications taken on an ongoing basis.

- The physician may **prescribe** medication by giving the patient a written order, called a prescription, to take to the pharmacy. A pharmacist will fill the order and give the medication to the patient. When medication is prescribed for a patient over the phone, the physician's office will either call the pharmacy or fax the prescription for the patient's convenience.

As a clinical medical assistant, you may be asked to write out the prescription (or "script") and give it to the physician for her signature. Every prescription must have a physician's signature.

## Maintaining Professional Records and Medications

As you learned in Chapter 1, the government classifies certain medications as controlled substances and closely monitors how they are prescribed and dispensed. One of the most important jobs you may be given in a medical office is to help complete and maintain the paperwork that enables the physician to administer these controlled substances.

Some medications in the controlled substance category need special handling because they contain narcotics. Narcotics are habit-forming, and patients may become dependent on medications that contain them. Physicians need specific permissions and licenses both to prescribe such drugs and to keep them in the office.

To prescribe or handle controlled substances, a physician must register with the Drug Enforcement Administration (DEA). The registration period lasts 3 years after the DEA accepts the application.

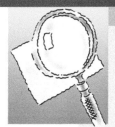

## Closer Look

### LEARNING MORE ABOUT DRUG DEPENDENCE AND ADDICTION

Patients who are taking prescription pain medications or other powerful medications can become dependent on them. Drug dependence is sometimes called drug **addiction**. Patients may develop a dependence that is physical, psychological, or both.

- **Physical dependence** causes mild to severe physiological, or bodily, reactions to the medication. These symptoms may decrease or disappear after the patient stops taking the drug.

- **Psychological dependence** means that the patient has developed a need for the feelings the drug gives him.

Medical personnel should closely monitor any patient who is given controlled substances for signs of dependence. The patient may have a problem if he displays some or all of the following behaviors:

- asking for refills because he "lost the medications" or "dropped them in the toilet"
- requesting higher and more frequent doses
- exhibiting tremors
- behaving increasingly irritable
- displaying physical difficulty when walking, writing a check, etc.
- slurring his speech
- dozing off in the waiting room
- smelling of alcohol or requesting narcotic drugs

## Running Smoothly

### KEEPING UP WITH THE DRUG ENFORCEMENT ADMINISTRATION

*What if you're assigned the task of keeping up with the physician's DEA registration?*

A DEA number is valid for 3 years, after which the physician's registration must be renewed. The DEA does not send out reminders to renew soon-to-expire registrations. As a medical assistant, you may be responsible for maintaining registration or reminding the physician or practitioner about registering with the DEA. You can do this by tracking the physician's DEA registration and submitting a renewal application at the appropriate time. The DEA's Office of Diversion Control handles renewal applications. These applications can now be completed online by visiting the Office of Diversion Control's website at www.deadiversion.usdoj.gov.

## THE DEA NUMBER

When the physician registers with the DEA, he is assigned a special identification number, called a DEA number, to use on prescription forms. The number belongs to the physician personally, *not* to the physician's office. This registration limits the drugs that a physician or practitioner may handle.

> Do not wait until the physician's DEA number expires to look into updating the registration. A lapse in registration means that the physician won't be allowed to prescribe controlled substances to patients.

## CONTROLLED SUBSTANCES IN THE MEDICAL OFFICE

Some medical offices keep controlled substances on hand to be administered or dispensed to patients in the office. These drugs must be handled very carefully for legal reasons.

### Ordering Controlled Substances

There is a federal order form (DEA Form 222) that must be completed to place an order for controlled substances. A copy of this form is kept on file with the DEA.

### Monitoring Inventory

When a shipment of any controlled substance arrives at the medical office, you may be given the job of logging the shipment in the office's records. For this you'll use a special controlled sub-

## Closer Look — DEA DRUG SCHEDULES

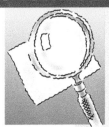

As you learned in Chapter 1, the DEA classifies controlled substances into five "schedules," or categories, depending on their potential for abuse. Drugs on Schedule I are highly abused and have no approved medical use. These include narcotics such as heroin, ecstasy or MDMA, and LSD.

Cannabis (marijuana) also appears on Schedule I, which means that according to the DEA, it has no medical use. However, the DEA deals with major drug trafficking, not individual medical users. Twenty percent of U.S. states have decriminalized marijuana use. Patients with medical need use marijuana openly in those places.

Drugs on Schedule II also have potential for abuse but have important medical applications as well. These include drugs such as oxycodone hydrochloride (OxyContin), acetaminophen and oxycodone hydrochloride (Percocet), morphine, methylphenidate hydrochloride (Ritalin), and dronabinol (Marinol), a marijuana derivative that is used to stimulate the appetite in patients with terminal cancer or HIV.

When a drug supplier sends Schedule II controlled substances to the physician's office, the supplier must include a Federal Triplicate Order Form DEA 222 with the shipment.

Controlled substances on Schedules III through V have less potential for abuse. Examples include acetaminophen and codeine (Tylenol with Codeine), diazepam (Valium), and phenobarbital (Solfoton). These drugs do not require a DEA Form 222, but the medical office must keep invoices for receipt of the substances for a period of 2 years.

> When you receive a shipment of Schedule II drugs, check the package to make sure the supplier included a DEA Form 222.

> It's essential that all inventory forms and receipts related to controlled substances are filed correctly. The DEA may request copies of these forms within 2 years.

stances inventory form like the one shown on page 81. Both you and another witness must sign the log-in form.

Furthermore, every time a controlled substance leaves the office's inventory, that fact must also be recorded. You'll need to include the following information:

- the name of the drug
- the patient's name

- the size of the dose
- the date
- the name of the physician who ordered the administration or dispensing of the drug
- the name of the person at the medical office who handled the transaction

Ask your instructor about the record-keeping requirements in your state.

These inventory forms must be kept on file for 2 years.

Not every medical office administers or dispenses controlled substances. Sometimes, the physician just writes a prescription to be filled by a pharmacist. In this case, record-keeping requirements vary from state to state. The first few times you handle a prescription for a controlled substance, be sure to ask what the laws of your state require until you have a full understanding.

## Disposing of Controlled Substances

The physician may ask you to dispose of medications or samples, for example, when they have expired. There are federal, state, and local regulations that you should follow whenever disposing of controlled substances to prevent these powerful substances from getting into the wrong hands.

First, you must complete four copies of the DEA Form 41 (Registrants Inventory of Drugs Surrendered). Then, the physician must sign these forms. The information required for this form is similar to the information required for dispensing controlled substances. After completing the form, two copies are sent to the nearest DEA office.

The DEA will notify you about how to dispose of the drugs. Disposal methods may include incineration or shipping drugs to the DEA office by registered mail. Once the controlled substances are disposed of, the DEA will issue the physician a receipt. Make sure you store this receipt with the inventory records for controlled substances.

## WRITING A PRESCRIPTION

In a busy medical office, the physician you're assisting might ask you to write out a prescription for a patient based on information entered in the patient's chart. After entering the data on the form, you must then give it to the physician for his or her signature.

## Parts of a Prescription

There is a customary *protocol*, or set of rules, for the order in which the information is provided on a prescription form. The printed portions of the prescription form are sometimes

**Controlled Substance:** ___Meperidine (Demerol) 50mg Injection___

**Amount Ordered:** ___five___ 50 mg vials/ampules    **Rec'd by:** _____    **Rec'd on:** 02/10/XX

**Distribution:** _____

| Date | Patient Name | Ordering Physician | Dose Given | Amount Discarded | Employee Signature | Remaining Inventory |
|------|-------------|-------------------|-----------|-----------------|-------------------|--------------------|
| 02/22/XX | John Jones | Dr. Smith | 25 mg | 25 mg | Marie Masters/Sally Lee | |
| | | | | | | |
| | | | | | | |
| | | | | | | |
| | | | | | | |
| | | | | | | |
| | | | | | | |
| | | | | | | |
| | | | | | | |

*If you're discarding a narcotic, a witness should co-sign the controlled substances inventory form.*

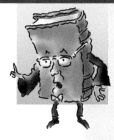

## Legal Brief    REPORTING ILLEGAL BEHAVIOR

If you suspect that a physician or other health care professional is diverting controlled substances illegally, you must report your suspicions to the proper authorities (usually the local police). Before making your report, be sure to gather and document evidence and the reasons why you suspect substances are being diverted illegally. It's important to present a clear and compelling case to the authorities.

If you suspect that a physician is involved, you also have a legal and ethical responsibility to report any evidence to the:

- DEA
- American Medical Association (AMA)
- state board of medicine

However, if you suspect a health care worker *other* than the physician, you should report your concerns to the appropriate supervisor. Most states have programs to assist health care professionals in dealing with addiction and dependency issues. Often, the individual who reports illegal activity remains anonymous.

arranged in a way different from the illustration on page 83. However, each of the following components will appear on the form and must be completed.

- *Heading.* The heading includes the patient's name and address as well as the date. It tells the pharmacist whom the prescription is written for. The date is also important because a prescription must be filled within 6 months of the date when it was written.

- *Superscription.* The symbol *Rx* introduces the medication information on the prescription. The letters are an abbreviation of the Latin word *recipe*, which means "take thou."

- *Inscription.* The information in this part gives the name of the medication, the form in which it is to be taken (liquid, tablet, capsule), and the strength of the individual dosage (for example, 250 mg, 500 mL).

- *Subscription.* This line tells the pharmacist how much of the medication to dispense to the patient (for example, 90 tablets, 150 mL).

- *Signature.* The signature provides information for taking the medication (for example, twice a day, before bedtime, with meals) as well as the route by which the medication is to be taken.

- *Generic.* Often, physicians allow patients to take a generic version of a medication if one exists. Insurance companies often urge the use of generic medications as a cost-saving measure. However, if the physician does *not* want the pharmacist to replace a medication with its generic equivalent, write or place a check mark next to the letters *DAW* (meaning "dispense as written"), or write *label* or *no substitution*, on the prescription form.

- *Refills.* This information tells the pharmacist how many times the prescription may be refilled. Generally, refills should not be done more than five times within 6 months. If the prescription should not be refilled at all, check or circle *none* or *0*.

- *Physician's signature.* The physician should check and sign all prescriptions written in his office.

- *DEA number.* For security's sake, the physician's DEA number should *not* be filled in unless the prescription is for a controlled substance.

All prescriptions must be documented in the patient's medical record. Remember that the patient's medical record is a legal

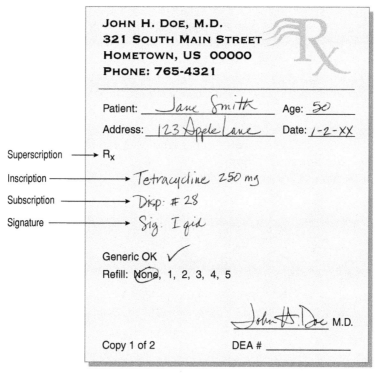

JOHN H. DOE, M.D.
321 SOUTH MAIN STREET
HOMETOWN, US 00000
PHONE: 765-4321

Patient: _Jane Smith_    Age: _50_

Address: _123 Apple Lane_    Date: _1-2-XX_

Superscription → Rx

Inscription → Tetracycline 250 mg

Subscription → Disp: # 28

Signature → Sig. I qid

Generic OK ✓

Refill: None, 1, 2, 3, 4, 5

John H. Doe M.D.

Copy 1 of 2    DEA # _____

The prescription form your office uses may look different, but the components should be the same as in this example.

document. If the medication order isn't included in the chart, it's as if it were never ordered.

## Prescriptions for Controlled Substances

The physician must follow certain rules when prescribing controlled substances. For example, the physician must use special prescription forms. These forms are tamper resistant and must be ordered from a government-approved security printer.

As a medical assistant, you may be given responsibility for ordering and safeguarding these prescription forms. You must keep careful track of them so they are not lost or stolen. They should be locked up until they're needed. Law enforcement officials recommend that the physician's DEA number not be preprinted on these prescription forms.

You'll also need to be familiar with the stipulations for prescribing controlled substances.

- Prescriptions for Schedule II drugs can't be called in to a pharmacy, but must be written on a prescription form. In extreme emergencies, the physician may call in a prescription; however, a handwritten prescription must be presented to the pharmacist within 72 hours. These prescriptions can't be refilled.

- Prescriptions for Schedule III drugs may be called in to a pharmacy by the physician and refilled up to six times in 6 months.
- Prescriptions for Schedule IV drugs may be called into a pharmacy by a medical office employee and refilled up to five times in 6 months.

## Running Smoothly

### WHEN THE PHYSICIAN PRESCRIBES A CONTROLLED SUBSTANCE . . .

*What if the physician asks you to write out a prescription for a controlled substance?*

If a prescription is for a controlled substance, the physician's DEA number must be filled in. In addition, several other guidelines must be followed.

- Never use prescription pads as scrap paper or leave them around where they could be stolen and used to forge prescriptions.
- Write any prescription in black ink.
- Use both words and numbers to write out the number of tablets or capsules prescribed. For example, write *twenty (20)*. Doing this will make it more difficult to change a quantity from, for example, 20 to 200.
- Be cautious if a prescription requires large amounts of controlled substances. Confirm the quantity with the physician.
- Never ask the physician to sign the prescription form before all the appropriate information has been filled in.
- Alert the physician if you know or suspect that a patient has also received controlled substances from a hospital or another physician.
- Be sure that you and/or the physician have correctly logged in all prescriptions for controlled substances as required by state and DEA regulations.

## Storing Prescription Pads and Medications

Because they are so important, prescription pads must be handled very carefully in the medical office. Prescription pads should not be left out where they are accessible to patients. They should always be stored in a locked drawer or cabinet.

The same rules apply to any medications stored in the medical office. It's likely that the physician frequently receives sample medications from drug manufacturers. Any sample drugs in the office should also be kept in a secure place so that only the physician may distribute them. Each office should have an inventory control book for any sample medications that are kept in the office.

---

**Ask the Professional**   **PRESCRIPTION PAD SAFETY PROCEDURES**

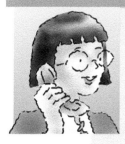

**Q:** *In the past week, I've found the cabinet where we store prescription pads unlocked on two separate occasions. I'm the newest medical assistant in the office and do not want to seem like a tattletale. But isn't this dangerous?*

**A:** You're right to be concerned! Not only is this practice dangerous, it's against the law in some states. Prescription pads are very powerful and need to be handled with care. Every medical office should have a special cabinet where prescription pads are stored, and the cabinet should always be locked. You definitely need to alert your supervisor to your finding so that she can remind the office staff about how important it is to keep that cabinet locked.

In addition to storing prescription pads in a locked cabinet, there are some other things your office can do to protect itself and its patients. Here are some tips:

- Remove prescription pads from the locked cabinet only when you need them. You should not leave pads unattended in the reception area or in an examination room—even for just a few minutes.

- If prescription pads are stolen from the office, your office should alert the police and local pharmacies.

- Keep track of the number of pads in the office. If a theft occurs, you'll be able to tell the police exactly how many pads are missing.

- Maintain a small inventory of prescription pads in the office. It may seem like a hassle to reorder frequently, but it's safer to have few prescription pads in the office.

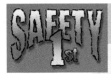

## THE SIX RIGHTS

To ensure patient safety, medical assistants and other medical office staff need to have a complete understanding of all aspects of medication administration, including the "six rights" (explained below). Medical assistants may also be called on to help patients and family members understand and remember instructions from the physician.

## Administering Medications

Physicians, physician assistants, nurse practitioners, and nurses are usually responsible for administering medications in the medical office. Some states also allow medical assistants, under some circumstances, to administer medications.

### THE "SIX RIGHTS" OF DRUG ADMINISTRATION

Do you want to be sure that patient safety is at the heart of what you do? Keep in mind the "six rights" of drug administration whenever you assist patients with their medications or administer them yourself:

- right patient
- right drug
- right dose
- right route
- right time
- right documentation

### Right Patient

If you're administering a medication, you must be sure that you're giving it to the person for whom the drug has been ordered. In a medical office, ask the patient for his date of birth as a way to double-check. Confirm that he is the right patient by checking his chart—the John Smith born on 2/15/78 must not receive the medicine prescribed for the John Smith born on 6/6/88!

### Right Drug

It's very easy to confuse the names of two medications. Their names may sound similar or have similar spellings. If you did not hear the full name of the medication or can't read what the patient's chart says, ask the prescribing physician. Further, to check that you have the correct medication in hand, compare the name of the medication, the label on the package or bottle, and the patient's medication record.

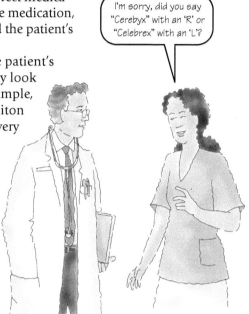

I'm sorry, did you say "Cerebyx" with an 'R' or "Celebrex" with an 'L'?

It's also very important to read the patient's chart carefully. Some drug names may look similar when written quickly. For example, the trade names for the drugs crotamiton (Eurax) and oxazepam (Serax) look very similar. Always ask the physician to clarify his order if you have even the slightest doubt. Handwritten orders can sometimes cause problems, too. For example, you may find yourself unsure if the physician has written *pc* or *po*. The difference can be significant. The abbreviation *pc* stands for "after meals," referring to when a drug should be administered; *po* means "by mouth," referring to how a drug should be taken. Always ask for clarification if you're unsure.

## Right Dose

The physician or other health care professional who prescribes a medication for a patient should write an order for administering it correctly. In an emergency, the physician may give a verbal order to administer a drug. She must then write and sign a formal order as soon as the emergency is over.

One of the most important pieces of information in the order is the dosage. Check or listen carefully for decimal points. There is a significant difference between 25 mg of a medication and 0.25 mg. Be sure to note precisely what was ordered.

## Right Route

Medications may be administered by a variety of routes. Tablets may be swallowed or placed under the tongue. Some injections are administered directly into a muscle (intramuscular), just under the skin (subcutaneous), or through the skin (intradermal). Other medications are inhaled or placed into a body cavity. Be sure that you clearly understand how a medication should be delivered.

### Right Time

Another important piece of information in a drug order tells when the patient should take the medication. Be sure that you know if it should be taken with food or on an empty stomach, in the morning or in the evening, with or apart from other medications, and other important facts, such as how many times a day it should be taken.

### Right Documentation

Any time a medication is administered, that fact should be noted immediately in the patient's chart. The purpose for this is to avoid duplication and to create an accurate and complete record of patient care.

## READING A MEDICATION ORDER

A licensed health care professional—a physician, a dentist, or, in some states, a physician's assistant or a nurse practitioner—must order a medication before it can be given to a patient. All medication orders should be recorded immediately in the patient's chart.

These are the medication orders you're most likely to encounter in the medical office:

- *Single order.* A single order means that a medication should be administered one time only. If it should be given immediately for an emergency condition, the term "STAT" will follow the order.

- *Standing order.* A standing order means that a patient is supposed to receive a prescribed medication on a regular basis. The drug should be given to the patient until the physician specifically discontinues it. The physician might order the medication for a specific number of days, after which it is to be discontinued, or stopped. The physician may also decide to renew the standing order for the drug.

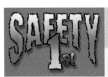

## ASK FOR CLARIFICATION

If you're unsure what any part of a medication order means, ask the physician who wrote it. If she is not present, ask another knowledgeable authority. Your concern should always be for the patient's safety. A "good guess" is not enough.

## Take Care with Abbreviations

Medical terminology is firmly based in Latin and ancient Greek. It should come as no surprise, then, that many medical abbreviations are shortened forms of Latin words or phrases. For example, the letters *NPO* are an abbreviation of the Latin phrase *nihil per os,* or "nothing through the mouth."

### The "Do Not Use" List

When medical personnel are working quickly or when someone's handwriting is unclear, it can be easy to misread some medical abbreviations. That's why The Joint Commission has acted. The Joint Commission has published an official "do not use" list—a compilation of abbreviations, acronyms, and symbols that should not be used in handwritten, printed, and electronic documents. The table on page 90 provides a listing of medical abbreviations that appear on The Joint Commission's "Do Not Use" List. Although certain abbreviations, such as those in the following table, have become outdated, it's important to be familiar with them as you may encounter these abbreviations in old medical records.

### Commonly Used Medication Abbreviations

The table on page 91 lists commonly used abbreviations related to medications. You need to know what they mean so that you can understand what the entries on the prescription and in a patient's chart mean. As a medical assistant, you'll also need to use them correctly if you're asked to enter medication data that a physician gives you.

## Practice Reading Labels

Remember that the physician is always the person who *dispenses* medication to patients in the office. However, you may be asked to retrieve a specific medication from the storage room at the physician's request. When retrieving medication, it's possible to make mistakes if you misread a package label and pick up the wrong medication or the wrong dosage of the right medication. For this reason, it's important to practice reading drug labels. Following are the labels from several common medications. (You'll learn more about drug labels in Chapter 8.)

## GENERAL SAFETY RULES FOR ADMINISTERING MEDICATIONS

It's important to follow some general safety rules when you're administering medications in the medical office. Doing so will reduce the risk of **drug errors**. These errors include any

### Official "Do Not Use" List[1]

| Do Not Use | Potential Problem | Use Instead |
|---|---|---|
| U (unit) | Mistaken for "0" (zero), the number "4" (four) or "cc" | Write "unit" |
| IU (International Unit) | Mistaken for IV (intravenous) or the number 10 (ten) | Write "International Unit" |
| Q.D., QD, q.d., qd (daily) | Mistaken for each other | Write "daily" |
| Q.O.D., QOD, q.o.d, qod (every other day) | Period after the Q mistaken for "I" and the "O" mistaken for "I" | Write "every other day" |
| Trailing zero (X.0 mg)* Lack of leading zero (.X mg) | Decimal point is missed | Write X mg Write 0.X mg |
| MS | Can mean morphine sulfate or magnesium sulfate | Write "morphine sulfate" Write "magnesium sulfate" |
| MSO$_4$ and MgSO$_4$ | Confused for one another | |

[1] Applies to all orders and all medication-related documentation that is handwritten (including free-text computer entry) or on pre-printed forms.

*Exception: A "trailing zero" may be used only where required to demonstrate the level of precision of the value being reported, such as for laboratory results, imaging studies that report size of lesions, or catheter/tube sizes. It may not be used in medication orders or other medication-related documentation.

### Additional Abbreviations, Acronyms and Symbols
(For possible future inclusion in the Official "Do Not Use" List)

| Do Not Use | Potential Problem | Use Instead |
|---|---|---|
| > (greater than) < (less than) | Misinterpreted as the number "7" (seven) or the letter "L" Confused for one another | Write "greater than" Write "less than" |
| Abbreviations for drug names | Misinterpreted due to similar abbreviations for multiple drugs | Write drug names in full |
| Apothecary units | Unfamiliar to many practitioners Confused with metric units | Use metric units |
| @ | Mistaken for the number "2" (two) | Write "at" |
| cc | Mistaken for U (units) when poorly written | Write "ml" or "milliliters" |
| μg | Mistaken for mg (milligrams) resulting in one thousand-fold overdose | Write "mcg" or "micrograms" |

## Commonly Used Medication Abbreviations

| Abbreviation | Meaning | Abbreviation | Meaning |
|---|---|---|---|
| ac | before meals | NKA | no known allergies |
| ad lib | as desired | Noc | night |
| ADL | activities of daily living | NPO | nothing by mouth |
| AM, a.m., A.M. | morning | NS | normal saline |
| amp | ampule | OD | right eye |
| amt | amount | OS | left eye |
| aq | aqueous | OU | both eyes |
| bid | twice a day | Os | mouth |
| BM | bowel movement | Oz | ounce |
| BRP | bathroom privileges | P | after |
| c̄ | with | Pc | after meals |
| cap | capsule | PM, p.m., P.M. | afternoon or evening |
| DC, disc, d/c | discontinue | po, PO | by mouth |
| disp | dispense | prn, PRN | whenever necessary |
| DW | distilled water | Pt | pint or patient |
| EDC | estimated date of confinement (date baby is due) | Q | every |
| | | Qh | every hour |
| | | q2h | every 2 hours |
| et | and | q3h | every 3 hours |
| ext | extract | qid | four times a day |
| FGW | full glass of water | qt | quart |
| FU | follow up | R | right, rectal |
| g, gm | gram | RTW | return to work |
| gr | grain | Rx | take, prescribe |
| gt(t) | drop(s) | s̄ | without |
| h, hr | hour | SC, subcu, subq, S/Q, SQ | subcutaneously |
| hs, HS | hour of sleep | | |
| Id, ID | intradermal | Sig | label |
| IM | intramuscular | SL | sublingual |
| IV | intravenous | sol | solution |
| Kg | kilogram | SOS | once if necessary |
| L, l | liter | ss | one-half |
| lb | pound | stat, STAT | immediately |
| LMP | last menstrual period | supp | suppository |
| mcg, μg | microgram | syr | syrup |
| mEq | milliequivalent | tab | tablet |
| ml, mL | milliliter | T, tb, tbs, tbsp | tablespoon |
| n | normal | t, tsp | teaspoon |
| NaCl | sodium chloride | tid | three times a day |
| NH | nursing home | WNL | within normal limits |

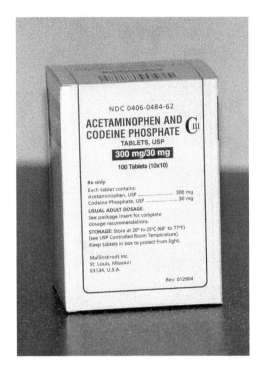

The label of a controlled substance must include a special symbol that shows its schedule category. The letter C and the Roman numeral *III* that appear on this label indicate that acetaminophen and codeine is a Schedule III controlled substance.

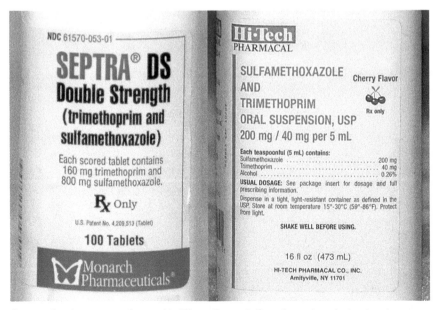

Some medications are manufactured in different forms. Sulfamethoxazole and trimethoprim (Septra, Septra DS) comes in the form of tablets or oral suspension.

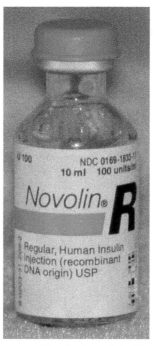

The strength of insulin is measured in units instead of milligrams. According to this label, regular insulin (Novolin R) contains 100 units of insulin per milliliter of solution (100 units/mL).

occurrence that causes a patient to receive the wrong dose, the wrong drug, a drug by the wrong route, or a drug given at the incorrect time.

Along with following the "six rights" and additional safety guidelines, it's also helpful to have some knowledge about the drugs you handle in the medical office. In the course of your work, you'll become familiar with the properties of the drugs that are commonly used or prescribed in your office. For less commonly used drugs or new drugs, you can read the drug package insert, which is very detailed, or consult a pharmaceutical reference book to obtain the information you need.

## Drug Information to Know

Before administering a medication to a patient, you should be familiar with the following information:

- the reason the drug is given
- how the drug works or acts on the body
- the drug's more common adverse reactions

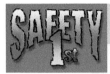

## AVOIDING DRUG ERRORS

Drug errors usually occur when one of the "six rights" has not been followed. To avoid drug errors, follow these additional safety guidelines:

- Confirm any questionable medication orders.
- If a dosage calculation is necessary, verify it with another qualified professional.
- If the patient questions a drug or prescribed dosage, listen up! Never administer a medication until the patient's questions have been researched and answered.
- Avoid multitasking; concentrate on only one task at a time.

## Ask the Professional  DRUG ERRORS

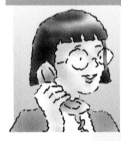

**Q:** *I gave 2 mL of diazepam (Valium) IM. After I gave the injection, I realized the order was for 5 mg of diazepam and the vial said: 10 mg/2 mL. I'd given twice as much as I should have given. I was so ashamed and scared, I didn't tell anyone. What should I have done?*

**A:** When a drug error occurs, you must report the error to the physician immediately. Depending on the error, the physician may need to take steps to counteract the action of the drug. Additionally, it may be necessary to monitor the patient for any adverse reactions. Even if the patient suffers no harm, it's vital to report the error.

Most drug errors are made during administration. The most common errors are a failure to administer a drug that has been ordered, administration of the wrong dose or strength of the drug, or administration of the wrong drug. In a busy medical office, mistakes can sometimes occur. You may be embarrassed to admit to a mistake, but when a patient's health is on the line, it's absolutely necessary!

- any special precautions you should take when you administer it
- the dosage typically given

## Patient Information to Know

You must be sensitive to the condition and needs of the patients who receive the medications. Before a medication is administered, you should know the following information about a patient:

- the patient's allergy history
- any history of adverse reactions to the drug
- any changes in the patient's condition
- other medications currently being taken by the patient

If the physician has ordered a medication, but the patient's condition changes before taking a dose, make sure the physician knows before giving any medication. For example, if you return to give a patient with a fever some acetaminophen (Tylenol) and the patient has begun to vomit, relay this information to the physician before proceeding with any medications. Also notify the physician first if a patient makes any statement about a medication, such as a physical reaction he has had to it. The physician may want to consider other options.

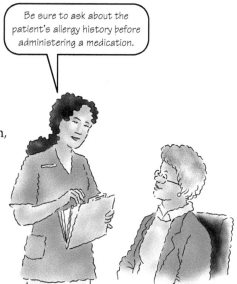

Be sure to ask about the patient's allergy history before administering a medication.

For patients who are taking a medication for the first time, also ask about the following factors:

- any known allergies to drugs
- any known allergies to food, pollen, animals, and other sources
- a family history of allergies

Patients with a personal or a family history of allergies are more likely to have an allergic reaction to a new medication. Because allergic reactions can cause a range of responses from discomfort to loss of life, patients with allergies should be closely monitored.

## Preparing a Medication for Administration

Follow these guidelines when you prepare a medication to be given to a patient:

- Check the physician's written order and ask any questions you may have about it.

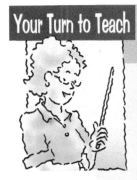

## Your Turn to Teach

## DISCUSSING ALLERGY HISTORIES WITH PATIENTS

Patients often do not know or can't remember which medications they have taken or the dosages that they were given. The problem is worsened if they had a bad reaction to a medication, often an antibiotic, and they can't recall its name. Help them gauge the severity of their reaction so that you can inform the physician you're assisting.

Here are some things to keep in mind when discussing allergy histories with patients.

- Explain that allergic reactions to drugs can happen immediately, or they can occur days and even weeks after the patient first takes the drug. Explain that the skin is the organ that is most commonly involved. Ask about rashes of any kind, hives (itchy, red swellings), and sensitivity to light.

- Explain that an allergic reaction might not have happened the first time they took a medication but during the second or third time they took it. Listen for responses that fit this pattern and inform the physician.

- Not every bad response to a medication is an allergic reaction. Explain that two medications may cause problems when they are taken together. Ask patients what other medications they were taking at the time. Ask about nonprescription medications and herbal remedies, too. Let the physician know.

- Sometimes, a bad response can result from an overdose. Gently probe how patients keep to a regimen of drug administration. Do they often or sometimes forget to take their medications and then do "catch-up" doses or take a few pills at a time?

- Sometimes, the reaction is one of the irritating but known adverse reactions of taking a drug, including nausea, vomiting, or diarrhea. Ask patients to recall how severe these responses were, and inform the physician.

- Work in a quiet, well-lit area.
- Check the label on the drug three times: first, when you take the drug from its storage area; second, immediately before you take the medication out of its package; and third, before returning the medication to its storage area.
- Never take a drug from an unlabeled container or from a container with an illegible label.
- Always wash your hands right before preparing the drug for administration.
- Do not touch capsules and tablets with your hands. Instead, shake the correct number of tablets or capsules into the cap of the container. Then, shake them from the cap into the medicine cup.
- Always follow aseptic technique when you prepare syringes and needles. Wear gloves for all procedures that might result in contact with blood or body fluids.
- Put the cap back on the drug container right after the drug is removed.
- Some drugs require special storage, such as refrigeration. Others must be protected from exposure to light. Immediately return these medications to their storage places after preparing them for administration.
- Never crush tablets or open capsules without first checking with the physician or a pharmacist.
- Never administer a drug that someone else has prepared. The person who prepared the drug should administer it.

> Read drug labels with care! Some drug names sound alike, but the chemicals inside are very different. Giving one drug when the physician ordered the other drug could cause serious problems.

## Documenting Medications

Most medical offices have a wall of filing cabinets containing patients' records. Every visit to the medical office, every treatment, and every medication is recorded in the patient's file, giving physicians an ongoing medical history of each patient who visits the office.

Everyone on the health care team who provides a medical service to a patient—including medical assistants—makes entries in these records. These confidential files are both a medical record and a legal record of the care given to a patient.

## VERBAL ORDERS

The sample chart entry below shows how to document a verbal order from a physician. The medical assistant used the abbreviation *VO* to indicate a "verbal order." She identified the medication and how often it was to be administered to the patient (pt). She did not need to identify the dosage because it's the standard 325-mg nonprescription tablet. Notice that the physician wishes to see the patient for a follow-up (FU) visit the next day.

| DATE | TIME | ORDERS |
|---|---|---|
| 06/30/XX | 9.35 AM | V.O. from Dr. Stuart: Tylenol 650 mg every 6–8 hrs for pain. Pt. to be seen tomorrow A.M. for FU in office. |
| | | ———————————— M. Smith, CMA |

The abbreviation *VO* indicates that this entry describes a verbal order from the physician.

As a medical assistant, when you receive a verbal order from a physician, here is the procedure to follow:

- Repeat the order back to the physician to be sure that you understand it fully.
- Write it correctly in the chart.
- Sign the order with your name and professional title.

You should follow the same procedure to document a phone order. See the chart entry below. Notice that the medical assistant documented exactly what she told the patient at Dr. Stuart's request—even though some of the information (the name of the medication) already appears in the chart. The phone call must be logged as a separate and complete entry in the patient's chart.

| DATE | TIME | ORDERS |
|---|---|---|
| 06/30/XX | 9.40 AM | Contacted pt. by phone. Instructed to use Tylenol 650 mg every 6–8 hr for pain and call us if pain increases or does not respond. Advised to seek help at ED if unable to reach our office. Given appointment for 07/01/XX at 10:00 A.M. |
| | | ———————————— M. Smith, CMA |

A second chart entry must be added after the medical assistant calls the patient to relay the physician's verbal order.

## PRESCRIPTIONS

All medications dispensed or prescribed to a patient should be recorded in the patient's chart. See the entry below. The prescription (Rx) is for an antibiotic that the patient is to take by mouth (po).

| DATE | TIME | ORDERS |
|------|------|--------|
| 02/01/XX | 10:30 AM | *Rx for ampicillin 500 mg po (#40) to be taken every 6 hrs x 10 days per Dr. Espinosa's orders called to Acme Pharmacy on Park Blvd.* |
| | | *T. Jones, CMA* |

The patient's prescription for ampicillin is entered in the chart.

Notice how complete the entry is. The medical assistant documents the name of the drug, the dosage, how often it should be taken, and for how many days the patient should take it. The medical assistant also phoned the prescription to the patient's pharmacy. He documents the name and location of the drug store as well.

## ADMINISTERED INJECTIONS

The following three entries show how to record injections.

- *Subcutaneous (SubQ) injection.* The entry below describes an injection of insulin just under the skin. It gives the amount of insulin (20 units) and the exact site where it was injected. This fact is important. If the patient later reported a sore left arm, the cause was probably *not* the injection, which was given in the upper right arm.

| DATE | TIME | ORDERS |
|------|------|--------|
| 12/02/XX | 11:00 AM | *20 units of regular insulin SubQ to dorsal aspect of (R) upper arm. Manufacturer Eli Lilly Lot # 355728-8A exp. 05/31/2010.* |
| | | *C. Lee, CMA* |

In documenting an injection, be sure to record the injection site (where the injection was given).

- *Intramuscular (IM) injection.* In the next entry, a patient's haloperidol (Haldol) injection is documented. Because all drugs, for example, haloperidol, may cause adverse reactions, the medical assistant also noted that the patient was observed for 20 minutes before being allowed to leave the office. No adverse reactions occurred, or the medical assistant would have listed them.

| DATE | TIME | ORDERS |
|------|------|--------|
| 05/29/XX | 2.45 PM | 5 mg Haldol IM given to (L) ventral gluteal area. Manufacturer Ortho McNeil Lot # 421CC9 exp. 04/31/2009. Pt. observed for 20 minutes before leaving office. No complaints or adverse reactions noted. ———— A. Alvarez, CMA |

Certain drugs can cause adverse reactions. If a patient was monitored after a drug was given, this should be recorded in the chart.

- *Intradermal (ID) injection.* The entry below documents a Mantoux test, which screens for tuberculosis. The Mantoux test is done as an injection of serum between the layers of the skin. The medical assistant records both the exact amount of serum and where it was injected (the patient's right forearm). The medical assistant also records the instructions to the patient to return in 48 to 72 hours to read the results of the test. In the next entry, the results of the test are recorded.

| DATE | TIME | ORDERS |
|------|------|--------|
| 07/19/XX | 3.30 PM | Mantoux test: 0.2 cc serum ID to (R) forearm. Manufacturer Sanofi Adventis Lot #3429A91 exp. 04/31/2009. Pt. given verbal and written instructions to RTO in 48–72 hours for reading the results. Pt. verbalized understanding and willingness to comply. ———— J. Khan, CMA |

Note the abbreviation *ID* in this entry, which indicates that the patient was given an intradermal injection.

| DATE | TIME | ORDERS |
|------|------|--------|
| 07/21/XX | 4:15 PM | Mantoux done 7/19. Results ≈3 mm wheal raised. |
| | | No induration. |
| | | ————————————————— J. Khan, CMA |

A separate entry is needed to document the results of the Mantoux test.

## ADMINISTERED ORAL MEDICATIONS

The following entry shows that a patient was given 10 mg of nifedipine (Procardia), which is used to treat high blood pressure. The abbreviation *SL* means the drug was administered sublingually (under the tongue). The capsule was pricked with a needle, and the contents were squeezed under the patient's tongue. When administered by this route, a drug can be absorbed directly into the bloodstream.

| DATE | TIME | ORDERS |
|------|------|--------|
| 01/24/XX | 9:00 AM | BP 220/110 (L) arm. Dr. Stuart notified and order |
| | | received to give 10 mg Procardia SL stat. Pt given |
| | | Procardia 10 mg SL (Manufacturer Pfizer Lot |
| | | # 366890-34 exp. 06/21/2010) and assisted to |
| | | recline in semi-fowlers position in darkened exam |
| | | room. Wife sitting quietly next to exam table. Will |
| | | recheck BP every 10 minutes. ————————— |
| | | ————————————————— M. Smith, CMA |

When documenting a medication administered in the office, be sure to include the name of the drug and the dose given to the patient.

## PATIENTS' REFUSALS TO ACCEPT MEDICATION

The entry on page 102 documents a patient's refusal to receive an injection of vitamin $B_{12}$. The medical assistant notified the physician and documented his notification in the patient's chart.

## APPLICATION OF A TRANSDERMAL PATCH

As you learned in Chapter 1, a transdermal patch is another way to deliver medication into the bloodstream. It's an adhesive pad that delivers a time-released dose of medication

| DATE | TIME | ORDERS |
|------|------|--------|
| 08/01/XX | 10.30 AM | Pt. refused B₁₂ injection. States: "I can't afford them." Dr. Watson notified. |
|  |  | ——————————————— D. Brooks, CMA |

If a patient refuses medication, this must be documented in the patient's chart as well.

through the skin. The entry below shows how to document the application of a patch containing nitroglycerin (NitroDur). This drug controls chronic angina, or chest pain, in heart patients. The medical assistant writes down the amount of medication and where the patch was placed on the patient's body.

| DATE | TIME | ORDERS |
|------|------|--------|
| 04/10/XX | 2.25 PM | Nitro-Dur 5 mg patch (Manufacturer Key Pharmaceuticals Lot # 211-445 exp. 03/01/2009) applied to (R) upper shoulder area of back. Pt advised to leave in place for 24 hours and to dispose of patch where pets and children cannot get it. |
|  |  | ——————————————— L. Johanson, CMA |

After applying a transdermal patch in the medical office, note the drug name, dosage, and application site in the patient's chart.

## IMMUNIZATIONS

When certain immunizations (vaccines) are given, the following information must be recorded in the patient's record:

- date the vaccine was administered
- lot number, manufacturer, and expiration date of the vaccine
- any adverse reactions to the vaccine
- name and title of the person who administered the vaccine

### Adult Immunizations

Signed consent forms and VIS statements usually aren't required for adult immunizations. However, the maker of the vaccine and the lot number of the batch it came from

## Closer Look    PAPERWORK, PAPERWORK!

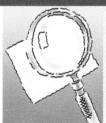

The law requires that a patient's chart show proof that patients are aware of the risks associated with certain vaccines. If you're assisting with immunizations, be sure to include references to the following paperwork:

- *Vaccine Information Statement.* Federal law requires that the medical office give patients an appropriate Vaccine Information Statement (VIS) before certain childhood vaccines are given. The purpose of this information sheet is to explain the risks and benefits of the vaccine. These statements are prepared by the Centers for Disease Control and Prevention (CDC), and physicians should not substitute their own. The patient's chart should state that the patient's parent or legal guardian has received the VIS for the vaccine the patient will receive.

- *Consent form.* Some states also require that the patients sign a form giving their informed consent before receiving a vaccination. The original purpose of this consent form was to protect vaccine makers from lawsuits. The patient's chart should state that the patient has signed a consent form. A parent or legal guardian will sign one for a child.

> Remind travelers that the CDC lists recommended and required vaccinations for people going to certain parts of the world. The CDC website (www.cdc.gov/travel) can help.

should be recorded. If the batch is found to have problems, physicians can track the patients who received injections from the bad batch.

### Childhood Immunizations

Children receive a series of immunizations against childhood diseases as they grow up. The chart entry on page 104 shows how to document the vaccination of a child. Note that the parent or guardian needs to be given a VIS every time a child is vaccinated in a multidose series, not just the first time.

| DATE | TIME | ORDERS |
|------|------|--------|
| 10/21/XX | 11.30 AM | MMR booster given. Info given to patient's mother, signed consent obtained. Manufacturer Merk Lab Lot # 322A61 exp. 04/31/2008. 0.5 cc IM. to (R) deltoid. Patient tolerated injection. |
| | | — G. McMillan, CMA |

Signed consent must be obtained before certain vaccinations may be administered. If the patient is a child, the child's parent or legal guardian must sign the consent form.

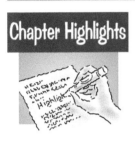

## Chapter Highlights

- Only some states allow clinical medical assistants to administer drugs under the direction of a physician. As a medical assistant, you must know what authority has been and can be delegated to you by state law and the professional in charge.

- Medications classified as controlled substances by the DEA require special prescriptions, special handling in the medical office, and special licensing (a DEA number) from the DEA both to prescribe them and to store them in the medical office.

- You may be required to help maintain professional medical records, such as the physician's DEA registration, controlled substances inventory forms, and prescriptions.

- When administering medications, it's important to observe the "six rights": the right patient, the right drug, the right dose, the right route of administration, the right time, and the right documentation. Observing these rights helps ensure patient safety.

- Aside from observing the "six rights," other ways to decrease medication errors include confirming questionable medication orders, asking someone to verify your dosage calculations, and concentrating on one task at a time.

- When reading and recording medication orders, it's important to ask for clarification from the physician, recognize appropriate medical abbreviations, and read medication labels closely.

- As a medical assistant, you should understand the information on drug labels, including the name of the medication, the strength of the medication, the amount of the drug in the package or container, and the expiration date.

- When medications are administered in the medical office, the necessary information must be documented in the patient's chart. The method used to administer the medication (orally, by injection, etc.) determines what information must be recorded in the patient's chart.

## Chapter 4

# HOW DRUGS WORK

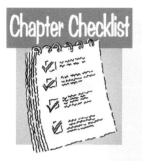

**Chapter Checklist**

- Differentiate between the local and systemic effects of drugs.
- Describe the roles of absorption, distribution, metabolism, and excretion in treating patients with medication.
- List four reasons why a drug might be contraindicated in a specific patient.
- Identify the symptoms of anaphylaxis and angioedema.
- Define synergism and antagonism.
- Explain the interactions that can occur between drugs and foods.
- List four factors that influence a drug's effects on the body.

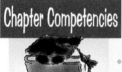

**Chapter Competencies**

- Practice standard precautions (CAAHEP Competency 3.b.1.e.)
- Recognize emergencies (ABHES Competency 4.e.)
- Practice standard precautions (ABHES Competency 4.r.)

As an important member of the medical team, it's important to understand how drugs treat illnesses and disorders. In this chapter, you'll discover how drugs work inside the body and which factors can cause a drug to be more or less effective. You'll also develop skills to help patients understand what the physician has told them about their medications during an office visit, as well as what adverse reactions to look for and how to handle such situations.

## Local and Systemic Effects

Drugs are meant to affect the body in one of two ways:
- locally
- systemically

### DRUGS WITH LOCAL EFFECTS

Drugs with local effects are used to treat one specific area of the body, for example:

- *Lidocaine (LidoPen Auto-Injector, Xylocaine) injection.* A dentist may give this medication to numb a patient's jaw before filling a cavity in a tooth.
- *Lidocaine patch.* A physician may prescribe this patch to relieve the pain of shingles.
- *Bacillus Calmette-Guérin (BCG) solution.* Physicians prescribe this medication to prevent and treat bladder cancer tumors. A catheter is used to place the BCG solution into the bladder.
- *Corticosteroid creams.* Physicians prescribe these creams to counteract inflammation caused by eczema, a skin rash.
- *Sunblocks.* These over-the-counter (OTC) medications protect the skin against ultraviolet rays.
- *Benzoyl peroxide (Acne-5, Benzac, Desquam-X 10% Wash, Dryox Wash, Exact, Loroxide, Neutrogena Acne Mask).* Physicians often recommend this OTC treatment to treat mild cases of acne.
- *Oxymetazoline hydrochloride (OcuClear, Visine L.R.).* These eye drops help relieve dry eyes.
- *Atropine sulfate (Atropine-1, Atropisol, Isopto Atropine).* Optometrists and ophthalmologists use a form of this drug as eye drops. The drops open, or dilate, the pupil of the eye so the physician can examine the inside of the eye.
- *Lindane.* Physicians may prescribe this insecticide to treat resistant cases of head lice.

Sometimes, however, a drug will have systemic side effects. For example, BCG immunotherapy can result in lung infection, and lidocaine injections can cause cardiac irregularities. Some medications can have both local and systemic effects, depending on the route of administration.

> Sunblock is an example of an over-the-counter drug with local effects.

## DRUGS WITH SYSTEMIC EFFECTS

Drugs with systemic effects travel through the bloodstream to reach specific body tissues. The body has nine major organ systems. Each system is made up of organs and tissues that work together as a unit. Drugs with systemic effects target specific systems, although they may have effects on other bodily systems as well. The table on page 108 lists the body's systems and identifies some drugs that target them.

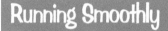

## Running Smoothly — USING OTHER PEOPLE'S MEDICATIONS

*I know it's inappropriate for one person to take another person's medication, but how do I explain to patients why that is the case?*

Suppose a patient who wants to save money asks you if it's safe to take medications prescribed for a friend or relative. "After all," this patient reasons, "I have high blood pressure just like my friend does."

Of course, you'll explain to this patient that it's not safe for him to take someone else's medications. Each patient's medical history and condition are unique, and medications are carefully prescribed for each individual's unique circumstances. In this case, the underlying medical reason why someone has high blood pressure can be different for each person. A drug that helps one person might actually harm another person. For example, some blood pressure medications are diuretics that alter the potassium level in the blood and can cause life-threatening cardiac arrhythmias. Also, a medication that was not prescribed specifically for a particular patient may interact with other medications being taken. Advise the patient to speak with the physician about obtaining the medication and dosage that's right for him.

## Common Drugs and the Body's Systems

| Body System | Main Organs | Medication |
|---|---|---|
| Central nervous system | brain and spinal cord | eszopiclone (Lunesta)—a sleeping pill<br>haloperidol (Haldol)—an antipsychotic<br>diazepam (Diastat, Diazepam Intensol, Valium)—an antianxiety drug<br>ibuprofen (Advil, Motrin, Nuprin)—relieves pain and swelling |
| Respiratory system | lungs and breathing passages | pseudoephedrine hydrochloride (Dimetapp, PediaCare Infants' Decongestant Drops, Sudafed, Triaminic)—relieves nasal congestion<br>albuterol (Proventil, Ventolin)—treats asthma<br>diphenhydramine hydrochloride (Benadryl, Benylin Cough)—an antihistamine |
| Cardiovascular system | heart, veins, arteries | milrinone lactate (Primacor)—for heart failure<br>nitroglycerin (Nitro-Bid, Nitro-Dur, Nitrogard)—prevents and relieves angina (chest pain)<br>isosorbide mononitrate (Imdur, ISMO, Isotrate ER, Monoket)—prevents angina attacks<br>carvedilol (Coreg)—controls high blood pressure (hypertension)<br>warfarin sodium (Coumadin, Jantoven)—prevents blood clots |
| Gastrointestinal system | stomach, large and small intestines | omeprazole (Prilosec, Zegerid)—treats stomach ulcers and acid reflux disease<br>cimetidine (Tagamet, Tagamet HB)—an antacid |
| Urinary system | kidneys, bladder | furosemide (Lasix)—controls fluid buildup from chronic heart failure<br>tolterodine tartrate (Detrol, Detrol LA)—controls overactive bladder |
| Endocrine system | hormone-releasing glands such as the thyroid, adrenal, and pituitary glands | rosiglitazone maleate (Avandia)—treats type 2 diabetes<br>somatropin (Genotropin, Genotropin MiniQuick, Humatrope, Norditropin, Nutropin, Nutropin AQ, Saizen, Serostim)—a synthetic human growth hormone<br>levothyroxine sodium (Levothroid, Levoxine, Levoxyl, Novothyrox, Synthroid)—a thyroid hormone<br>insulins (Humalin R, Humulin 70/30, Lantus)—decrease blood glucose in patients with type 1 or type 2 diabetes |
| Reproductive system | vagina, uterus; penis, testicles | ritodrine hydrochloride (Yutopar)—used to stop premature labor<br>tadalafil (Cialis)—treats erectile disorders<br>sildenafil (Viagra)—treats erectile disorders |
| Immune system | thymus, spleen, lymph nodes | amoxicillin (Amoxil, Trimox)—treats bacterial infections<br>tetracycline (Achromycin, Sumycin)—a broad-spectrum antibiotic<br>pneumococcal 7-valent conjugate vaccine (Prevnar)—immunizes infants and toddlers against pneumonia |
| Musculoskeletal system | the muscles and bones of the skeleton | alendronate sodium (Fosamax)—prevents brittle bones (osteoporosis)<br>etanercept (Enbrel)—treats inflammation and deformity of the joints caused by rheumatoid arthritis |

## *How Drugs Work in the Body*

The two most common forms in which medications are given are solid and liquid. Drugs in solid form include tablets and capsules that a patient takes by mouth. Drugs in liquid form can be taken by mouth or given by injection.

Drugs taken by mouth (except liquids) go through three phases after they are swallowed.

- pharmaceutic phase
- pharmacokinetic phase
- pharmacodynamic phase

Drugs swallowed as liquids or given by injection do not have to dissolve. They go through only two phases after they are swallowed.

- pharmacokinetic phase
- pharmacodynamic phase

### THE PHARMACEUTIC PHASE—ENTERING THE BODY

Tablets and capsules both go through the **pharmaceutic phase**. During this phase, the tablet or capsule breaks into small particles in the gastrointestinal tract, where it dissolves and releases the medication into the body.

---

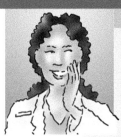

## Secrets for Success

### DO NOT BUY THE "PHARM" ON THESE TERMS!

Break these *pharma-* words into parts to help yourself remember what they mean.

pharmaco + kinetic

pharmaco + dynamic

- *Pharmaco* refers to the drug.
- *Kinetic* refers to motion and movement. Therefore, *pharmacokinetic* means the drug goes where it's supposed to go.
- *Dynamic* refers to force and power. Therefore, *pharmacodynamic* means the drug does what it's supposed to do.

During the pharmaceutic phase, drugs in solid form turn into a form the body can take in and use. Drug companies do a great deal of research to get the pharmaceutic phase right.

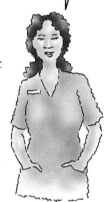

Enteric coated tablets are less likely to cause an upset stomach.

- Some tablets are made to dissolve, or break up, in stomach acids.
- Time-release capsules and extended-release capsules are made to dissolve very slowly in the stomach.
- Enteric coated tablets do not break apart until they pass through the stomach and reach the intestines. The enteric coating protects them from being dissolved by stomach acids, but allows them to dissolve in the alkaline environment of the small intestine.

Drugs that are already dissolved do not go through the pharmaceutic phase because they are already in a form the body can use. These medications include liquids that a patient swallows and drugs that are injected into the body.

## THE PHARMACOKINETIC PHASE— ENTERING THE BLOODSTREAM

After a patient swallows a pill or capsule, the medication dissolves and then moves into the next phase. That phase is the pharmacokinetic phase, during which the drug becomes available for use in the body. **Pharmacokinetics** refers to activities involving the drug within the body after it has been administered. One reason why injected medications can take effect so quickly is that they are ready for use immediately as liquids.

Once it's inside the body, a drug goes through four activities:

- absorption
- distribution
- metabolism
- excretion

### Absorption

When the body absorbs a drug, it takes the drug into the bloodstream through the walls of the stomach or intestines. The bloodstream carries the drug to the places in the body that the drug is meant to reach and affect.

The body does not absorb every drug with the same speed. The speed depends on how the drug is given.

- Drugs get absorbed fastest when they are inhaled, injected intravenously (directly into the bloodstream), or administered sublingually (placed under the tongue).

- The second-fastest way for a drug to be absorbed into the body is by intramuscular injection, which means by injecting the drug directly into a muscle.
- The third-fastest way is by subcutaneous injection, which means by injecting the drug below the skin.

Other factors besides the method of administration affect how quickly a drug is absorbed. Some drugs dissolve faster than other drugs, and conditions inside the body may also affect how quickly a drug can start to work.

## Distribution

The bloodstream carries the drug to the **target place**, the place within the body where the drug is supposed to go. Once the drug reaches the correct site, sometimes only part of the drug is available to do its job. This is called **bioavailability**. Portions of the drug may not be available because they have been bound to protein in the blood. Sometimes, drugs sent to target areas are not fat soluble, and they can't cross body tissues around the brain, placenta, or testes.

If the blood level in the body were reduced, as it would be if the patient were bleeding heavily, the medication might not work. Likewise, if the blood level is too high, the drug may have a harmful effect.

## Metabolism

You probably already know one meaning of the word **metabolism**. It refers to the process by which the body turns food into energy. Metabolism has another slightly different meaning when it's applied to medications. When the liver metabolizes a drug, it takes out all the important chemicals the body needs. These chemicals are the drug's active ingredients. Then, the liver turns what is left into inactive substances that the body can get rid of. Sometimes, the liver can't metabolize a drug fully. Patients who have liver disease may need lower dosages of a drug.

## Excretion

The liver gets rid of the inactive leftovers of a drug by sending them to the kidneys. The kidneys get rid of the leftovers in the urine. The name for this process is **excretion**.

Some medications bypass the liver and go directly through the kidneys and into the patient's urine. The physician may need to give patients with kidney disease lower dosages of the drug. Physicians may also need to monitor these patients' kidney (renal) functions to be sure there is no kidney failure.

Some medications bypass both the liver and the kidneys in leaving the body. These drugs are eliminated from the body through sweat, breast milk, breathing, and feces.

## Half-Life

The **half-life** of a drug is the time it takes the body to eliminate 50% of the drug.

- If a drug has a short half-life (2 to 4 hours), it may be necessary to administer the drug frequently. Aspirin (Bayer Aspirin, St. Joseph's Aspirin) and acetaminophen (Tylenol) are two OTC medications that have a short half-life.

- If a drug has a long half-life (21 to 24 hours), it may be administered less often. Many prescription medications generally require only daily dosages to stay effective.

Patients with liver or kidney disease may have problems eliminating a drug. For them, a drug may have a longer half-life. A drug may build up to toxic, or harmful, levels inside these patients because their bodies can't eliminate the drug fast enough. The physician must adjust dosages and order liver or kidney tests, as needed, to ensure that the medication won't harm the patient.

> Physicians often order blood tests to monitor liver and kidney functions. Kidney function tests are called KFTs. Liver function tests are called LFTs.

## THE PHARMACODYNAMIC PHASE— GOING INTO ACTION

**Pharmacodynamics** are a drug's actions and effects within the body. The pharmacodynamic phase of a drug is the phase when the drug begins to work. It includes the actions the drug takes

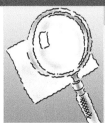

## Closer Look    KIDNEY FUNCTION IN OLDER AND YOUNGER PATIENTS

- Kidney function in children is not as developed as it is in adults. Thus, children often need lower dosages of a drug. The physician may also need to order tests to monitor children's kidney function.

- The kidneys of older adults may not work as well as they did earlier in adulthood. The physician may need to monitor the kidney function of older adult patients closely.

and the effects it has on the body before excretion. When a drug travels through the bloodstream, the whole body is exposed to its possible effects.

- The primary effect of a drug is what the active ingredient in the drug is intended to do. Some possible primary effects are to relieve pain, lower blood sugar, or lower cholesterol.
- All other effects of a drug are secondary effects. Some secondary effects are desirable, whereas others are not. For example, aspirin relieves pain but can also upset the stomach.

Most drugs are designed to work on specific bodily organs or tissues, which are the target sites for the drug. The drugs have their greatest effect on those areas. The drugs usually change how the cells in the target site behave or react.

## DRUG REACTIONS

Drugs produce many chemical reactions in the body. In Chapter 1, you learned about how the United States Food and Drug Administration (FDA) approves and monitors drugs. During clinical trials and testing, the drug manufacturers try to identify all of the beneficial and harmful effects a drug can have on different groups of people. During the approval stage, the data they gather are given to the FDA for further review. From this research, the FDA and the manufacturer determine who benefits most from taking the drug. An important result of this process is identifying those individuals whom the drug will *not* help and whom it could potentially harm. These findings are listed on the package inserts that accompany medications under the heading *contraindications*.

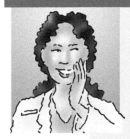

**Secrets for Success**    *CONTRA- WHAT?*

Breaking the word *contraindication* into its word parts can help you decipher its meaning.

- contra = "against"
- indication = "sign"

*Contra-* has the same meaning—"against"—as in the words *contradict* and *contraception*. A *contraindication* is a "sign against" prescribing the drug.

## What Are Contraindications?

**Contraindications** are the circumstances under which a drug or treatment should *not* be used. As a clinical medical assistant, you should become familiar with the contraindications of drugs commonly prescribed in your office. Likewise, you need to be aware of special circumstances in patients' lives that can affect their use of a drug. Be ready to remind the physician about those circumstances if the patient forgets to mention them.

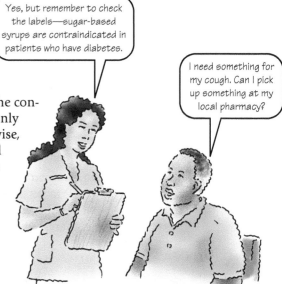

Yes, but remember to check the labels—sugar-based syrups are contraindicated in patients who have diabetes.

I need something for my cough. Can I pick up something at my local pharmacy?

## Adverse Reactions

Patients may experience harmful side effects, or adverse reactions, when they take a drug. As a medical assistant, you need to be vigilant, because these undesirable effects are often not predictable. Depending on the patient and the medication,

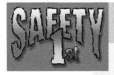

### MAKE SURE THE PHYSICIAN KNOWS

Some patients think that a physician knows or can notice everything important about them. It's impossible for that to be true.

- Remind the physician if a patient is in recovery from alcohol abuse. The physician can prescribe the patient medications that do not have an alcohol base.

- Certain drugs can be harmful to a fetus. If you know that a patient has been trying to get pregnant, be sure she lets the physician know.

- If you know a new patient has young children at home, be sure the physician knows. Aspirin is safe for most adults to take, but it's contraindicated in children. Studies have shown a possible link between aspirin use in children and Reye syndrome, a brain disease that can be fatal.

adverse reactions can include any combination of the following. They may:

- be mild, severe, or even life threatening
- happen after the first dose, after several doses, or after many doses
- happen in a predictable way or without warning

### Allergic Reactions

Patients can be allergic to medications, just as they can be allergic to other substances. An **allergic reaction** happens when the patient's immune system responds to the drug as if it were

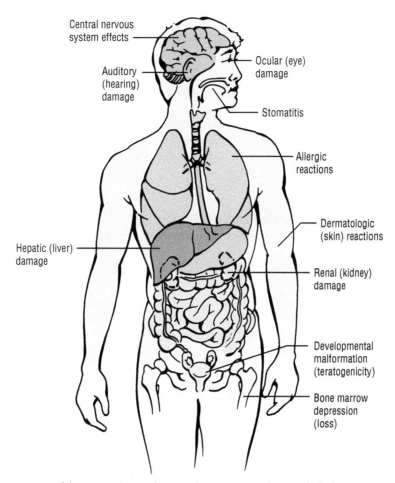

Adverse reactions to drugs can happen in many places in the body.

## Your Turn to Teach

### WHEN TO CONTACT THE PHYSICIAN'S OFFICE

Patients' responses to any medication may differ from the known adverse reactions. Thus it's always wise to remind patients to contact the physician's office if they experience any of the following:

- upset stomach
- chest pain
- hot flashes
- blurred vision
- weakness
- dizziness
- any other symptom not specified as a known adverse reaction

The cause of the patient's response could be an adverse reaction to the medication. If you're the one who speaks to the patient over the phone, bring these symptoms to the attention of the physician. Under no circumstances should you offer medical advice to the patient; only a physician may adjust a patient's prescription.

being invaded by a foreign substance, or **antigen**. The immune system produces antibodies to combat the invader.

Allergic reactions to drugs usually take time to build up. Remember these facts when you take a patient's medication history:

- Most allergic drug reactions occur after the patient has received more than one dose of a drug.
- If the patient experiences an allergic reaction after taking a medication for the first time, it's possible that the patient may have taken the drug at some time in the past but does not remember it.
- Find out how allergies or reactions are flagged in the patients' charts (that is, the method your office uses, such as a red pen or bright orange sticker).

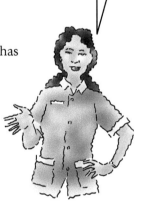

Another name for an allergic reaction is a **hypersensitivity** reaction.

### Signs and Symptoms of Drug Allergies

Look and listen for the following signs and symptoms of drug allergies. Both over-the-counter and prescription drugs can cause them.

- itching
- skin rash
- urticaria (hives)—one or more pale, itchy, pink swellings of the skin that may burn or sting
- **dyspnea**—difficulty breathing
- wheezing
- **cyanosis**—a bluish discoloration of the lips, face, fingertips, or other body parts
- swelling of the eyes, lips, or tongue
- sudden loss of consciousness

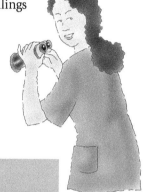

If a patient experiences a reaction, be sure to report it to the physician.

## Running Smoothly

### RESPONDING TO ALLERGIC REACTIONS

*What if a patient begins having difficulty breathing shortly after you administer an injection?*

Any health care professional who administers medications to patients needs to be cautious about allergic reactions. As a medical assistant, you'll be the backup "eyes and ears" for the physician and other medical staff members.

A patient who begins experiencing difficulty breathing may be having an allergic reaction to the drug. A more serious allergic reaction, **anaphylactic shock**, is life-threatening. (Anaphylactic shock is a severe allergic reaction that may result in death.) All drug reactions should be taken seriously.

Allergic reactions that occur immediately after a drug has been administered are usually the most serious. That's one reason why patients are asked to wait for 20 minutes before leaving the office after an injection. It's important to report any suspected allergic reactions to the physician because the patient may need emergency treatment. Signs and symptoms of severe allergic reactions are often related to breathing problems and tissue swelling. Check the patient for wheezing, cyanosis, itching, hives, sweating, and swelling of the eyes, lips, mouth, or throat. If you notice any of these symptoms after administering a drug to a patient, alert the physician immediately!

### Angioedema

Angioedema is another type of allergic reaction to a medication. Edema is an abnormal build-up of fluid. Patients with angioedema look like they have welts, or ridges, below the skin. The painless welts usually appear around the eyes, lips, mouth, and throat, and sometimes other parts of the body.

Angioedema can be dangerous when the patient's mouth is affected, because the swelling can block the patient's airway and cause asphyxia (suffocation). If you notice that a patient has difficulty breathing or has swelling in any part of her body, tell the physician immediately.

### Anaphylactic Shock

The most serious allergic reaction a patient may have to a drug is anaphylactic shock. This type of reaction requires immediate medical attention. Anaphylactic shock usually occurs soon after a patient is given a drug to which he is extremely sensitive. Teach yourself to look for the signs and symptoms of anaphylactic shock listed in the table below.

## Idiosyncratic Reactions

Sometimes a drug acts on a patient in a way other than the drug manufacturer intended. The response to the drug is unusual and different from what is normally expected. This type of response

### Signs and Symptoms of Anaphylactic Shock

| | |
|---|---|
| Respiratory system | • bronchospasm (severe narrowing of the airways into the lungs)<br>• dyspnea (difficulty breathing)<br>• feeling of fullness in the throat<br>• cough<br>• wheezing |
| Cardiovascular system | • extremely low blood pressure<br>• tachycardia (rapid heart rate—greater than 100 beats per minute)<br>• palpitations (irregular or forceful beating of the heart)<br>• syncope (fainting)<br>• cardiac arrest (heart attack) |
| Skin | • urticaria (skin rash)<br>• angioedema (welts below the skin)<br>• pruritus (itching)<br>• sweating |
| Gastrointestinal system | • nausea<br>• vomiting<br>• abdominal pain |

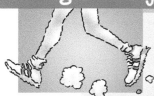

## Running Smoothly

### TREATING ANAPHYLACTIC SHOCK

*What if a patient under your care goes into anaphylactic shock and the physician isn't in the room?*

Anaphylactic shock is life threatening. Your first step should be to notify the physician immediately. Here are several other steps you may take until the physician or another qualified health care professional arrives:

- Take the patient's blood pressure, pulse, and respirations.
- If a patient needs assistance with an epinephrine hydrochloride (EpiPen) injection that has been prescribed for a severe reaction, it would be appropriate to assist the patient if requested.
- If the patient is having difficulty breathing, loosen any tight clothing.
- Do not give the patient anything to drink.
- If the patient is feeling lightheaded, have him lie on his back with his legs elevated higher than his head. This position helps blood flow to the brain.
- If the patient starts to vomit or bleed from the mouth, turn him on his side to help avoid choking.
- If the patient stops breathing, start CPR.

is called **drug idiosyncrasy**. For example, suppose a patient is given a sleeping pill to relax her and help her sleep. But instead, the drug has the opposite effect, and the patient remains wide awake and shows signs of nervousness and excitement.

Why do some patients have an idiosyncratic response (a response peculiar to that individual) to a drug? It's not clear. Some researchers speculate that a person's genetic makeup may make them unable to tolerate certain drugs.

### Drug Tolerance

Some patients build up a tolerance to a drug. **Drug tolerance** is a decreased response to a drug; taking the same dosage no longer has the same effect. These patients may need a larger dosage of the painkiller, sleep medication, or other drug to get the desired results.

Patients may, on their own, decide to increase the dose of a medication so they will get relief. Counsel them to follow the

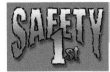

## UNUSUAL DRUG RESPONSES

Listen with care to what patients tell you about their experiences with medications. If a patient mentions any kind of drug response that is out of the ordinary or other than what is expected, be sure the physician is aware.

> Hmmm, that sounds unusual. I'll let the physician know that you had an unusual reaction to the medication.

physician's orders. Let the physician know that the patient's response to a medication has changed.

### Cumulative Drug Effect

The liver and kidneys are the organs that metabolize and excrete medications from the body. Patients with liver or kidney disease may develop problems with the active ingredients in the drugs they take. They may become unable to fully metabolize and excrete one dose of a medication before they take the next one. A part of the first dose remains active in the body, and a **cumulative drug effect** may happen. Too much of the drug can build up in the body and cause a harmful reaction.

### Toxic Reactions

Drugs are designed to be safe for most patients. However, most drugs can produce toxic, or harmful, reactions under the following circumstances:

- The dosages are too large.
- An unsafe amount of the drug remains in the bloodstream. An amount is unsafe if it's greater than the **therapeutic level**, which is the level usually used to treat the patient's condition.
- The kidneys are not working correctly and can't excrete the drug in the patient's urine.

Be aware of the signs and symptoms of toxicity of the drugs that the physicians in your office commonly prescribe.

## Closer Look

## DRUG TOXICITY AND PATIENT AWARENESS

As a medical assistant, the short-term and long-term well-being of patients must always be your priority. Remember these facts about drug toxicity.

- Certain drugs can cause toxic reactions in some patients even when the drugs are given at the recommended dose.
- Some toxic effects happen immediately, and some build up over time. They may not be seen for weeks or even months.
- Some toxic drug effects can be reversed depending on the organ involved. For example, liver cells can regenerate, or grow back, after being damaged. Full liver function can be restored.
- There are some toxic drug effects that can't be reversed. A toxic reaction to streptomycin is an example. Streptomycin, an antibiotic, is used to control infections. However, a toxic reaction to it can do irreversible damage to the eighth cranial nerve and cause hearing loss.

Any medication allergies should be carefully recorded in the patient's medication history.

## DRUG INTERACTIONS

Medications work by interacting with the chemistry of the human body to produce their results. They also interact with the things people put into their bodies, including foods and other drugs. As a clinical medical assistant, you need to be aware of these interactions so that you can help to keep patients safe.

### Drug–Drug Interactions

The patients you encounter in the medical office probably take more than just the drugs and medications prescribed by the physician. It's likely that they are also taking over-the-counter medications such as acetaminophen or ibuprofen (Advil, Motrin, Nuprin) for pain; famotidine (Pepcid, Pepcid AC, Pepcid RPD), calcium carbonate (Maalox Antacid Caplets, Oscal, Rolaids Calcium Rich, Tums, Viactiv), or other antacids for heartburn; as well as herbal supplements and vitamins for nutrition. They may be taking medications prescribed by other physicians, such as specialists who treat them for chronic diseases. Additionally, they may be taking antibiotics after dental surgery.

Drug–drug interactions occur when one drug interacts with or interferes with the action of another drug. There are scientific terms for these interactions.

- **Synergism** occurs when two drugs work together.

- **Antagonism** is when one drug reduces the effects of the other drug.

- **Potentiation** occurs when one drug increases or prolongs the effects of the other drug.

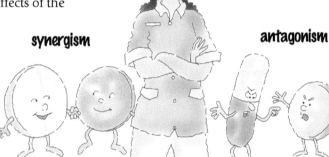

*Synergism occurs when two drugs work together. But when one drug interferes with the other's effects, it's called antagonism.*

synergism

antagonism

### Synergistic Drug Reactions

Drug synergism happens when two or more drugs work together to produce an effect that is greater than what each drug would have produced by itself.

Combination medications take advantage of the positive aspects of synergism. For example, a physician or dentist might prescribe acetaminophen mixed with codeine (Tylenol with Codeine No. 3) for pain relief after minor surgery. The acetaminophen enhances the effect of codeine as a pain reliever.

However, negative effects of synergism can occur, such as when tranquilizers are combined with alcohol intake. The increased effects of sedation can lead to severely impaired judgment or death.

### Antagonistic Drug Reactions

When two drugs have an antagonistic effect on each other, one drug interferes with the action of the other drug. Either they cancel each other out, or one drug makes the other drug less powerful.

For example, the drug heparin (Heparin Sodium Injection) is sometimes called a blood thinner because it keeps blood

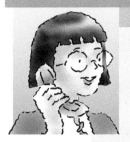

## Ask the Professional    OBTAINING COMPLETE MEDICATION HISTORIES

**Q:** *I've had a difficult time obtaining complete medication histories from patients. Some patients aren't able to remember all the medications they take. Other patients become offended when I ask about alcohol or recreational drug use. I know it's my job to gather this information, but what should I do when patients can't or won't provide it?*

**A:** Encourage patients to be forthcoming and complete. Explain that, because of the harmful nature of certain drug interactions, it's important for the physician to be aware of all the medications patients are currently taking.

If a patient is unable to remember which medications he's taking, start by asking him for a complete listing of the physicians, dentists, and other health care professionals he is seeing. This may help the patient recall which physicians prescribed his medications. Next, if the patient can't think of the names of the drugs he takes, have the patient or a family member collect the patient's prescription and OTC medications in a plastic bag and bring them to the patient's next appointment. Finally, ask the patient when he takes each medication and whether he has adjusted drug dosages on his own. Explain that the physician needs to know whether the patient has been taking his medication the correct way.

If a patient is uncomfortable with discussing his alcohol or drug use, gently remind him that the information will remain confidential. Explain that the physician needs to know this information because alcohol and certain drugs can interact with medications. However, harmful interactions can be avoided if the physician has thorough and accurate information about the patient's medication history.

from clotting. It's used to treat blood clots and is often used in heart surgery. To treat a heparin overdose, physicians use protamine sulfate. This drug, a heparin antagonist, totally neutralizes, or cancels out, heparin's effects. Another example is that certain antibiotics may render hormone-based contraceptives ineffective.

Patients sometimes need to be warned about antagonistic reactions. For example, a patient who is taking the antibiotic tetracycline (Achromycin, Sumycin) by mouth should be warned not to use antacids because they decrease the effectiveness of tetracycline.

## Food–Drug Interactions

The foods we eat also affect how drugs act in the body. Foods, like drugs, contain chemicals that affect us. The caffeine in soft drinks and coffee is a stimulant. The glucose in Halloween candy can cause a "sugar rush" in trick-or-treaters. Candy can also be used as a medical therapy. Patients with type 1 diabetes who are experiencing hypoglycemia (low blood sugar levels) are told to suck on some hard candy to quickly treat the condition.

Patients need to know about any interactions between the foods they eat and the medications the physician prescribes. They may need to adjust their diets in order to get the most from their medications. By being aware of these issues, you'll be able to provide patients with the correct information.

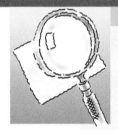

## Closer Look  MORE ABOUT FOOD-DRUG INTERACTIONS

Learn as much as you can about the medications commonly prescribed by the physician you assist. Here is some information about several common medications.

| Food Caution | Drug Name | Category |
|---|---|---|
| Do not take with dairy products. | doxycycline (Vibramycin) tetracycline hydro-chloride (Achromycin, Sumycin) oxytetracycline (Terramycin) | Antibiotic (tetracycline) |
| Do not take with fruit juice. | nafcillin (Unipen, Nallpen) ampicillin (Omnipen, Principen) cloxacillin (Tegopen) penicillin G benzathine (Bicillin L-A) | Antibiotic (penicillin) |

| Food Caution | Drug Name | Category |
|---|---|---|
| Do not take with caffeine. | ciprofloxacin (Cipro) | Antibiotic (fluoroquinolone) |
| Do not take with tyramine-rich foods: | phenelzine (Nardil) tranylcypromine (Parnate) isoniazid (Nydrazid) | monoamine oxidase (MAO) inhibitors Antituberculars |
| • avocados | | |
| • bananas | | |
| • raisins | | |
| • cheese | | |
| • chocolate | | |
| • yeast | | |
| • wine | | |
| • salami/ pepperoni | | |
| • bologna | | |
| • hot dogs | | |
| • sausage | | |
| • beer | | |
| • sour cream | | |
| • yogurt | | |
| • fava or broad beans | | |

## When an Empty Stomach Is Best

Medicine taken on an empty stomach gets absorbed into the bloodstream faster than when food is in the stomach. Some medications are most effective when they are taken on an empty stomach. For example, food may interfere with the body's absorption of the antibiotics ampicillin (Principen) and nafcillin (Unipen).

## When Food Is the Key

Always know about a drug's peculiarities. Some medications irritate the stomach and cause nausea, vomiting, or epigastric irritation (irritation in the upper central part of the abdomen). The following medications can be taken with food to make an upset stomach less likely:

Certain medications should be taken with food to avoid upset stomach.

- ibuprofen (Motrin, Advil, Nuprin)—an analgesic and anti-inflammatory drug
- amoxicillin (Amoxil)—an antibiotic
- verapamil (Calan)—a heart medication

Other drugs, when taken with certain foods, produce enhanced effects in the body. For example, orange juice helps increase the body's absorption of iron.

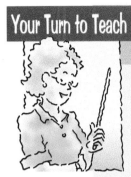

## "TAKE THIS MEDICATION WITH . . ." STICKERS ON MEDICINE BOTTLES

**Your Turn to Teach**

Patients may ask you about the food-related stickers that pharmacists sometimes place on medicine bottles. These are some of the stickers in common use:

- With Food
- Take on Empty Stomach
- No Grapefruit Juice
- No Orange Juice
- With or Without Food

Explain to patients that these stickers tell them how to get the most from their medications. Explain that food can change the effects of certain medications. Encourage patients to follow the instructions on the sticker.

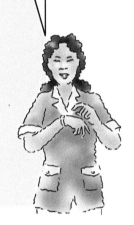

"Take on empty stomach" means one hour before eating or two hours after eating.

## Factors Influencing Drug Responses

Every patient is an individual from a medical point of view. This means that all patients will not react to the same drug in exactly the same way. These are some of the factors that influence an individual's response to a drug:

- age
- weight
- gender
- pre-existing disease or condition

### AGE

A patient's age can affect how well a drug can do its intended job. Infants and children usually require smaller doses of a medication than adults need. Furthermore, some drugs are not even tested for use in children. The kidneys, liver, and other organs are immature in children, which affects a child's ability to metabolize, or take what it needs from, a drug.

Elderly patients may also require smaller doses of a drug, although this may depend on the type of drug. For instance,

## Closer Look

### MULTIPLE MEDICATIONS AND ADVERSE REACTIONS

Elderly patients are often treated for more than one long-term, or chronic, medical condition. These patients may be taking a variety of medications to keep their conditions under control. They may be receiving medications from several specialists as well as from their primary care physician. **Polypharmacy**, or the taking of multiple drugs, is common in elderly patients. The danger of polypharmacy is that it increases the risk of adverse reactions.

As a medical assistant, you should encourage elderly patients who are starting a new treatment plan to be very explicit with each physician about all of the medications they are taking. Also, patients should be encouraged to use only one pharmacist who has a history of their past medication use.

> When it comes to drug responses, age matters!

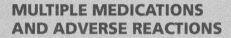

an elderly patient may need a smaller dose of a sleeping aid than a 20- or 30-year-old patient. Both, however, will require the same sized dose of an antibiotic.

### WEIGHT

The dosages for medications are generally calculated for a person of average weight, or 150 pounds in both men and women. If a patient weighs significantly more or less than 150 pounds, the physician may adjust the dosage to produce the desired effect.

> Average medication dosages are calculated for a person weighing 150 pounds.

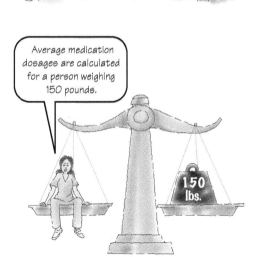

### GENDER

The patient's gender may affect how some drugs work. A female patient may require a smaller dose of some medications than a male patient because of differences in the makeup of their bodies. Adult men and women differ in the average amount of body fat they have and in the ratio of body mass to body water.

## PRE-EXISTING DISEASE OR CONDITION

The presence of liver or kidney disease in a patient may also affect a physician's decision to prescribe a specific drug. Disease in these organs can prevent a patient from metabolizing a drug or excreting it through the kidneys.

Pregnancy can also affect the physician's choice of medications because the drugs may pass into the bloodstream of the unborn child, injuring the fetus. If you're aware that a patient is pregnant or might become pregnant, remind her to tell the physician immediately.

## Chapter Highlights

- Drugs are meant to affect the body either locally or systemically. Drugs with local effects affect only one spot or part of the body. Drugs with systemic effects, such as high blood pressure medications, travel through the bloodstream to reach specific body tissues or target sites.

- The body absorbs a drug by taking it into the bloodstream through the walls of the stomach or intestines. The bloodstream distributes the drug by carrying it to the target site.

- When the liver metabolizes a drug, it takes out the active ingredients and turns what is left into inactive substances that the body can get rid of through the kidneys in a process called excretion.

- Reasons a drug might be contraindicated include the drug's known adverse reactions, allergic reactions caused by the drug, harmful cumulative effects, and possible toxic reactions in certain individuals.

- Angioedema and anaphylactic shock are two serious allergic reactions. When a patient experiences angioedema, the eyes, lips, or tongue may become swollen. Symptoms of anaphylactic shock can include difficulty breathing, irregular or rapid heart rate, fainting, skin rash, sweating, and vomiting. Both types of allergic reactions require immediate medical attention.

- Synergistic drug reactions occur when two drugs together produce an effect that is greater than what each drug would have produced by itself. Antagonistic drug reactions occur when one drug interferes with the action of another drug, canceling it out or making it less powerful.

- Age, weight, gender, and pre-existing diseases or medical conditions, including pregnancy, can affect a patient's response to a drug. Dosages may need to be adjusted to meet each patient's specific circumstances.

- Drugs also interact with foods. Some medications need to be taken with food to avoid irritating the stomach. Others should be taken on an empty stomach because food interferes with their absorption. Some drugs interact with certain foods that lessen or cancel the drugs' effects.

## Chapter 5

# COMMONLY PRESCRIBED DRUGS

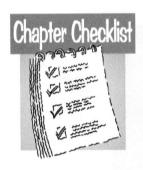

**Chapter Checklist**

- Explain how drugs are classified

- Identify the uses for antibiotics and discuss the therapeutic actions of these drugs

- Recognize the conditions topical drugs are commonly used to treat and explain how these medications are thought to work

- List the uses for anti-inflammatory drugs and describe how they work

- List the uses for analgesics and antipyretics and describe how these drugs work

- Explain why muscle relaxants may be prescribed and discuss the two ways these drugs work in the body

- Identify the various conditions cardiac drugs are used to treat and describe the different therapeutic actions of these drugs

- List the uses for respiratory medications and explain the various ways in which these medications work

- Recognize the indications for digestive drugs and discuss how these drugs work

- Explain why urinary drugs may be used and identify the therapeutic actions of these drugs

- Discuss the main use for diuretic drugs and how these drugs accomplish their purpose

- Identify the uses for nervous system medications and recognize where these drugs work in the body

- List the various conditions endocrine drugs are used to treat and describe the therapeutic actions of these drugs

- Explain why oncology medications are used and how these drugs work

Your work as a clinical medical assistant puts you in daily contact with the medications that physicians in your office prescribe. Some categories of drugs may be prescribed more frequently at certain times of the year, such as during the flu season. Other drugs are prescribed year-round to patients with cardiac problems, diabetes, and other chronic conditions. It's important to be familiar with the drugs that are most commonly used in your individual work setting. It's also important to rely on your supervisor and know where to reference the most current and accurate drug information.

Remember also that most drugs cause certain adverse reactions (side effects). When you're familiar with the most commonly prescribed drugs in your office, you can teach patients what to watch for and how to respond to possible adverse reactions to a drug. Remember, however, that these reactions may or may not occur.

## General Drug Classifications

As you know, there are many prescription and over-the-counter drugs available to patients. There are also several ways to classify these drugs. To make them easier to understand, drugs are classified according to their primary action on the body. For example, antiviral medications work to resist viruses; muscle relaxants work to help muscles relax; decongestants work to reduce congestion, and so on. Throughout this chapter, each group of drugs is described according to its purpose. You'll also learn about how these drugs work.

Immediately after a drug class is introduced, an icon shows you which body system (or systems) the drugs in that class work upon. Within each class of drugs, a table is used to identify the generic and trade names and to describe the action, use, and possible adverse reactions to that drug. As you read through each of these tables, remember that the primary use of a particular drug may have effects and actions on other systems of the body. For example, a drug classified as a diuretic may also be used as an antihypertensive drug. It takes time to understand not only the basic classification of a particular drug but also the many secondary uses and effects each drug has on the human body.

You'll notice that the names of many prescription drugs include suffixes, such as the letters *DS, HS, SR,* or *XR.* In some cases, these suffixes describe a chemical that has been added to the drug. For example, Robitussin DM contains the drug dextromethorphan (DM for short). In other cases, these suffixes refer to the strength or release of the drug, such as:

- DS = double strength
- HS = half strength
- SR = sustained release
- XR = extended release

By becoming familiar with these suffixes, you'll have a better understanding of the drugs you encounter on a daily basis.

## *Antibiotics*

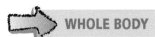 **WHOLE BODY**

Your body does a terrific job of fighting off germs. But, sometimes, microbes (germs) multiply faster than the body can cope with them. You get sick. You develop an infection from the bacteria. Infection-fighting drugs, however, treat the infection itself.

There are several major classes of antibiotics that physicians in your office may prescribe. The names of some of these medications might be somewhat familiar, whereas other names may be new. The classes of antibiotics described in this chapter are:

- penicillins
- cephalosporins
- tetracyclines
- macrolides
- aminoglycosides
- sulfonamides
- quinolones
- miscellaneous antibiotics

## WHY YOU USE THEM

Physicians use **antibiotics** to treat systemic bacterial infections. (A systemic infection is an infection that involves the whole body, not just one area of it.)

As a clinical medical assistant, you'll see this situation happen many times: A patient comes into the office complaining of a sore throat. The physician examines the patient's throat, and, sure enough, there are clear signs of inflammation. But what kind of infection is causing that inflammation? Is it a virus? Is it a bacterial infection? Before the physician can choose the right drug to treat the inflammation, she needs to know what is causing it.

### Culture

"Strep throat" is an infection that's common among children and teenagers. It responds very well to antibiotics—if that's the kind of infection the patient has. If a virus is the cause of the sore throat, antibiotics won't help at all. Fluids, rest, and acetaminophen will be the best treatment.

The way the physician can diagnose strep throat for certain is to take a throat culture, which usually takes 24 hours to grow.

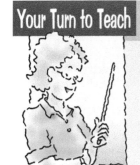

## Your Turn to Teach    FOLLOWING THE PHYSICIAN'S ORDERS

Remind patients that antibiotics work best when:
- the amount of medication is kept at a constant level in the body
- the antibiotics are taken for the full course of treatment

Remind patients to take their antibiotics on schedule during the day and for the number of days the physician said to take them. Explain that stopping the medication early may allow the bacteria that caused the infection to begin growing again. The infection could come back!

Urge patients to read the label on the medicine bottle and the written information provided by the pharmacist. The pharmacist's instructions will tell patients what to do if they accidentally forget to take a dose on time.

A positive test means that the *Streptococcus* bacteria are present. Newly developed tests can detect a strep infection in 15 minutes. The physician may often do both tests and reevaluate treatment plans when the results of the tests are in.

## Sensitivity

The physician must then match the drug she chooses to the patient's condition. One antibiotic might have a greater effect on the strain of bacteria than another. The patient's medication history is important, too. A child might tolerate one antibiotic better than he tolerates another one.

## HOW THEY WORK

Antibiotics work in one of two ways. Some antibiotics work to kill bacteria (bacteriocidal), whereas others simply interrupt the way the bacteria reproduce (bacteriostatic).

## TYPES AND EXAMPLES

| DRUG SPOTLIGHT | Antibiotics |
|---|---|

| Penicillins | | | | |
|---|---|---|---|---|
| **Drug Name Generic (Trade)** | **Typical Form and Route of Administration** | **Indications** | **Therapeutic Action** | **Adverse Reactions and Drug Interactions** |
| amoxicillin (Amoxil, Disper-Mox, Trimox) | oral: tablets, capsules, suspension | wide variety of bacterial infections | kills sensitive bacteria | *Adverse reactions:* nausea vomiting diarrhea *Drug interactions:* reduces the effectiveness of oral contraceptives |
| amoxicillin and clavulanate potassium (Augmentin) | oral: tablets, suspension | wide variety of bacterial infections | kills sensitive bacteria | *Adverse reactions:* diarrhea or loose stools nausea and vomiting skin rashes and urticaria vaginitis |

**DRUG SPOTLIGHT**    **Antibiotics (continued)**

### Cephalosporins

| Drug Name Generic (Trade) | Typical Form and Route of Administration | Indications | Therapeutic Action | Adverse Reactions and Drug Interactions |
|---|---|---|---|---|
| cephalexin monohydrate (Keflex) | oral: tablets, capsules, suspension | staph and strep infections including pneumonia, cellulitis, and osteomyelitis | kills bacteria by interfering with the bacteria's cell wall formation, which weakens the cell wall and causes it to rupture | *Adverse reactions:* confusion bleeding diarrhea nausea • vomiting |
| ceftriaxone sodium (Rocephin) | injection | wide variety of bacterial infections, including those affecting the lower respiratory tract, ears, skin, urinary tract, and bones/joints | kills bacteria by interfering with the bacteria's cell wall formation, which weakens the cell wall and causes it to rupture | *Adverse reactions:* diarrhea nausea vomiting |
| cefaclor (Ceclor) | oral: tablets, capsules, suspension | wide variety of bacterial infections, including pharyngitis and tonsillitis, skin infections, chronic bronchitis, ear infections, lower respiratory tract infections, and urinary tract infections | kills bacteria by interfering with the bacteria's cell wall formation, which weakens the cell wall and causes it to rupture | *Adverse reactions:* headache rhinitis diarrhea nausea vaginitis vaginal moniliasis abdominal pain increased cough pharyngitis pruritus back pain |

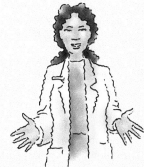

Be careful! A patient who has had a reaction to penicillin may also have a reaction to cephalosporins.

*(continued)*

**DRUG SPOTLIGHT** **Antibiotics (continued)**

### Tetracyclines

| Drug Name Generic (Trade) | Typical Form and Route of Administration | Indications | Therapeutic Action | Adverse Reactions and Drug Interactions |
|---|---|---|---|---|
| tetracycline hydrochloride (Achromycin, Sumycin) | oral: capsules, suspension | wide variety of bacterial infections<br>acne<br>acute intestinal amebiasis (as adjunct therapy) | slows the growth of sensitive bacteria by interfering with the production of proteins needed by the bacteria to grow<br>allows the body's defense mechanisms (such as white blood cells) to destroy the bacteria | *Adverse reactions:*<br>black hairy tongue<br>bulky loose stools<br>diarrhea<br>difficulty swallowing<br>headache<br>hoarseness<br>indigestion<br>inflammation of the mouth<br>inflammation of the skin<br>inflammation or redness of tongue<br>joint pain<br>anorexia<br>mouth sores<br>nausea<br>sensitivity to sunlight<br>swelling and itching of the rectum<br>• vomiting |
| doxycycline (Vibramycin) | oral: tablets, capsules, suspension, syrup<br>injection | pneumonia and other respiratory tract infections<br>Lyme disease<br>acne<br>infections of skin, genital, and urinary systems<br>anthrax<br>also used to prevent malaria | slows the growth of bacteria, allowing the body's immune system to destroy it | *Adverse reactions:*<br>nausea<br>vomiting<br>abdominal distress and distention<br>diarrhea<br>photosensitivity reactions (red rash on areas exposed to sunlight)<br>*Drug interactions:*<br>Antacids containing aluminum, calcium, or magnesium make it harder for the body to absorb the drug in its oral form.<br>Unlike other tetracyclines, doxycycline does not interact with milk or milk products.<br>Barbiturates, phenytoin, and carbamazepine make it less effective. |

**DRUG SPOTLIGHT** | **Antibiotics (continued)**

## Macrolides

| Drug Name Generic (Trade) | Typical Form and Route of Administration | Indications | Therapeutic Action | Adverse Reactions and Drug Interactions |
|---|---|---|---|---|
| azithromycin (Zithromax) | oral: tablets, suspension injection | mild to moderate bacterial infections, such as certain pneumonias, strep infections, and minor staph infections of the skin | slows the growth of, or sometimes kills, sensitive bacteria by reducing the production of important proteins needed by the bacteria to survive | *Adverse reactions:* diarrhea or loose stools nausea abdominal pain |
| clarithromycin (Biaxin) | oral: tablets, suspension | mild to moderate bacterial infections, such as certain pneumonias, strep infections, and minor staph infections of the skin | slows the growth of, or sometimes kills, sensitive bacteria by reducing the production of important proteins needed by the bacteria to survive | *Adverse reactions (adults):* diarrhea nausea abnormal taste *Adverse reactions (children):* diarrhea vomiting abdominal pain rash headache |

## Aminoglycosides

| gentamicin (Garamycin) | injection ophthalmic: ointment, solution topical: ointment, cream | serious infections caused by sensitive strains of *Escherichia coli (E. coli)*, *Staphylococcus*, or several other types of bacteria | slows the growth of, or kills, sensitive bacteria | *Adverse reactions:* nerve toxicity ototoxicity kidney toxicity |
|---|---|---|---|---|

> Aminoglycosides are usually given by injection because they're absorbed poorly from the gastrointestinal tract.

*(continued)*

**DRUG SPOTLIGHT** **Antibiotics (continued)**

### Aminoglycosides

| Drug Name Generic (Trade) | Typical Form and Route of Administration | Indications | Therapeutic Action | Adverse Reactions and Drug Interactions |
|---|---|---|---|---|
| tobramycin (Tobrex) | injection inhalation: nebulizer solution ophthalmic: solution, ointment | serious infections caused by sensitive strains of *Escherichia coli (E. coli)*, *Staphylococcus*, or several other types of bacteria | kills sensitive bacteria | *Adverse reactions:* diarrhea headache nausea vomiting |

### Sulfonamides

| | | | | |
|---|---|---|---|---|
| trimethaprim and sulfamethoxazole (Bactrim DS, Septra DS) | oral: tablets, suspension injection | infections of the urinary tract, lungs, ears, and intestines traveler's diarrhea | kills sensitive bacteria | *Adverse reactions:* crystals in the urine photosensitivity scarlet rash all over body |

### Quinolones

| | | | | |
|---|---|---|---|---|
| ciprofloxacin (Cipro) | oral: tablets, suspension injection | bacterial infections patients who have been exposed to airborne anthrax germs | kills sensitive bacteria by stopping the production of essential proteins needed by the bacteria to survive | *Adverse reactions:* nausea vomiting diarrhea abdominal pain |
| ofloxacin (Floxin) | oral: tablets ophthalmic: solution otic: solution | mild to moderate bacterial infections conjunctivitis ear infections | kills sensitive bacteria by stopping the production of essential proteins needed by the bacteria to survive | *Adverse reactions:* diarrhea dizziness headache anorexia nausea vomiting photosensitivity insomnia |

### Miscellaneous Antibiotics

| | | | | |
|---|---|---|---|---|
| vancomycin (Vancocin, Vancoled) | oral: solution injection | drug of choice to treat serious resistant staph infections in patients who are hypersensitive to penicillins | kills sensitive bacteria | *Adverse reactions:* anaphylactic reactions |

| DRUG SPOTLIGHT | Antibiotics (continued) | | | |
| --- | --- | --- | --- | --- |
| **Miscellaneous Antibiotics** | | | | |
| **Drug Name Generic (Trade)** | **Typical Form and Route of Administration** | **Indications** | **Therapeutic Action** | **Adverse Reactions and Drug Interactions** |
| metronidazole (Flagyl) | oral: tablets, capsules injection topical: lotion, cream, gel vaginal: gel | intestinal infections caused by amebas (amebiasis) infections, such as vaginitis, caused by trichomonads (trichomoniasis) | thought to work by entering the bacterial cell, acting on some components of the cell, and destroying the bacteria | *Adverse reactions:* nausea vomiting anorexia diarrhea abdominal cramps turns urine dark or brown and gives a metallic taste in the mouth *Drug interactions:* causes flushing, weakness, light-headedness, and sweating when taken with alcohol increases the effect of oral anticoagulants (which slow clotting of the blood), increasing the tendency to bleed |

## *Antifungal Drugs*

 **SKIN/MUCOUS MEMBRANES**

### WHY YOU USE THEM

**Antifungal drugs,** also known as **antimycotic drugs,** are used to treat fungus infections such as diaper rash, oral thrush, and other infections of the skin and mucous membranes.

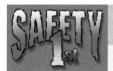 **PREVENTING CRYSTALLURIA**

Sulfonamide use can lead to the development of *crystalluria,* a condition in which crystals form in the body and are excreted in the urine. These crystals can cause kidney irritation. Patients who are taking sulfonamides should be advised to increase their fluid intake to prevent crystals from forming in the body.

## HOW THEY WORK

The antifungal medicine is administered orally or applied to the affected area. The medicine works by killing the invading fungus.

## TYPES AND EXAMPLES

| DRUG SPOTLIGHT | Antifungals | | | |
| --- | --- | --- | --- | --- |
| **Drug Name Generic (Trade)** | **Typical Form and Route of Administration** | **Indications** | **Therapeutic Action** | **Adverse Reactions and Drug Interactions** |
| fluconazole (Diflucan) | oral: tablets, suspension injection | candidal infections, such as vaginal candidiasis (yeast infections) | kills sensitive fungi by interfering with the formation of the fungal cell membrane | *Adverse reactions:* nausea headache skin rash vomiting abdominal pain diarrhea |
| miconazole (Monistat) | topical: cream, ointment, powder, spray powder, spray liquid, solution, gel vaginal: suppositories, cream | vulvovaginal candidiasis external vulvar itching and irritation associated with yeast infections fungal infections such as tinea pedis (athlete's foot), tinea cruris (jock itch), and tinea corporis (ringworm) | weakens the cell membrane of the fungus, resulting in the death of the fungus | *Adverse reactions:* headache mild vaginal burning, irritation, or itching stomach cramps |
| ketoconazole (Nizoral) | oral: tablets topical: cream, foam, gel, shampoo | systemic fungal infections such as candidiasis and oral thrush fungal infections such as tinea pedis (athlete's foot), tinea cruris (jock itch), and tinea corporis (ringworm) dandruff tinea versicolor (an infection characterized by lighter or darker patches of skin) | kills sensitive fungi by interfering with the formation of the fungal cell membrane | *Adverse reactions:* nausea or vomiting abdominal pain pruritus |

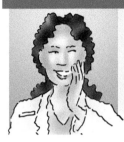

## Secrets for Success — *FUNGI*-TASTIC!

- If a drug is a *fungicide,* it destroys the fungus; *-cidus* is a Latin term for "killing."
- If a drug is *fungistatic,* it keeps the fungus from growing and multiplying; *-stasis* is a Greek term that means "halting."

## Antiviral Drugs

**WHOLE BODY**

### WHY YOU USE THEM

A viral infection is caused by the presence of a virus in the body. Viruses are responsible for a wide range of illnesses ranging from the common cold and chicken pox to the human immunodeficiency virus (HIV). Physicians prescribe a variety of **antiviral drugs** to treat infections caused by viruses.

> Drugs used to treat viral illnesses such as herpes and HIV usually have the letters *vir* or *hiv* as part of their name.

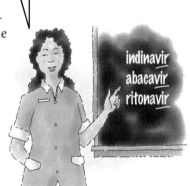

indinavir
abacavir
ritonavir

### HOW THEY WORK

Antiviral drugs block the way certain viruses reproduce. Some antivirals also help the body's immune system fight the invading virus.

### TYPES AND EXAMPLES

| DRUG SPOTLIGHT | Antivirals | | | |
| --- | --- | --- | --- | --- |
| **Drug Name Generic (Trade)** | **Typical Form and Route of Administration** | **Indications** | **Therapeutic Action** | **Adverse Reactions and Drug Interactions** |
| acyclovir (Zovirax) | oral: tablets, capsules, suspension injection | severe HSV (herpes simplex virus) type 2 infections | stops viral replication, although does not eliminate the virus | *Adverse reactions:* may cause headache, nausea, vomiting, and diarrhea (if taken orally) |

*(continued)*

**DRUG SPOTLIGHT** **Antivirals (continued)**

| Drug Name Generic (Trade) | Typical Form and Route of Administration | Indications | Therapeutic Action | Adverse Reactions and Drug Interactions |
|---|---|---|---|---|
| | topical: ointment, cream | herpes zoster infections (shingles) varicella (chicken pox) infections in patients with weakened immune systems | causes minimal damage to cells | |
| oseltamivir (Tamiflu) | oral: capsules, suspension | prevention or treatment of influenza | stops the virus from reproducing in the body | *Adverse reactions:* nausea vomiting |
| zidovudine (Retrovir) | oral: tablets, capsules, solution, syrup injection | HIV infection prevention of maternal-fetal HIV transmission | blocks the reproduction of the HIV virus | *Adverse reactions:* headache anorexia nausea vomiting fatigue |

## Topical Drugs

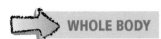 **WHOLE BODY**

### WHY YOU USE THEM

A **topical** drug is a cream or ointment used to treat mild to severe itching. The itching could be caused by an insect bite, allergic reaction, diaper rash, or other skin condition. Topicals are rubbed or applied to the skin or to mucous membranes.

### HOW THEY WORK

Once the topical drug comes into contact with the skin or other surface, the medicine is absorbed into the body. Topicals are thought to interfere with the body's inflammation response.

## TYPES AND EXAMPLES

| DRUG SPOTLIGHT | Topicals | | | |
|---|---|---|---|---|
| **Drug Name Generic (Trade)** | **Typical Form and Route of Administration** | **Indications** | **Therapeutic Action** | **Adverse Reactions and Drug Interactions** |
| hydrocortisone | topical: ointment, cream, lotion, liquid, gel, solution, spray, roll-on stick | relief of inflammation from various skin conditions relief of itching associated with minor skin irritations, inflammation, and rash due to insect bites, poison ivy, eczema, detergents, etc. | depresses the formation, release, and activity of different cells and chemicals that cause swelling, redness, and itching | *Adverse reactions:* mild, temporary stinging skin irritation or dryness |
| betamethasone valerate (Valisone) | topical: ointment, cream, lotion, foam, powder | reduces itching, redness, and swelling associated with many skin conditions | depresses the formation, release, and activity of different cells and chemicals that cause swelling, redness, and itching | *Adverse reactions:* acne cracking and stinging of the skin dryness excessive hair growth inflamed hair follicles itching skin irritation |
| 1% silver sulfadiazine (Silvadene) | topical: cream | prevents bacterial infection in second- and third-degree burns | kills bacteria by working on the cell membrane and cell wall | *Adverse reactions:* burning hives itching rash redness skin discoloration |

## *Anti-inflammatory Drugs*

 **SKIN AND MUSCULOSKELETAL SYSTEM**

### WHY YOU USE THEM

Some of the most commonly used over-the-counter (OTC) medications are **anti-inflammatory** drugs that people use to reduce inflammation or swelling and the discomfort of minor aches and pains. These drugs are often combined with aspirin or codeine for greater results.

## HOW THEY WORK

Anti-inflammatory drugs work by controlling the part of the brain that produces redness, heat, swelling, pain, and discomfort in the affected body part.

## TYPES AND EXAMPLES

### DRUG SPOTLIGHT  Anti-Inflammatory Drugs

| Drug Name Generic (Trade) | Typical Form and Route of Administration | Indications | Therapeutic Action | Adverse Reactions and Drug Interactions |
|---|---|---|---|---|
| aspirin (Bayer Aspirin, St. Joseph's Aspirin) | oral: tablets rectal: suppositories | to relieve pain to reduce fever to reduce inflammation to increase blood flow during a heart attack or to prevent one from happening | inhibits several different chemical processes within the body that cause pain, inflammation, and fever reduces the tendency for blood to clot | *Adverse reactions:* gastrointestinal (GI) bleeding tinnitus slowed clotting time Reye syndrome |
| betamethasone valerate (Valisone) | topical: ointment, cream, lotion, foam, powder | reduces itching, redness, and swelling associated with many skin conditions | depresses the formation, release, and activity of different cells and chemicals that cause swelling, redness, and itching | *Adverse reactions:* acne cracking and stinging of the skin dryness excessive hair growth inflamed hair follicles itching skin irritation |

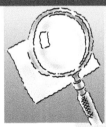

## Closer Look  WHO NOT TO TREAT WITH ASPIRIN

- *Teenagers and children.* Aspirin or salicylates should not be used to treat chicken pox or flu-like symptoms. The drugs may trigger Reye syndrome, a lethal disease of the brain and liver, in young people.
- *Pregnant women.* Aspirin is classified as pregnancy risk category D due to its potential to harm the fetus. Other salicylates pose a category C risk to pregnant patients.

- *Nursing mothers.* Salicylates can get into breast milk.
- *Asthma sufferers.* People with asthma are more likely than others to be sensitive to aspirin. It can cause breathing difficulties, urticaria, angioedema, or shock.

## Nonsteroidal Anti-Inflammatory Drugs

 **MUSCULOSKELETAL SYSTEM**

### WHY YOU USE THEM

Nonsteroidal anti-inflammatory drugs (NSAIDs) are used most commonly to treat mild to severe acute and chronic pain caused by inflammation. In some situations, inflammation causes so much stiffness that the patient can't move the inflamed body part. NSAIDs help reduce stiffness and may also reduce the pain resulting from the inflammation.

### HOW THEY WORK

When some infections occur, the body responds by causing the affected area to become inflamed. NSAIDs block the messenger molecules that make the inflammation response happen.

### TYPES AND EXAMPLES

| DRUG SPOTLIGHT | Anti-Inflammatory Drugs | | | |
|---|---|---|---|---|
| **Drug Name Generic (Trade)** | **Typical Form and Route of Administration** | **Indications** | **Therapeutic Action** | **Adverse Reactions and Drug Interactions** |
| ibuprofen (Advil, Motrin, Nuprin) | oral: tablets, capsules, suspension, drops | pain fever inflammation | exact therapeutic action is unknown; may block certain substances in the body that are linked to inflammation | *Adverse reactions:* GI bleeding |

*(continued)*

| DRUG SPOTLIGHT | Anti-Inflammatory Drugs (continued) | | | |
|---|---|---|---|---|
| **Drug Name Generic (Trade)** | **Typical Form and Route of Administration** | **Indications** | **Therapeutic Action** | **Adverse Reactions and Drug Interactions** |
| celecoxib (Celebrex) | oral: capsules | rheumatoid arthritis, osteoarthritis, ankylosing spondylitis, and juvenile arthritis menstrual pain pain | exact therapeutic action is unknown; may block certain substances in the body that are linked to inflammation | *Adverse reactions:* GI bleeding |
| naproxen (Naprosyn) | oral: tablets, suspension | rheumatoid arthritis, osteoarthritis, ankylosing spondylitis, and juvenile arthritis tendonitis, bursitis, and gout menstrual cramps mild to moderate pain | exact therapeutic action is unknown; may block certain substances in the body that are linked to inflammation | *Adverse reactions:* GI bleeding |

## *Analgesic and Antipyretic Drugs*

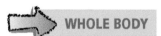 **WHOLE BODY**

### WHY YOU USE THEM

**Analgesics** are prescribed to patients for relief of mild to severe pain. Because fever is often also seen in patients suffering from pain, **antipyretics** may also be prescribed.

### HOW THEY WORK

The exact way that analgesics work is unknown. However, scientists think that analgesics probably work on the central nervous system to prevent the pain response from occurring.

## TYPES AND EXAMPLES

| DRUG SPOTLIGHT   Analgesics and Antipyretics | | | | |
|---|---|---|---|---|
| **Drug Name Generic (Trade)** | **Typical Form and Route of Administration** | **Indications** | **Therapeutic Action** | **Adverse Reactions and Drug Interactions** |
| oxycodone (Percodan, OxyContin) | oral: tablets, capsules, solution | moderate to severe pain sedation immediately before surgery | dulls the pain perception center in the brain at higher doses, may also affect other body systems (such as the respiratory and circulatory systems) | *Adverse reactions:* constipation dizziness drowsiness headache nausea sleeplessness vomiting weakness can be addictive |
| meperidine (Demerol) | oral: tablets, syrup, solution injection | to treat severe pain in acute, chronic, and terminal (fatal) illnesses | dulls the pain perception center in the brain | *Adverse reactions:* decreased rate and depth of breathing with increased dosage tremors palpitations tachycardia delirium can be addictive |

# Otic Drugs

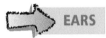 **EARS**

> When administering otic drops, make sure the solution or suspension is at body temperature. If not, the patient may experience pain and vertigo when the drops are administered.

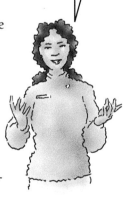

### WHY YOU USE THEM

**Otic drugs** are antibiotics used specifically to treat middle ear infections and infections of the ear canal.

### HOW THEY WORK

Because otics are antibiotics, they act by killing the bacteria that are causing the infection. It's important to know that otics are specifically used to treat ear infections only. Some otics are combined with a steroid that helps reduce the symptoms of the infection. For example, the brand-name drug Ciprodex is a combination of ciprofloxacin (an antibiotic) and dexamethasone (a steroid).

## TYPES AND EXAMPLES

| DRUG SPOTLIGHT | Otics | | | |
|---|---|---|---|---|
| **Drug Name Generic (Trade)** | **Typical Form and Route of Administration** | **Indications** | **Therapeutic Action** | **Adverse Reactions and Drug Interactions** |
| ciprofloxacin and dexamethasone (Ciprodex) | otic: suspension | ear infections caused by certain bacteria | kills bacteria by stopping the production of essential proteins needed by the bacteria to survive | *Adverse reactions:* discomfort, pain, or itching in the ear |
| ofloxacin (Floxin Otic) | otic: solution | outer ear infections some middle ear infections | kills bacteria | *Adverse reactions:* itching of the ear taste changes |

## *Ophthalmic Drugs*

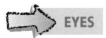 EYES

### WHY YOU USE THEM

**Ophthalmic drugs** are used to treat bacterial infections of the eye only. It's important to note that ophthalmics should **never** be used to treat fungal or viral infections.

### HOW THEY WORK

Like otics, ophthalmics are also a combination of one or more antibiotics and a steroid. The antibiotic weakens or kills the bacteria causing the infection, and the steroid reduces the symptoms that result from the infection.

### TYPES AND EXAMPLES

| DRUG SPOTLIGHT | Ophthalmics | | | |
|---|---|---|---|---|
| **Drug Name Generic (Trade)** | **Typical Form and Route of Administration** | **Indications** | **Therapeutic Action** | **Adverse Reactions and Drug Interactions** |
| polymyxin B, neomycin, and hydrocortisone (Cortisporin Ophthalmic) | ophthalmic: suspension | eye infections and associated symptoms, including redness, | slow the growth of, or kill, the infection-causing bacteria in the eye | *Adverse reactions:* burning or stinging when the medication is first put into the eye dry, flaky skin |

| Drug Name Generic (Trade) | Typical Form and Route of Administration | Indications | Therapeutic Action | Adverse Reactions and Drug Interactions |
|---|---|---|---|---|
| | | irritation, and discomfort | (polymyxin B and neomycin) reduces inflammation (hydrocortisone) | irritation itching redness swelling |
| chloramphenicol (Chloromycetin Ophthalmic) | ophthalmic: solution, ointment | serious bacterial infections for which less potentially dangerous drugs are ineffective or contraindicated | kills or slows the growth of certain bacteria | *Adverse reactions:* temporary burning or stinging sensations severe blood problems (such as anemia, low blood platelets, and low white blood cell count) |

# Muscle Relaxant Drugs

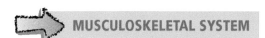 **MUSCULOSKELETAL SYSTEM**

### WHY YOU USE THEM

**Muscle relaxants** are used to relax certain muscles in the body. Physicians prescribe these drugs to treat a variety of conditions that range from stiffness to muscle spasms. A spasm is an involuntary muscle contraction. Muscle spasms are sometimes called reflex contractions because they happen automatically in response to an outside stimulus. For example, any of these three conditions can cause a muscle spasm:

- exposure to severe cold
- lack of blood flow to the muscle
- overexertion

When the body senses what's happening, nerves in the affected part send a signal to the spinal cord and the central nervous system (CNS), which causes a muscle contraction to occur. The first muscle contraction can stimulate the muscle to contract again and again, setting up a cycle of contractions.

Muscle relaxants are also used to treat spasticity (stiff, awkward movements) associated with stroke, cerebral palsy, and multiple sclerosis.

## HOW THEY WORK

Muscle relaxant drugs that act on the CNS are believed to break the cycle of muscle contractions by depressing the CNS. Centrally acting skeletal muscle relaxants act on the central nervous system, whereas direct-acting skeletal muscle relaxants act directly on skeletal muscles. The drugs that act directly on skeletal muscles cause fewer adverse reactions than those that act on the central nervous system.

> Patients taking centrally acting muscle relaxants need to know that they might not want to drive, climb ladders, or sign important contracts, because these medications affect the brain!

## TYPES AND EXAMPLES

| DRUG SPOTLIGHT | Muscle Relaxants | | | |
| --- | --- | --- | --- | --- |
| **Drug Name Generic (Trade)** | **Typical Form and Route of Administration** | **Indications** | **Therapeutic Action** | **Adverse Reactions and Drug Interactions** |
| cyclobenzaprine hydrochloride (Flexeril) | oral: capsules, tablets | acute (brief and severe) muscle spasm | works in parts of the brain and central nervous system to help reduce muscle spasms | *Adverse reactions:* urinary retention dizziness drowsiness ataxia mental sluggishness |
| orphenadrine citrate (Norflex) | oral: tablets injection | short-term painful musculoskeletal conditions | exact therapeutic action is unknown, but may be related to the drug's analgesic properties also possesses anticholinergic actions | *Adverse reactions:* agitation blurred vision constipation dizziness or light-headedness drowsiness dry mouth headache enlarged pupils nausea stomach irritation or upset vomiting weakness |

## *Antihypertensive Drugs*

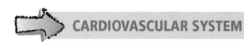 **CARDIOVASCULAR SYSTEM**

### WHY YOU USE THEM

**Antihypertensive drugs** reduce blood pressure and are therefore used to treat **hypertension** (high blood pressure). Hypertension affects approximately one in three Americans and causes stroke, heart attack, and heart failure if left untreated.

### HOW THEY WORK

There are numerous drugs for treating hypertension, including:

- diuretics
- vasodilating drugs
- adrenergic blocking drugs
- antiadrenergic blocking drugs
- calcium channel blocking drugs
- angiotensin-converting enzyme (ACE) inhibitors
- angiotensin II receptor antagonists

Although these drugs work in different ways, the goal—to reduce blood pressure—is the same. Often, combinations of two drugs from different classes are used to improve the drugs' effectiveness. In addition, treatment with antihypertensive drugs is often combined with diet and exercise.

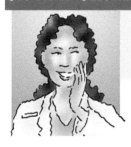

**Secrets for Success** **TOO MUCH OR TOO LITTLE?**

Remember that the word part *hyper-* tells you there's too much of something. The word part *hypo-* tells you there is too little of it.

## TYPES AND EXAMPLES

**DRUG SPOTLIGHT** Antihypertensive Drugs

| Drug Name Generic (Trade) | Typical Form and Route of Administration | Indications | Therapeutic Action | Adverse Reactions and Drug Interactions |
|---|---|---|---|---|
| metoprolol (Lopressor) | oral: tablets injection | hypertension angina myocardial infarction | reduces the amount of work the heart has to do (reduces chest pain) and the amount of blood the heart pumps out (lowers high blood pressure) | *Adverse reactions:* blurred vision cold hands and feet confusion constipation depression diarrhea dizziness dry mouth or eyes gas hair loss headache heartburn itching light-headedness mild drowsiness muscle aches nausea nightmares ringing in the ears short-term memory loss sleeplessness stomach pain unusual tiredness or weakness |
| carvedilol (Coreg) | oral: tablets | hypertension certain types of heart failure | decreases blood pressure by relaxing the blood vessels, slowing the heart rate, and decreasing the amount of blood pumped out by the heart | *Adverse reactions:* diarrhea dizziness dry eyes headache fatigue light-headedness nausea numbness or tingling of the hands or feet weakness vomiting |

Patients should be aware that suddenly stopping metoprolol or carvedilol can trigger angina, hypertension, arrhythmias, or heart attack.

# Calcium Channel Blocker Drugs

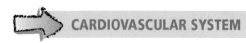
**CARDIOVASCULAR SYSTEM**

### WHY YOU USE THEM

**Calcium channel blockers** may be prescribed for patients who suffer from both hypertension and chronic stable angina (chest pain). The tightness associated with angina is the result of the heart not getting enough oxygen. The coronary arteries supply oxygen to the heart muscle. But if these arteries are constricted, the heart is "starved" of oxygen and tries to work harder. This increases blood pressure.

### HOW THEY WORK

Calcium is needed for muscles to contract. In patients with hypertension and angina, the coronary arteries and the heart muscle work harder by contracting more. Calcium channel blockers block calcium from reaching the muscle and prevent the smooth muscle walls of the arteries from contracting as much. This helps keep coronary arteries open, which, in turn, decreases the burden on the heart.

### TYPES AND EXAMPLES

| DRUG SPOTLIGHT | Calcium Channel Blockers | | | |
| --- | --- | --- | --- | --- |
| **Drug Name Generic (Trade)** | **Typical Form and Route of Administration** | **Indications** | **Therapeutic Action** | **Adverse Reactions and Drug Interactions** |
| amlodipine besylate (Norvasc) | oral: tablets | angina hypertension | • relaxes (dilates) blood vessels, lowers blood pressure, and decreases the heart rate<br>• dilates coronary arteries, increasing blood flow to the heart | *Adverse reactions:* edema headache |

*(continued)*

| **DRUG SPOTLIGHT** | **Calcium Channel Blockers (continued)** | | | |
|---|---|---|---|---|
| **Drug Name Generic (Trade)** | **Typical Form and Route of Administration** | **Indications** | **Therapeutic Action** | **Adverse Reactions and Drug Interactions** |
| diltiazem hydrochloride (Cardizem) | oral: tablets, capsules injection | angina hypertension supraventricular tachycardia atrial fibrillation and flutter | • relaxes (dilates) blood vessels, lowers blood pressure, and decreases the heart rate<br>• dilates coronary arteries, increasing blood flow to the heart<br>• slows electrical conduction in the heart, which slows heart rate and/or normalizes heart rhythm | *Adverse reactions:*<br>edema<br>dizziness<br>flushing<br>headache<br>asthenia<br>first-degree AV block<br>bradycardia<br>nausea<br>rash |

## *Vasodilating Drugs*

 **CARDIOVASCULAR SYSTEM**

### WHY YOU USE THEM

**Vasodilating drugs** are commonly prescribed to patients with hypertension. Hypertension is an indicator that the heart is working harder than it should. When veins or arteries become constricted, they have to contract harder to move the blood through the body. This causes blood pressure to go up, which is hypertension. When coronary arteries become constricted, they also have to contract harder to supply blood to the heart muscle.

### HOW THEY WORK

Vasodilators relax the muscles in veins and arteries, which allows them to open wider, or dilate. This lowers blood pressure because there is more room in the blood vessels for the blood to move through.

## TYPES AND EXAMPLES

**DRUG SPOTLIGHT**    Vasodilators

| Drug Name Generic (Trade) | Typical Form and Route of Administration | Indications | Therapeutic Action | Adverse Reactions and Drug Interactions |
|---|---|---|---|---|
| nitroglycerin (Nitro-Bid, Nitrostat) | oral: capsules sublingual: tablets lingual: aerosol spray injection topical: ointment transdermal: patch | chronic angina (preventative) acute angina perioperative hypertension | relaxes blood vessels, allowing them to dilate more blood flows through blood vessels more easily, which reduces the workload on the heart | *Adverse reactions:* headache hypotension increased heart rate and dizziness |
| clonidine hydrochloride (Catapres) | oral: tablets transdermal: mineral oil | hypertension | relaxes blood vessels and decreases heart rate, which lowers blood pressure | *Adverse reactions:* dry mouth drowsiness sedation dizziness constipation |

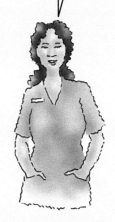

Remind patients to dispose of nitrate patches and creams safely so that children and pets won't be exposed to the drug.

## Antiarrhythmic Drugs

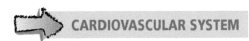 **CARDIOVASCULAR SYSTEM**

### WHY YOU USE THEM

For some patients, the heart beats too fast, too slowly, or irregularly. An arrhythmia can be life threatening or simply an annoyance. Medicines that are prescribed to treat arrhythmias are called **antiarrhythmic drugs.** These drugs must be used cautiously because they can cause or worsen the arrhythmias they're supposed to cure.

### HOW THEY WORK

There are four different classes of antiarrhythmics. The medication prescribed is determined by which area of the heart is being affected by the arrhythmia. The most commonly prescribed antiarrhythmics are propranolol hydrochloride (Inderal) and digoxin (Lanoxin). These drugs work by slowing the heart rate, which allows the heart to pump more efficiently.

### TYPES AND EXAMPLES

| DRUG SPOTLIGHT | Antiarrhythmics | | | |
| --- | --- | --- | --- | --- |
| **Drug Name Generic (Trade)** | **Typical Form and Route of Administration** | **Indications** | **Therapeutic Action** | **Adverse Reactions and Drug Interactions** |
| propranolol hydrochloride (Inderal) | oral: tablets, capsules, solution injection | hypertension angina myocardial infarction arrhythmias migraine headaches tumors | slows down the heart and decreases the amount of blood it pumps out, which decreases blood pressure and helps the heart pump more efficiently | *Adverse reactions:* arrhythmias bradycardia heart failure hypotension nausea vomiting diarrhea bronchoconstriction |
| digoxin (Lanoxin) | oral: tablets, capsules, elixir injection | congestive heart failure (CHF) arrhythmias, such as atrial fibrillation and atrial flutter | increases the force of contraction of the heart and slows the heart rate | Regular monthly blood level should be drawn and patients should be monitored for the signs and symptoms of toxicity, including: |

| DRUG SPOTLIGHT | Antiarrhythmics (continued) | | | |
|---|---|---|---|---|
| Drug Name Generic (Trade) | Typical Form and Route of Administration | Indications | Therapeutic Action | Adverse Reactions and Drug Interactions |
| | | | | nausea abdominal pain vomiting diarrhea headache irritability depression insomnia confusion vision changes arrhythmias complete heart block |

## Antilipemic Drugs

 **CARDIOVASCULAR SYSTEM**

### WHY YOU USE THEM

A rich diet puts many Americans at risk of developing high levels of fatty substances called **lipids**—cholesterol, triglycerides, and phospholipids—in their blood. High serum lipid levels increase a person's chances of developing coronary artery disease.

Lifestyle changes, such as proper diet, exercise, weight loss, and treatment of any underlying disorders, can bring lipid levels under control. When these changes do not have enough of an effect, physicians prescribe **antilipemic drugs** as the next step.

### HOW THEY WORK

Antilipemic drug choices today are often **cholesterol synthesis inhibitors,** which lower lipid levels by slowing the liver's production of cholesterol. These drugs are sometimes called *statins* because their generic names end in the letters *statin.*

## TYPES AND EXAMPLES

**DRUG SPOTLIGHT    Antilipemics**

| Drug Name Generic (Trade) | Typical Form and Route of Administration | Indications | Therapeutic Action | Adverse Reactions and Drug Interactions |
|---|---|---|---|---|
| atorvastatin (Lipitor) | oral: tablets | reduces cholesterol and other fatty substances in the blood slows the production of cholesterol decreases the risk of heart disease, angina, stroke, and myocardial infarction | reduces the production of certain fatty substances in the body, including cholesterol | *Adverse reactions:* diarrhea, gas, bloating muscle pain flu-like symptoms |
| simvastatin (Zocor) | oral: tablets | hypercholesterolemia in adolescents hyperlipidemia decreases the risk of stroke and myocardial infarction | reduces the production of certain fatty substances in the body, including cholesterol | *Adverse reactions:* constipation |

## Anticoagulant Drugs

 **CARDIOVASCULAR SYSTEM**

### WHY YOU USE THEM

**Anticoagulants**—sometimes called "blood thinners"—help reduce the risk of blood clots. Heparin and warfarin sodium are two of the most common anticoagulants prescribed for patients.

### HOW THEY WORK

Heparin slows the time blood takes to clot. It comes in a variety of dosages and must be checked closely before administration. In fact, before administering heparin, the dose should *always* be double-checked by another health care professional. Warfarin works by inhibiting the synthesis of certain factors in the blood clotting process.

> Tell patients who are taking oral anticoagulants to notify the physician immediately if they notice any signs of bleeding or bruising.

## TYPES AND EXAMPLES

**DRUG SPOTLIGHT**    **Anticoagulants**

| | | Anticoagulants | | |
|---|---|---|---|---|
| **Drug Name Generic (Trade)** | **Typical Form and Route of Administration** | **Indications** | **Therapeutic Action** | **Adverse Reactions and Drug Interactions** |
| heparin (Caliparine) | injection | preventing or treating blood clots in the veins or arteries preventing clots from forming in patients with atrial fibrillation (a condition that causes blood to pool in the atria, the two upper chambers of the heart) preventing more clots from forming in patients who have suffered a heart attack preventing clotting during orthopedic surgery | prevents or slows blood clot formation in the veins, arteries, or heart | *Adverse reactions:* bleeding *Drug interactions:* Warn patients who smoke that nicotine may inactivate heparin. Tell heart patients who might be taking nitroglycerin (a drug used to treat angina) that it may reduce the effects of heparin. Tell patients who are taking oral anticoagulants to notify the physician immediately if they notice any signs of bleeding or bruising. Heparin increases the effects of oral anticoagulants, such as warfarin sodium. |
| warfarin sodium (Coumadin) | oral: tablets injection | to prevent clots deep in the veins to treat patients with artificial or diseased heart valves to prevent thromboemboli to prevent clot formation in patients with atrial fibrillation | blocks the formation of certain blood clotting factors | *Adverse reactions:* • bruising • nosebleeds • GI bleeds • possible excessive bleeding with shaving, brushing teeth, dental surgery, etc. |

# Antitubercular Drugs

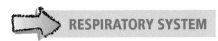 **RESPIRATORY SYSTEM**

### WHY YOU USE THEM

Tuberculosis, or TB, is a chronic and deadly infectious disease that affects the lungs. It may also affect the central nervous system and other parts of the body. It is caused by an organism called *Mycobacterium tuberculosis*. Although it's no longer common in the United States, TB is still a leading cause of death for young adults worldwide. **Antitubercular drugs** can't always cure the disease, but they may halt its progress.

> Drugs used to treat tuberculosis are very powerful and must be monitored by a physician. Blood dyscrasias, liver toxicity, kidney failure, and pancreatitis are common side effects.

### HOW THEY WORK

Because many drug-resistant strains of TB exist, physicians now use a four-drug "cocktail" to treat it.

- isoniazid (Nydrazid)
- rifampin (Rifadin, Rimactane)
- pyrazinamide (Tebrazid, Zinamide)
- ethambutol (Myambutol)

These drugs work by killing or stopping the growth of TB bacteria. Isoniazid is the most important drug for treating TB. People who have been exposed to TB, but who are not actively ill, can be treated with isoniazid without concern that the TB bacteria will become resistant. People with active TB, however, may need combinations of drugs such as isoniazid and rifampin for long periods of time. If the bacteria become resistant, different drug combinations may be necessary.

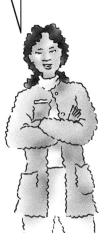

### TYPES AND EXAMPLES

| DRUG SPOTLIGHT | Antituberculars | | | |
|---|---|---|---|---|
| **Drug Name Generic (Trade)** | **Typical Form and Route of Administration** | **Indications** | **Therapeutic Action** | **Adverse Reactions and Drug Interactions** |
| isoniazid (Nydrazid) | oral: tablets, syrup injection | tuberculosis | kills the bacteria that cause tuberculosis | *Adverse reactions:* peripheral neuropathy mild hepatic dysfunction |

| DRUG SPOTLIGHT | Antituberculars (continued) | | | |
|---|---|---|---|---|
| **Drug Name**<br>**Generic (Trade)** | **Typical Form**<br>**and Route of**<br>**Administration** | **Indications** | **Therapeutic**<br>**Action** | **Adverse Reactions**<br>**and Drug Interactions** |
| rifampin (Rifadin) | oral: capsules<br>injection | tuberculosis | kills or stops the<br>growth of<br>tuberculosis<br>bacteria | *Adverse reactions:*<br>• cramps<br>• diarrhea<br>• dizziness<br>• drowsiness<br>• gas<br>• headache<br>• heartburn<br>• joint pain<br>• anorexia<br>• menstrual changes<br>• nausea<br>• stomach pain or bloating<br>• vomiting |

## *Bronchodilator Drugs*

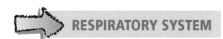 **RESPIRATORY SYSTEM**

### WHY YOU USE THEM

The job of **bronchodilators** is to improve bronchial airflow into and out of the lungs. These drugs are prescribed for various forms of asthma.

### HOW THEY WORK

Bronchodilators work by relaxing the bands of muscles that tighten up around airways. Once these breathing passages are open, air flows more smoothly into and out of the lungs. Bronchodilators also help clear mucus from the lungs.

Depending on the patient's needs, there are:

- *Fast-acting inhalers.* These medications relieve symptoms quickly, often within 20 minutes. Many asthma sufferers use them as "rescue" medications for sudden attacks. They also use these inhalers 15 or 20 minutes before exercising to prevent asthma attacks that can be triggered by exercise.

- *Long-acting bronchodilators.* These medications control asthma but do not provide quick relief. However, their effects last as long as 12 hours.

## TYPES AND EXAMPLES

**DRUG SPOTLIGHT** **Bronchodilators**

| Drug Name Generic (Trade) | Typical Form and Route of Administration | Indications | Therapeutic Action | Adverse Reactions and Drug Interactions |
|---|---|---|---|---|
| albuterol (Proventil, Ventolin) | oral: tablets, syrup inhalation: aerosol, solution | prevents and treats bronchospasm caused by asthma prevents exercise-induced asthma | fast acting relaxes the smooth muscle in the airway, which allows air to flow in and out of the lungs more easily | *Adverse reactions:* palpitations tachycardia hypertension tremor dizziness shakiness nervousness nausea vomiting |
| theophylline (Theo-Dur, Slo-Bid) | oral: tablets, capsules, elixir injection | asthma chronic bronchitis emphysema | long acting relaxes the smooth muscle in the bronchial tubes of the lungs, allowing the tubes to widen, making breathing easier improves contraction of the diaphragm | *Adverse reactions:* nausea vomiting abdominal cramping epigastric pain anorexia diarrhea headache irritability restlessness insomnia dizziness tachycardia palpitations arrhythmias |
| fluticasone propionate and salmeterol (Advair) | inhalation: powder, aerosol spray | chronic asthma chronic obstructive pulmonary disease (COPD) associated with chronic bronchitis | long acting improves lung function and makes breathing easier by reducing airway swelling and irritation and by causing muscle relaxation | *Adverse reactions:* headache dizziness menstrual changes nausea nervousness throat irritation tremor vomiting |

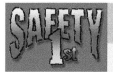

## OXYGEN SAFETY

Patients with reduced lung function (for example, those with emphysema) may have trouble getting the oxygen their bodies need from inhaled air alone, which only contains about 20 percent oxygen. For these patients, the physician may prescribe supplemental (extra) oxygen, which is pure, 100% oxygen.

Supplemental oxygen can be given continuously, such as in a hospital setting, or it can be given on an as-needed basis. For example, some patients may need supplemental oxygen only when they are physically active. These patients may receive oxygen from a pressurized tank, which can be small enough to be wheeled around with the person, or from an oxygen concentrator that can be used at home. Oxygen concentrators are devices that take in air and filter out nitrogen, leaving behind pure oxygen. The oxygen is then delivered to the patient at a rate that has been programmed into the unit.

Regardless of the method by which patients receive supplemental oxygen, they should be aware of several safety tips.

- Do not light matches or cigarette lighters when oxygen is in use. Remember that the better the air supply, the better a fire will burn.

- Do not smoke when oxygen is in use. The use of oxygen therapy can increase the oxygen content of clothing and any other fabrics in the immediate area. If burning ashes from a cigarette should fall on the patient's clothing, a fire would be more likely to start and would burn much faster as a result of the added oxygen.

- Make sure any electrical equipment, such as electric razors, are in good working order, and that cords are not frayed. A patient who is receiving supplemental oxygen should use a battery-operated razor or a blade razor when shaving. Electrical equipment that is not properly maintained can be the source of a spark, which could start a fire.

## *Antitussive, Mucolytic, and Expectorant Drugs*

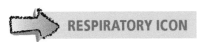 **RESPIRATORY ICON**

### WHY YOU USE THEM

Respiratory infections are often accompanied by a cough. But not all coughs are alike. **Antitussives, mucolytics,** and **expectorants** are medicines that treat specific types of cough in different ways.

### HOW THEY WORK

Antitussives control or suppress coughing. The physician might prescribe this type of medicine to treat a dry, unproductive cough. It's the kind of cough that brings up no sputum from the lungs or breathing passages. Antitussives work either by coating the throat or by acting on the cough center in the brain.

Mucolytics act directly on mucus. They break down sticky, thick secretions of mucus so that they can be eliminated more easily.

Expectorants make mucus thinner so clearing the airways is easier. These drugs also soothe the mucous membranes in the respiratory tract.

### TYPES AND EXAMPLES

| DRUG SPOTLIGHT | Antitussives, Mucolytics, and Expectorants | | | |
|---|---|---|---|---|
| **Drug Name Generic (Trade)** | **Typical Form and Route of Administration** | **Indications** | **Therapeutic Action** | **Adverse Reactions and Drug Interactions** |
| **Narcotic Drugs** | | | | |
| hydrocodone polistirex and chlorphenira-mine polistirex (Tussionex) | oral: syrup | relief of cough and rhinorrhea provides symptomatic relief of cough and runny nose caused by cold or allergy | suppresses cough reflex; stimulates opiate receptors in the CNS and blocks pain impulse generation (hydrocodone) blocks histamine by competing for histamine receptor sites in the CNS (chlorpheniramine) | *Adverse reactions:* drowsiness nausea |

| DRUG SPOTLIGHT | Antitussives, Mucolytics, and Expectorants (continued) | | | |
|---|---|---|---|---|
| **Drug Name Generic (Trade)** | **Typical Form and Route of Administration** | **Indications** | **Therapeutic Action** | **Adverse Reactions and Drug Interactions** |
| **Non-narcotic Drugs** | | | | |
| dextromethorphan (Benylin DM) | oral: capsules, lozenges, disintegrating strips, liquid, syrup, suspension, solution, freezer pops | dry, unproductive cough | acts on the cough center in the brain to suppress coughing loosens mucus and lung secretions in the chest, making coughs more productive | *Adverse reactions:* drowsiness dizziness nausea vomiting stomach pain |
| guaifenesin (Humibid) | oral: tablets, granules, syrup, liquid | cough | thins mucus in the lungs, making it easier to cough up reduces chest congestion by making coughs more productive | Adverse reactions are rare. |

# Decongestant Drugs

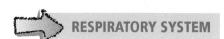 **RESPIRATORY SYSTEM**

### WHY YOU USE THEM

**Decongestants** are used to relieve symptoms of swollen nasal membranes caused by:

- hay fever
- the common cold
- allergic rhinitis (runny nose, sneezing, and congestion caused by allergens)
- vasomotor rhinitis (runny nose, sneezing, and congestion from other causes)
- acute coryza (profuse discharge from the nose)
- sinusitis (inflammation of the sinuses)

## HOW THEY WORK

Decongestants can be classified as *topical* or *systemic*, depending on how they're administered. Topical decongestants are sprayed directly onto the swollen lining of the nose to relieve symptoms. These drugs often come in the form of nasal sprays. Systemic decongestants, however, stimulate the sympathetic nervous system. These powerful drugs reduce swelling in the network of blood vessels in the respiratory tract.

## TYPES AND EXAMPLES

**DRUG SPOTLIGHT** **Decongestants**

| Drug Name Generic (Trade) | Typical Form and Route of Administration | Indications | Therapeutic Action | Adverse Reactions and Drug Interactions |
|---|---|---|---|---|
| pseudoephedrine (Sudafed) | oral: tablets, capsules, liquid, syrup, drops, suspension | nasal congestion | reduces swelling and constricts blood vessels in the nasal passages, making breathing easier | *Adverse reactions:* nervousness restlessness insomnia nausea palpitations difficulty urinating elevations in blood pressure |
| phenylephrine hydrochloride (Neo-Synephrine) | oral: tablets, liquid, solution, strip intranasal: solution | nasal congestion | shrinks swollen and congested nasal tissues by constricting blood vessels | *Adverse reactions:* nervousness insomnia restlessness headache nausea giddiness gastric irritation hypersensitivity reactions |

Because of the potential for misuse, federal law now dictates that patients must request a decongestant that contains pseudoephedrine from the pharmacist.

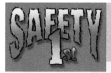

## CONTROLLED SALES OF PSEUDOEPHEDRINE

The good side of products that contain pseudoephedrine is the relief they bring many patients. The bad side is that these drugs are also used to manufacture methamphetamine, or "meth," a highly addictive street drug.

Federal and state laws now control the sale of decongestants that contain pseudoephedrine. Access is restricted. These medications are now sold "behind the counter" or from a locked cabinet rather than from open shelves. Quantities are limited, and the pharmacist must obtain proof of identify from the buyer.

State and local laws may be stricter than federal laws. Be sure you know how these products are sold in your community, and remind patients about these restrictions.

## Antihistamine Drugs

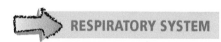 **RESPIRATORY SYSTEM**

### WHY YOU USE THEM

An allergic response to something causes your nose and throat to swell and produce mucus. You end up with an itchy, sneezy, runny nose, among other symptoms. The chemical responsible for these symptoms is histamine. Many patients use **antihistamines** for relief from these symptoms.

### HOW THEY WORK

Antihistamines work by blocking the action of histamines. These drugs can also reduce the nausea and vomiting brought on by motion sickness.

## TYPES AND EXAMPLES

| DRUG SPOTLIGHT | Antihistamines | | | |
| --- | --- | --- | --- | --- |
| **Drug Name Generic (Trade)** | **Typical Form and Route of Administration** | **Indications** | **Therapeutic Action** | **Adverse Reactions and Drug Interactions** |
| fexofenadine hydrochloride (Allegra) | oral: tablets, suspension | seasonal allergic rhinitis chronic idiopathic urticaria | blocks histamine in the body, which helps decrease allergy symptoms | *Adverse reactions:* headache dizziness stomach upset |
| cetirizine hydrochloride (Zyrtec) | oral: tablets, solution | urticaria allergies and hay fever | blocks the actions of histamine and reduces the symptoms of an allergic reaction | *Adverse reactions:* drowsiness dry mouth stomach pain (in children) insomnia (in children) |

## Antacid Drugs

 **GASTROINTESTINAL SYSTEM**

> It's important to note that antacids can interfere with the absorption of other orally administered drugs. Make sure the physician knows what other medications the patient is taking.

### WHY YOU USE THEM

**Antacids** are OTC medications. They are used alone or with other drugs to treat heartburn, acid reflux, and peptic or duodenal ulcers.

### HOW THEY WORK

Some of the cells in the stomach secrete hydrochloric acid, a substance that aids in the initial digestive process. Antacids neutralize or reduce the acidity of stomach and duodenal contents by combining with hydrochloric acid and producing salt and water.

### TYPES AND EXAMPLES

| DRUG SPOTLIGHT | Antacids | | | |
| --- | --- | --- | --- | --- |
| **Drug Name Generic (Trade)** | **Typical Form and Route of Administration** | **Indications** | **Therapeutic Action** | **Adverse Reactions and Drug Interactions** |
| ranitidine hydrochloride (Zantac) | oral: tablets, capsules, solution injection | duodenal and gastric ulcers gastro-esophageal reflux disease (GERD) heartburn | blocks histamine from entering stomach cells, which reduces stomach acid production | Adverse reactions are uncommon, but may include: vertigo malaise headache |

| DRUG SPOTLIGHT | Antacids (continued) | | | |
|---|---|---|---|---|
| **Drug Name Generic (Trade)** | **Typical Form and Route of Administration** | **Indications** | **Therapeutic Action** | **Adverse Reactions and Drug Interactions** |
| | | | | blurred vision jaundice burning and itching at injection site (if administered by injection) anaphylaxis angioedema |
| sucralfate (Carafate) | oral: tablets, suspension | duodenal ulcers | forms a protective layer on the ulcer to serve as a barrier against acid, bile salts, and enzymes in the stomach | *Adverse reactions:* constipation |

## *Antiemetic Drugs*

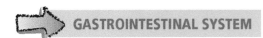

### GASTROINTESTINAL SYSTEM

### WHY YOU USE THEM

Many patients with gastrointestinal distress try a variety of OTC preparations before they seek treatment from their physicians. One of the most popular class of drugs used for gastrointestinal distress is the **antiemetics**. Antiemetics decrease nausea and reduce the urge to vomit.

### HOW THEY WORK

Most antiemetics work in the brain stem to reduce the urge to vomit and to decrease nausea. The antiemetic ondansetron is often prescribed to cancer patients to counteract the nausea that occurs as the result of chemotherapy or radiation therapy.

## TYPES AND EXAMPLES

**DRUG SPOTLIGHT** **Antiemetics**

| Drug Name Generic (Trade) | Typical Form and Route of Administration | Indications | Therapeutic Action | Adverse Reactions and Drug Interactions |
|---|---|---|---|---|
| ondansetron hydrochloride (Zofran) | oral: tablets, solution injection | nausea and vomiting caused by cancer chemotherapy, radiation therapy, and surgery | blocks the action of serotonin, a natural substance that may cause nausea and vomiting | *Adverse reactions:* confusion anxiety euphoria agitation depression headache insomnia restlessness weakness |
| prochlorperazine (Compazine) | oral: tablets, spansules, syrup injection rectal: suppositories | severe nausea and vomiting | blocks dopamine in the brain | *Adverse reactions:* blurred vision chills constipation dizziness drowsiness dry mouth jitteriness nasal congestion insomnia |
| meclizene (Antivert) | oral: tablets, capsules | nausea, vomiting, or dizziness associated with motion sickness | blocks a chemical messenger in the brain, which helps to reduce or prevent vomiting | *Adverse reactions:* drowsiness dry mouth |

## *Anticholinergic Drugs*

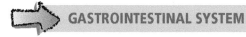 **GASTROINTESTINAL SYSTEM**

### WHY YOU USE THEM

For patients who suffer from peptic ulcers, the activity of stomach muscles contributes to the increased production of stomach acid. For relief of the symptoms associated with peptic ulcers, patients may be prescribed an anticholinergic.

## HOW THEY WORK

**Anticholinergics** work directly in the nervous system to inhibit the action of the neurotransmitter acetylcholine. Anticholinergics work to decrease muscular activity in the stomach and also lower the production of stomach acid.

## TYPES AND EXAMPLES

| DRUG SPOTLIGHT | Anticholinergics | | | |
|---|---|---|---|---|
| **Drug Name Generic (Trade)** | **Typical Form and Route of Administration** | **Indications** | **Therapeutic Action** | **Adverse Reactions and Drug Interactions** |
| methartheline bromide (Pro-Banthine) | oral: tablets | peptic ulcers | • decreases the motion of muscles in the stomach, intestines, and bladder<br>• decreases acid production in the stomach | *Adverse reactions:* bloated feeling<br>blurred vision<br>clumsiness<br>constipation<br>dry mouth<br>decreased sweating<br>dizziness<br>drowsiness<br>enlarged pupils<br>excitement<br>headache<br>nausea<br>nervousness<br>insomnia |

## *Antispasmodic Drugs*

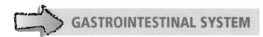 **GASTROINTESTINAL SYSTEM**

### WHY YOU USE THEM

Patients who have irritable bowel syndrome or other bowel disorders experience great discomfort. When the bowel becomes irritated, the smooth muscle walls can sometimes go into spasms. To counteract this effect, **antispasmodics** are prescribed.

### HOW THEY WORK

Antispasmodics slow down or stop smooth muscle contractions of the intestines. They do this by inhibiting the action of acetylcholine in the nervous system and by acting directly on smooth muscle to decrease contractions.

## TYPES AND EXAMPLES

| DRUG SPOTLIGHT | Antispasmodics | | | |
| --- | --- | --- | --- | --- |
| **Drug Name Generic (Trade)** | **Typical Form and Route of Administration** | **Indications** | **Therapeutic Action** | **Adverse Reactions and Drug Interactions** |
| dicylomine hydrochloride (Bentyl) | oral: capsules, tablets, syrup injection | irritable bowel syndrome | blocks a chemical in the smooth muscle of the stomach and intestines, causing them to relax, which reduces cramping | *Adverse reactions:* blurred vision constipation decreased sweating insomnia dizziness drowsiness dry mouth headache light-headedness loss of taste nausea nervousness |
| atropine, scopolamine, hyoscyamine, and phenobarbital (Donnatal) | oral: tablets, elixir | irritable bowel syndrome colitis | decreases the motion of the muscles of the stomach and intestine provides mild sedation | *Adverse reactions:* bloated feeling blurred vision clumsiness constipation decreased sweating dizziness drowsiness dry mouth excessive daytime drowsiness headache light-headedness nausea nervousness insomnia |

## *Antidiarrheal Drugs*

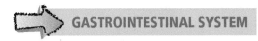 GASTROINTESTINAL SYSTEM

### WHY YOU USE THEM

Diarrhea and constipation are the two major symptoms of disturbances of the large intestine. **Antidiarrheals** are used to treat these conditions.

## HOW THEY WORK

Antidiarrheals slow down peristalsis. These drugs also decrease the contractions throughout the colon that expel the waste matter.

## TYPES AND EXAMPLES

| DRUG SPOTLIGHT | Antidiarrheals | | | |
|---|---|---|---|---|
| **Drug Name Generic (Trade)** | **Typical Form and Route of Administration** | **Indications** | **Therapeutic Action** | **Adverse Reactions and Drug Interactions** |
| diphenoxylate hydrochloride and atropine sulfate (Lomotil) | oral: tablets, liquid | acute, nonspecific diarrhea | decreases the motion of muscles in the intestine increases the time needed for food to move through the GI tract | *Adverse reactions:* drowsiness constipation lethargy confusion CNS depression paralytic ileus |
| loperamide hydrochloride (Imodium) | oral: tablets, capsules, liquid | acute, nonspecific diarrhea chronic diarrhea traveler's diarrhea | slows the movement of bowel contents | Loperamide may cause symptoms of the underlying diarrheal syndrome, including: abdominal pain/ discomfort nausea vomiting dry mouth fatigue drowsiness dizziness constipation flatulence |

# *Laxatives*

 **GASTROINTESTINAL SYSTEM**

## WHY YOU USE THEM

**Laxatives** are the opposite of the antidiarrheal drugs. They increase the urge to defecate. Laxatives are a multimillion-dollar business in the United States. Many people could benefit from increasing their fiber, fluid, and water intake to avoid constipation. No laxative—including the old standby, prune juice—should be taken longer than 1 week without a physician's advice.

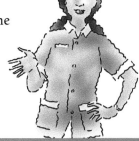

One important thing to remember about all laxatives: they have the potential for abuse, particularly by patients with eating disorders. This is a very serious health hazard.

## HOW THEY WORK

Various types of laxatives work in different ways. These drugs may work by:

- absorbing liquid in the intestines and forming a bulky, easy-to-pass stool
- using the water and the fats in the feces to soften the stool and make it easier to pass
- irritating the intestinal lining or stimulating nerve endings in the intestines to produce a bowel movement

## TYPES AND EXAMPLES

| DRUG SPOTLIGHT | Laxatives | | | |
|---|---|---|---|---|
| **Drug Name Generic (Trade)** | **Typical Form and Route of Administration** | **Indications** | **Therapeutic Action** | **Adverse Reactions and Drug Interactions** |
| **Bulk-Forming Laxatives** | | | | |
| psyllium (Metamucil) | oral: capsules, powder, granules, wafers | constipation | added fiber increases movement of matter through the bowel | *Adverse reactions:* wheezing and shortness of breath (after inhaling dust from preparation) stomach pain difficulty swallowing skin rash itching upset stomach vomiting |
| **Emollient Laxatives** | | | | |
| docusate sodium (Colace) | oral: capsules, tablets, syrup, liquid | constipation | softens the stool | *Drug interactions:* should not be used with mineral oil |

| DRUG SPOTLIGHT | Laxatives (continued) | | | |
| --- | --- | --- | --- | --- |
| **Drug Name Generic (Trade)** | **Typical Form and Route of Administration** | **Indications** | **Therapeutic Action** | **Adverse Reactions and Drug Interactions** |
| **Stimulant Laxatives** | | | | |
| bisacodyl (Dulcolax) | oral: tablets rectal: suppositories | treats constipation caused by prolonged bed rest, use of narcotics, and certain colon problems empties the bowel before general surgery and various examinations of the bowel | acts directly on the bowels, stimulating the bowel muscles to cause a bowel movement | *Adverse reactions:* weakness nausea abdominal cramps mild inflammation of the rectum and anus (when administered by rectal suppository) |

# H$_2$-Receptor Antagonist and Proton Pump Inhibitor Drugs

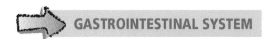 **GASTROINTESTINAL SYSTEM**

## WHY YOU USE THEM

Physicians often prescribe **H$_2$-receptor antagonists** and **proton pump inhibitors** to heal gastric and duodenal ulcers. Both types of drugs act to reduce the amount of acid produced by the stomach.

## HOW THEY WORK

H$_2$-receptor antagonists work by blocking histamine from getting into stomach cells. This decreases how much acid the stomach makes. Proton pump inhibitors also decrease how much acid the stomach makes because of the way the drugs bind to stomach cells. This lessens irritation and allows peptic ulcers to heal.

## TYPES AND EXAMPLES

| DRUG SPOTLIGHT | H$_2$-Receptor Antagonists and Proton Pump Inhibitors | | | |
|---|---|---|---|---|
| **Drug Name Generic (Trade)** | **Typical Form and Route of Administration** | **Indications** | **Therapeutic Action** | **Adverse Reactions and Drug Interactions** |
| **H$_2$-Receptor Antagonists** | | | | |
| ranitidine hydrochloride (Zantac) | oral: tablets, capsules, solution injection | duodenal and gastric ulcers GERD heartburn | blocks histamine from entering stomach cells, which reduces stomach acid production | Adverse reactions are uncommon, but may include: vertigo malaise headache blurred vision jaundice burning and itching at injection site (if administered by injection) anaphylaxis angioedema |
| cimetidine (Tagamet) | oral: tablets, solution injection | duodenal and gastric ulcers GERD heartburn certain hypersecretory conditions, such as Zollinger-Ellison syndrome GI bleeding (IV only) | blocks histamine, the chemical that stimulates the release of acid into the stomach | *Adverse reactions:* diarrhea dizziness drowsiness headache |
| **Proton Pump Inhibitors** | | | | |
| esomeprazole magnesium (Nexium) | oral: capsules, powder for suspension injection | short-term treatment of active gastric ulcers active duodenal ulcers erosive esophagitis symptoms of GERD that don't respond to other treatments | decreases the amount of acid produced in the stomach | Adverse reactions are uncommon, but may include: headache dry mouth diarrhea abdominal pain nausea flatulence vomiting constipation |
| omeprazole (Prilosec) | oral: capsules, tablets | duodenal ulcers erosive esophagitis gastric ulcers GERD heartburn certain hypersecretory conditions, such as Zollinger-Ellison syndrome | decreases the amount of acid produced in the stomach | *Adverse reactions:* diarrhea headache |

# Contraceptive Drugs

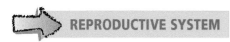 **REPRODUCTIVE SYSTEM**

## WHY YOU USE THEM

Physicians prescribe **contraceptive drugs** to prevent pregnancy or to help manage certain menstrual disorders. The contraceptive can be a tablet that is taken according to a prescribed schedule, or an injectable form. There are also transdermal patches that can be worn on the skin.

## HOW THEY WORK

Contraceptive drugs work by preventing ovulation and by thickening the mucus produced in the cervix. Because contraceptives consist of a specific mixture of hormones, the menstrual cycle is affected.

## TYPES AND EXAMPLES

**DRUG SPOTLIGHT    Contraceptives**

| Drug Name Generic (Trade) | Typical Form and Route of Administration | Indications | Therapeutic Action | Adverse Reactions and Drug Interactions |
|---|---|---|---|---|
| birth control pills (Progestin-only pill, Monophasic oral, Tri-phasic oral contraceptive pills) | oral: tablets | contraception | thickens cervical mucus to make implantation of sperm difficult prevents ovulation | *Adverse reactions:* headache dizziness nausea breakthrough bleeding spotting |
| Medroxyprogesterone acetate (Depo-Provera) | injection | contraception | thickens cervical mucus prevents ovulation | *Adverse reactions:* bloating abdominal pain breakthrough bleeding amenorrhea |
| etonogestrel-ethinyl estradiol (NuvaRing) | worn internally within the vagina | contraception | prevents ovulation | *Adverse reactions:* headache sinusitis nausea vaginitis leucorrhea upper respiratory infection |

## Urinary Antiseptic, Antibacterial, and Analgesic Drugs

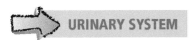 **URINARY SYSTEM**

### WHY YOU USE THEM

**Urinary antiseptic, antibacterial, and analgesic drugs** may be prescribed:

- to treat urinary tract infections (UTIs)
- to relieve pain and other symptoms associated with UTIs
- to relieve the symptoms of an overactive bladder

### HOW THEY WORK

**Phenazopyridine hydrochloride** is a kind of dye that is used in commercial coloring operations. Taken orally as a medication, phenazopyridine hydrochloride is used to relieve the symptoms of UTIs. Although this drug does not rid the body of infection, it lessens pain and burning and helps decrease the frequent or urgent need to urinate. Relief usually comes 24 to 48 hours after the patient starts taking the drug.

**Nitrofurantoin** is used to treat acute and chronic UTIs. After it's absorbed, the drug collects in the urine and works best when the urine is acidic. However, it does not work against systemic, or body-wide, bacterial infections.

### TYPES AND EXAMPLES

| DRUG SPOTLIGHT | Urinary Antiseptics, Antibacterials, and Analgesics | | | |
|---|---|---|---|---|
| **Drug Name Generic (Trade)** | **Typical Form and Route of Administration** | **Indications** | **Therapeutic Action** | **Adverse Reactions and Drug Interactions** |
| phenazopyridine hydrochloride (Pyridium) | oral: tablets | relieves symptoms of UTIs | exact mechanism of action is unknown; thought to work by relieving pain on the lining of the urinary tract | *Adverse reactions:* yellow skin and whites of the eyes acute liver or kidney failure reddish-orange urine |

| DRUG SPOTLIGHT | Urinary Antiseptics, Antibacterials, and Analgesics (continued) | | | |
| --- | --- | --- | --- | --- |
| **Drug Name Generic (Trade)** | **Typical Form and Route of Administration** | **Indications** | **Therapeutic Action** | **Adverse Reactions and Drug Interactions** |
| nitrofurantoin (Macrodantin) | oral: capsules, suspension | acute and chronic UTIs | interferes with various chemical processes in the bacteria causing the infection, which results in the death of the bacteria | *Adverse reactions:* gastrointestinal irritation anorexia nausea vomiting diarrhea dark yellow or brown urine abdominal pain chills fever joint pain |

## *Diuretic Drugs*

 **URINARY AND CARDIOVASCULAR SYSTEMS**

### WHY YOU USE THEM

When patients retain fluid or exhibit edema (the accumulation of an excessive amount of watery fluid in cells or intercellular tissues), the doctor may prescribe a diuretic. **Diuretics** decrease edema by increasing the flow of urine.

### HOW THEY WORK

Diuretics help the kidneys remove water and electrolytes from the body. Doing so allows these drugs to play a major role in treating hypertension and other cardiovascular conditions.

## TYPES AND EXAMPLES

**DRUG SPOTLIGHT    Diuretics**

| Drug Name Generic (Trade) | Typical Form and Route of Administration | Indications | Therapeutic Action | Adverse Reactions and Drug Interactions |
|---|---|---|---|---|
| **Thiazide Diuretics** | | | | |
| hydrochloro-thiazide (Hydro-diuril) | oral: capsules, tablets | hypertension | helps the kidneys remove fluid from the body | *Adverse reactions:* diabetes gout hypokalemia photosensitivity |
| **Loop Diuretics** | | | | |
| furosemide (Lasix) | oral: tablets, solution injection | reduces swelling and fluid retention from heart and liver disease treats hypertension | makes the kidneys eliminate larger amounts of electrolytes (especially sodium and potassium salts) and water than normal | *Adverse reactions:* too great a loss of fluid volume (especially in elderly patients) orthostatic hypotension hyperuricemia hypokalemia hypochloremia hyponatremia hypocalcemia hypomagnesemia |
| **Potassium-Sparing Diuretics** | | | | |
| triamterene (Dyre-nium, Maxzide, Diazide) | oral: capsules | edema hypokalemia in patients who are taking diuretics for heart failure cirrhosis of the liver nephrotic syndrome (abnormal condition of the kidneys) hypertension | makes the kidneys eliminate sodium and water from the body while retaining potassium | *Adverse reactions:* hyperkalemia |

## Anticonvulsant Drugs

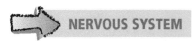

NERVOUS SYSTEM

### WHY YOU USE THEM

When a person goes into **convulsions,** the person's body shakes in a rapid, out-of-control way. Muscles keep contracting and relaxing without stopping. Convulsions can be alarming to watch.

The term *convulsion* often refers to **seizures** of any kind. Seizures are caused by a sudden burst of disorganized electrical activity in the brain. They often last from 30 seconds to 2 minutes. However, if a patient has severe seizures or if she experiences many seizures in a row and does not wake up in between, it becomes a medical emergency called *status epilepticus.*

Many different factors can cause seizures to occur. Among the causes are brain injuries, drug or alcohol abuse, electric shock, overheating, high fevers (in children), and stroke. A very common cause, however, is epilepsy.

**Anticonvulsants** are used to treat:

- chronic epilepsy (recurrent seizures)
- acute isolated seizures not caused by epilepsy, such as those occurring as a result of trauma or brain surgery

### HOW THEY WORK

Anticonvulsants work to keep nerve cells from firing rapidly enough to cause a seizure. They do this by blocking certain neurotransmitters from passing between nerve cells.

### TYPES AND EXAMPLES

| DRUG SPOTLIGHT | Anticonvulsant Drugs | | | |
| --- | --- | --- | --- | --- |
| **Drug Name Generic (Trade)** | **Typical Form and Route of Administration** | **Indications** | **Therapeutic Action** | **Adverse Reactions and Drug Interactions** |
| phenytoin sodium (Dilantin) | oral: tablets, capsules, suspension injection | tonic-clonic seizures psychomotor seizures | affects the motor cortex of the brain to inhibit seizure activity | *Adverse reactions:* gingival hyperplasia *Drug interactions:* interacts with many drugs *(continued)* |

**DRUG SPOTLIGHT**   **Anticonvulsant Drugs (continued)**

| Drug Name Generic (Trade) | Typical Form and Route of Administration | Indications | Therapeutic Action | Adverse Reactions and Drug Interactions |
|---|---|---|---|---|
| carbamazepine (Tegretol) | oral: tablets, capsules, suspension | mixed seizures partial seizures | controls seizures by blocking certain nerve impulses in the brain | *Adverse reactions:* may cause absence seizures to worsen will affect mood |
| clonazepam (Klonopin) | oral: tablets | panic disorder seizure disorders | increases the activity of a naturally occur-ring chemical in the brain | *Adverse reactions:* drowsiness ataxia behavior problems |

## Antiparkinsonian Drugs

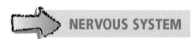 **NERVOUS SYSTEM**

### WHY YOU USE THEM

Parkinson disease belongs to a group of conditions called movement disorders. The disease occurs when the brain does not produce enough of a chemical called dopamine. Patients with Parkinson disease often have the following symptoms:

- muscle rigidity (inflexibility)
- **akinesia** (loss of muscle movement)
- tremors (involuntary shaking) when the body is at rest
- unstable posture, which leads to impaired balance and falls

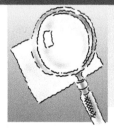

## Closer Look   AVOIDING DRUG INTERACTIONS

Drugs such as phenytoin sodium are very popular, but can interact with a number of other drugs. This is, again, an illustration of why it's important for medical assistants to obtain a updated medical history from patients each time they come into the office.

Drug therapy that includes **antiparkinsonian drugs** is an important part of the treatment plan for patients with Parkinson disease. The goals of drug therapy are to relieve the patient's symptoms and to help the patient remain mobile and independent.

## HOW THEY WORK

Currently, there is no cure for Parkinson disease. As a result, treatment is usually restricted to decreasing the symptoms associated with the disease. Antiparkinsonian drugs affect the brain to decrease tremors and other parkinsonian symptoms.

## TYPES AND EXAMPLES

| DRUG SPOTLIGHT | Antiparkinsonian Drugs | | | |
|---|---|---|---|---|
| **Drug Name Generic (Trade)** | **Typical Form and Route of Administration** | **Indications** | **Therapeutic Action** | **Adverse Reactions and Drug Interactions** |
| levodopa and carbidopa (Sinemet) | oral: tablets | symptoms of Parkinson disease | Levodopa is transformed by the body and the brain into a substance that helps decrease tremors and other symptoms of Parkinson disease. Carbidopa helps levodopa reach the brain. | *Adverse reactions:* vomiting constipation diarrhea confusion dizziness drowsiness dry mouth headache increased sweating anorexia nausea taste changes insomnia upset stomach urinary tract infection |
| benzotropine mesylate (Cogentin) | oral: tablets injection | Parkinson disease drug-induced extrapyramidal symptoms (except tardive dyskinesia) acute dystonic reaction | decreases the effects of acetylcholine, a chemical in the brain, resulting in decreased tremors or muscle stiffness | *Adverse reactions:* dry mouth constipation |

## *Antidepressant Drugs*

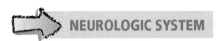 NEUROLOGIC SYSTEM

### WHY YOU USE THEM

Everyone feels sad or "down in the dumps" from time to time. But **depression** is a mood disorder in which feelings of sadness, loss, hopelessness, and helplessness get in the way of everyday life for periods of time.

Depression can be caused by personal problems; medical conditions; medication, alcohol, or drug abuse; social isolation; and other causes. Depression often runs in families.

Manic depression, also called **bipolar disorder,** is a serious mental illness. People who suffer from bipolar disorder experience dramatic mood swings. Researchers do not yet understand the causes of bipolar disorder. However, they agree that there is no single cause. The current thinking is that it's a disorder of the brain that the person's genes and personal experiences both have a role in causing.

Physicians use **antidepressants** to treat mood disorders characterized by depression.

### HOW THEY WORK

Scientists do not fully understand how antidepressants work. It is believed that these drugs prevent the reuptake of neurotransmitters such as norepinephrine and serotonin—two chemicals that play an important role in the way the body reacts to stress and in inhibiting anger and aggression. In other words, when these chemicals are secreted into the spaces between neurons, the chemicals are prevented from being reabsorbed. This helps keep the levels high for longer periods of time.

### TYPES AND EXAMPLES

| DRUG SPOTLIGHT | Antidepressants | | | |
| --- | --- | --- | --- | --- |
| **Drug Name Generic (Trade)** | **Typical Form and Route of Administration** | **Indications** | **Therapeutic Action** | **Adverse Reactions and Drug Interactions** |
| amitriptyline hydrochloride (Elavil) | oral: tablets | depression | exact mechanism of action is not fully under- | *Adverse reactions:* orthostatic hypotension sedation |

| Drug Name Generic (Trade) | Typical Form and Route of Administration | Indications | Therapeutic Action | Adverse Reactions and Drug Interactions |
|---|---|---|---|---|
| | | | stood; thought to increase the activity of certain chemicals in the brain (norepinephrine and serotonin), which help improve mood | jaundice rashes photosensitivity reactions a fine resting tremor (a tremor that is worse at rest) decreased sexual desire difficulty ejaculating reduced white blood cell count transient eosinophilia |
| venlafaxine hydrochloride (Effexor) | oral: tablets, capsules | depression generalized anxiety disorder social anxiety disorder panic disorder | restores the balance of certain natural substances in the brain (norepinephrine and serotonin), which help improve mood | *Adverse reactions:* anorexia anxiety asthenia blurred vision constipation dizziness dry mouth nausea nervousness somnolence sweating tremor vomiting abnormal ejaculation/ orgasm and impotence (men) |
| imipramine (Tofranil) | oral: tablets | depression | increases the activity of certain chemicals in the brain that help elevate mood | *Adverse reactions:* dizziness drowsiness dry mouth excitement headache impotence nausea nightmares pupil dilation photosensitivity sweating fatigue epigastric distress vomiting weakness weight loss or gain |

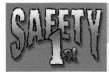

## STOPPING ANTIDEPRESSANTS

It's important to warn patients not to stop taking antidepressants abruptly. Instead, they should work with the physician to follow a plan for gradually weaning themselves off the drugs.

## *Selective Serotonin Reuptake Inhibitor Drugs*

 **NEUROLOGIC SYSTEM**

### WHY YOU USE THEM

Serotonin is a natural substance in the brain that helps maintain mental balance. Changes in the amount of this hormone can alter a person's moods. Companies have developed a group of antidepressants with fewer adverse reactions. These drugs are called **selective serotonin reuptake inhibitors (SSRIs).**

### HOW THEY WORK

SSRIs allow serotonin to build up in the neurosynapses. Although they cause fewer adverse reactions, these drugs take 7 to 21 days to begin relieving depression.

### TYPES AND EXAMPLES

| **DRUG SPOTLIGHT** | **Selective Serotonin Reuptake Inhibitors** | | | |
|---|---|---|---|---|
| **Drug Name Generic (Trade)** | **Typical Form and Route of Administration** | **Indications** | **Therapeutic Action** | **Adverse Reactions and Drug Interactions** |
| fluoxetine (Prozac) | oral: tablets, capsules, solution | depression obsessive-compulsive disorder some eating disorders panic attacks | restores the balance of serotonin, a natural substance in the brain, which helps improve certain mood problems | *Adverse reactions:* nervousness somnolence anxiety insomnia headache drowsiness tremor dizziness asthenia nausea diarrhea |

**DRUG SPOTLIGHT**    **Selective Serotonin Reuptake Inhibitors (continued)**

| Drug Name Generic (Trade) | Typical Form and Route of Administration | Indications | Therapeutic Action | Adverse Reactions and Drug Interactions |
|---|---|---|---|---|
| | | | | dry mouth anorexia suicidal behavior (uncommon but life threatening) |
| sertraline hydro-chloride (Zoloft) | oral: tablets, solution | depression obsessive-compulsive disorder panic disorder posttraumatic stress disorder premenstrual dys-phoric disorder social anxiety disorder | restores the balance of serotonin, a natural substance in the brain, which helps improve certain mood problems | *Adverse reactions:* anxiety constipation decreased sexual desire or ability diarrhea dizziness drowsiness dry mouth increased sweating anorexia nausea nervousness stomach upset tiredness insomnia vomiting weight loss |
| paroxetine hydro-chloride (Paxil) | oral: tablets, suspension | depression generalized anxi-ety disorder obsessive-compulsive disorder panic disorder posttraumatic stress disorder premenstrual dys-phoric disorder social anxiety disorder | restores the balance of serotonin, a natural substance in the brain, which helps improve certain mood problems | *Adverse reactions:* anxiety blurred vision constipation decreased sexual desire or ability diarrhea dizziness drowsiness dry mouth gas increased sweating increased urination anorexia nausea nervousness stomach upset trouble concentrating insomnia unusual skin sensations weakness yawning |

Adverse reactions to SSRIs may include anxiety, insomnia, and palpitations. With paroxetine, orthostatic hypotension may occur.

## Monoamine Oxidase Inhibitor Drugs

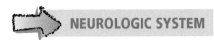 NEUROLOGIC SYSTEM

### WHY YOU USE THEM

**Monoamine oxidase inhibitors (MAOIs)** are another type of drug prescribed to treat depression. However, because of the serious interactions with certain foods and other drugs, MAOIs usually aren't considered unless all other antidepressants have proven to be ineffective.

### HOW THEY WORK

MAOIs block a chemical in the brain that affects the nervous system. Physicians prescribe MAOIs when the patient shows symptoms of atypical depression, or a type of depression that produces signs opposite those of typical depression.

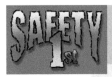

### USE CAUTION WITH MONOAMINE OXIDASE INHIBITORS

Be aware of drug interactions associated with MAOIs! For example, administering them with meperidine (Demerol) may result in excitation, hypertension or hypotension, extremely elevated body temperature, coma, and even death.

Certain foods can interact with MAOIs and produce severe reactions. The most serious reactions involve tyramine-rich foods, such as:

- red wine
- chocolate
- aged cheeses
- fava beans
- yeast
- olives
- sausage
- pepperoni
- beer
- sympathomimetic drugs

Patients taking MAOIs must follow a low-tyramine diet. However, they may occasionally eat foods with moderate tyramine content, such as ripe bananas and yogurt.

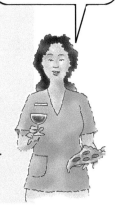

Tyramine-rich foods, such as red wine and pizza, can produce severe reactions if taken with MAOIs.

## TYPES AND EXAMPLES

**DRUG SPOTLIGHT**  **Monoamine Oxidase Inhibitors**

| Drug Name Generic (Trade) | Typical Form and Route of Administration | Indications | Therapeutic Action | Adverse Reactions and Drug Interactions |
|---|---|---|---|---|
| Tranylcypromine (Parnate) | oral: tablets | depression | blocks the action of the enzyme (monoamine oxidase) that breaks down the body's mood-elevating chemicals (dopamine, norepinephrine, and serotonin), producing an increase in these mood-elevating chemicals | *Adverse reactions:* blurred vision constipation diarrhea dizziness drowsiness dry mouth stomach pain tremors upset stomach weakness |

## *Antianxiety Drugs*

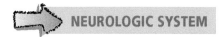 **NEUROLOGIC SYSTEM**

### WHY YOU USE THEM

**Anxiety** is a feeling of extreme worry or uneasiness that may or may not be based on reality. **Antianxiety drugs** reduce agitation or excitement and allow the patient to become drowsy. They are some of the most commonly prescribed drugs in the United States.

### HOW THEY WORK

Antianxiety drugs work by depressing, or slowing down, the central nervous system.

## TYPES AND EXAMPLES

| DRUG SPOTLIGHT | Antianxiety Drugs | | | |
|---|---|---|---|---|
| **Drug Name Generic (Trade)** | **Typical Form and Route of Administration** | **Indications** | **Therapeutic Action** | **Adverse Reactions and Drug Interactions** |
| diazepam (Valium) | oral: tablets, solution injection | anxiety disorders relief of anxiety and tension prior to surgical procedures (injectable form only) | slows the movement of chemicals in the brain, resulting in a reduction in anxiety and muscle spasm also causes sedation | *Adverse reactions:* sedation confusion ataxia weakness nystagmus |
| lorazepam (Ativan) | oral: tablets, solution injection | anxiety insomnia from anxiety | slows the movement of chemicals in the brain, resulting in a reduction in anxiety causes little sedation | *Adverse reactions:* sedation drowsiness amnesia weakness nausea dizziness unsteadiness rebound insomnia |
| alprazolam (Xanax) | oral: tablets, solution | anxiety disorders panic disorder | slows the movement of chemicals in the brain, resulting in a reduction in anxiety | *Adverse reactions:* changes in appetite changes in sexual desire constipation dizziness drowsiness dry mouth increased saliva production light-headedness tiredness trouble concentrating unsteadiness weight changes |

At low doses, benzodiazepines, such as lorazepam, decrease anxiety without causing drowsiness.

# Antipsychotic Drugs

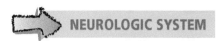

**NEUROLOGIC SYSTEM**

## WHY YOU USE THEM

A **psychotic disorder** is a severe mental disorder that can have many causes. People who are in a psychotic state are not in touch with reality. They experience delusions and hallucinations. **Antipsychotic drugs** can control the thought disorders associated with schizophrenia, mania, and other altered mental states.

## HOW THEY WORK

The specific way antipsychotics work is not known. However, they are believed to somehow change the way certain neurotransmitters are absorbed by neurons.

## TYPES AND EXAMPLES

| DRUG SPOTLIGHT | Antipsychotic Drugs | | | |
| --- | --- | --- | --- | --- |
| **Drug Name Generic (Trade)** | **Typical Form and Route of Administration** | **Indications** | **Therapeutic Action** | **Adverse Reactions and Drug Interactions** |
| haloperidol (Haldol) | • oral: tablets, concentrate<br>• injection | psychotic disorders<br>nonpsychotic behavior disorders<br>Tourette syndrome | exact mechanism of action is unknown; may work by blocking certain chemicals in the brain | *Adverse reactions:*<br>tardive dyskinesia<br>drowsiness<br>headache<br>dry mouth<br>orthostatic hypotension<br>akathisia<br>dystonia |
| chlorpromazine (Thorazine) | • oral: tablets<br>• injection | manic depression<br>schizophrenia<br>behavioral problems and hyperactivity (in children) | blocks dopamine receptors in the brain, which helps treat certain mental disorders | *Adverse reactions:*<br>agitation<br>dizziness<br>drowsiness<br>dry mouth<br>enlarged pupils<br>jitteriness<br>nausea<br>stuffy nose |

## Closer Look

### ANTIPSYCHOTIC DRUGS AND EXTRAPYRAMIDAL SYMPTOMS

The extrapyramidal portion of the nervous system controls body posture and muscle movement. When antipsychotic drugs affect this portion of the nervous system, they can cause extrapyramidal symptoms (EPS). These symptoms are the most significant adverse reactions to antipsychotic drugs.

EPS usually occurs in patients taking typical antipsychotic drugs such as haloperidol. The most common symptoms are:

- tardive dyskinesia—unusual, involuntary movements of the mouth, face, jaw, or tongue
- Parkinson-like symptoms—tremors, muscle rigidity, slurred speech, and an unsteady gait
- akathisia—extreme restlessness and increased motor activity
- dystonia—facial grimacing and twisting of the neck into unnatural positions

Some of these symptoms may appear after the first few days of therapy. Others may not occur until after several years of treatment.

EPS can usually be treated by reducing the patient's dosage of the antipsychotic drug. The physician may also prescribe an antiparkinsonian drug, such as benzotropine (Cogentin), to treat the Parkinson-like symptoms.

## Hormones

 **REPRODUCTIVE AND ENDOCRINE SYSTEMS**

### WHY YOU USE THEM

Although the body naturally produces hormones, many **hormones** are used in the treatment of certain disorders, such as:

- blood glucose imbalances
- male or female hormone deficiency

- menstrual disorders
- thyroid disorders

## HOW THEY WORK

Some hormones mimic the effects of naturally occurring hormones. For example, physicians prescribe estrogens to correct estrogen deficiencies and, along with oral contraceptives, to prevent pregnancy. Other hormones replace or supplement an underactive gland in the endocrine system.

## TYPES AND EXAMPLES

**DRUG SPOTLIGHT**    **Hormones**

| Drug Name Generic (Trade) | Typical Form and Route of Administration | Indications | Therapeutic Action | Adverse Reactions and Drug Interactions |
|---|---|---|---|---|
| glucagon | injection | hypoglycemia | stimulates the liver to release glucose into the blood | *Adverse reactions:* nausea |
| levothyroxine sodium (Synthroid) | • oral: tablets • injection | drug of choice for thyroid hormone replacement and thyroid-stimulating hormone suppression therapy (the treatment of nodules growing on the thyroid) | replaces or supplements natural thyroid hormones | *Adverse reactions:* • diarrhea • abdominal cramps • weight loss • increased appetite • palpitations • sweating • tachycardia • headache • tremor • insomnia • nervousness • fever • heat intolerance • menstrual irregularities |
| conjugated estrogens (Premarin) | • oral: tablets • injection | certain symptoms associated with menopause postmenopausal osteoporosis (preventative) female castration ovarian failure palliative treatment for breast and prostate cancer abnormal uterine bleeding | replaces natural estrogens in women who can no longer produce enough estrogen used for advanced prostate cancer because it antagonizes male hormones | *Adverse reactions:* • breast pain or tenderness • gas • headache • hair loss • mild nausea or vomiting • spotting or breakthrough bleeding • stomach cramps or bloating |

*(continued)*

| DRUG SPOTLIGHT | Hormones (continued) | | | |
|---|---|---|---|---|
| **Drug Name Generic (Trade)** | **Typical Form and Route of Administration** | **Indications** | **Therapeutic Action** | **Adverse Reactions and Drug Interactions** |
| oxytocin (Pitocin) | injection | to increase or start contractions of the uterus during labor | causes uterine contractions by changing calcium concentrations in the uterine muscle cells | *Adverse reactions:* nausea vomiting more intense or abrupt contractions of the uterus |
| medroxyprogesterone (Provera) | oral: tablets injection | endometrial hyperplasia menstrual problems abnormal uterine bleeding contraception (injectable form only) | alters the lining of the uterus | *Adverse reactions:* acne changes in menstrual flow, including breakthrough bleeding, spotting, or missed periods dizziness drowsiness fever headache hot flashes nausea nervousness pain rash insomnia stomach pain weakness weight gain or loss |

## *Corticosteroid Drugs*

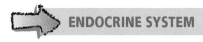 ENDOCRINE SYSTEM

### WHY YOU USE THEM

The group of drugs known as **corticosteroids** are often used to treat allergic reactions, skin conditions, rheumatic disorders, and other conditions. The body produces several corticosteroid substances that are essential for good health. When the natural production of these chemicals decreases, corticosteroids may be prescribed.

> Natural corticosteroids have a wide range of effects. When corticosteroids are used to supplement the body's natural levels, the dosage must be closely monitored.

## HOW THEY WORK

Corticosteroids enter target cells and bind to receptors, initiating many complex reactions in the body. These drugs influence or regulate functions such as the immune response and control of the anti-inflammatory response. Some of these actions are undesirable, depending on the indication for which these drugs are being used. However, the anti-inflammatory activity of these hormones makes them valuable as anti-inflammatories and as immunosuppressants to suppress inflammation and modify the immune response.

## TYPES AND EXAMPLES

**DRUG SPOTLIGHT    Corticosteroids**

| Drug Name Generic (Trade) | Typical Form and Route of Administration | Indications | Therapeutic Action | Adverse Reactions and Drug Interactions |
|---|---|---|---|---|
| prednisone (Deltasone) | oral: tablets, solution | wide variety of conditions, including endocrine disorders, rheumatic disorders (adjunctive therapy), allergic states, ophthalmic diseases, and respiratory diseases | decreases or prevents tissues from responding to inflammation modifies the body's response to certain immune stimulation | *Adverse reactions:* insomnia vertigo increased appetite increased sweating indigestion mood changes nervousness |
| dexamethasone (Decadron) | oral: tablets, elixir, solution | wide variety of conditions, including endocrine disorders, rheumatic disorders (adjunctive therapy), allergic states, ophthalmic diseases, and respiratory diseases | decreases or prevents tissues from responding to inflammation modifies the body's response to certain immune stimulation | *Adverse reactions:* insomnia vertigo increased appetite increased sweating indigestion mood changes nervousness |

# Hypoglycemic Drugs

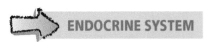 **ENDOCRINE SYSTEM**

### WHY YOU USE THEM

Antidiabetic drugs, or **hypoglycemic drugs,** are prescribed for patients with type 2 diabetes or who can't control their blood sugar levels with diet and exercise.

**Diabetes** is a chronic disease of insulin deficiency or resistance. In one type of diabetes, the body does not make enough insulin. In the other kind, the body makes enough insulin, but responds to it sluggishly. Type 2 diabetes is sometimes called adult-onset diabetes. People who have type 2 diabetes do not respond correctly to the insulin their bodies make. Their cells become insulin resistant. To compensate, the pancreas secretes more and more insulin. Over time, glucose levels in the blood become high—a condition called hyperglycemia. Hypoglycemic drugs act to lower glucose levels that are too high.

### HOW THEY WORK

The pancreas gland secretes the hormone **insulin,** which allows cells to absorb glucose (sugar). The cells use glucose as fuel. Without the help of insulin, the cells can't access the calories that glucose supplies.

Hypoglycemic drugs act to lower blood glucose levels. They do this by stimulating the pancreas to release more insulin, or by decreasing the absorption or production of glucose in the digestive system.

### TYPES AND EXAMPLES

| DRUG SPOTLIGHT | Hypoglycemic Drugs | | | |
|---|---|---|---|---|
| **Drug Name Generic (Trade)** | **Typical Form and Route of Administration** | **Indications** | **Therapeutic Action** | **Adverse Reactions and Drug Interactions** |
| glyburide (Micronase, DiaBeta) | oral: tablets | along with diet, lowers glucose levels in patients with type 2 diabetes in some patients, can replace insulin therapy | causes the pancreas to release insulin, which helps lower blood glucose | *Adverse reactions:* nausea epigastric fullness potential for hypoglycemia water retention rash hyponatremia photosensitivity |

**DRUG SPOTLIGHT**    Hypoglycemic Drugs (continued)

| Drug Name Generic (Trade) | Typical Form and Route of Administration | Indications | Therapeutic Action | Adverse Reactions and Drug Interactions |
|---|---|---|---|---|
| metformin (Glucophage) | oral: tablets, solution | used alone or with other medications, including insulin, to lower glucose level in patients with type 2 diabetes | decreases glucose production in the liver decreases glucose absorption in the intestines | *Adverse reactions:* metallic aftertaste nausea and vomiting abdominal discomfort urgent and explosive diarrhea |

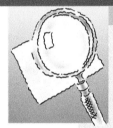

## Closer Look

### EXENATIDE: A LITTLE HELP FROM GILA MONSTERS

Exenatide (Byetta) is a new synthetic medication for treating type 2 diabetes. Scientists studying hormones found that the peptide exendin-4 found in the Gila monster's saliva was able to lower blood sugar. Based on their research, synthetic exendin-4 has been produced and is used to achieve the same effect.

- It's used with metformin (Fortamet, Glucophage, Glucophage XR, Riomet, Glumetza) and/or medications in the sulfonylurea family, such as glyburide (DiaBeta, Glynase PresTab, Micronase) and glipizide (Glucotrol, Glucotrol XL).

- Exenatide stimulates the pancreas to secrete insulin when blood sugar is high.

- The drug also slows down how fast the stomach empties and can decrease a patient's appetite.

- Exenatide is available only as an injectable. However, another incretin mimetic is now available in tablet form and is known as sitagliptin phosphate (Januvia) or vildagliptin (Galvus).

- It's the first of a new class of drugs called incretin mimetics that help the body make the right amount of insulin at the right time.

## Antineoplastic Drugs

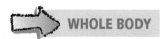 WHOLE BODY

### WHY YOU USE THEM

Tumors, or neoplasms, can grow quickly. Drugs used to slow or stop neoplastic growth are called **antineoplastics.** These chemicals are most successful when used to slow or stop the growth of breast cancer cells and certain skin cancers.

### HOW THEY WORK

Antineoplastics work by interfering, slowing, or preventing tumor cells from reproducing and/or repairing. Because tumor cells grow so rapidly, antineoplastics are able to specifically alter the chemical steps needed for cell multiplication and repair.

### TYPES AND EXAMPLES

**DRUG SPOTLIGHT** **Antineoplastics**

| Drug Name Generic (Trade) | Typical Form and Route of Administration | Indications | Therapeutic Action | Adverse Reactions and Drug Interactions |
|---|---|---|---|---|
| tamoxifen (Nolvadex) | oral: tablets, solution | breast cancer | blocks the effect of estrogen on certain tumors, possibly preventing tumor growth | *Adverse reactions:* bone pain constipation coughing hot flashes muscle pain nausea tiredness vaginal discharge weight loss |
| fluorouracil (Efudex) | topical: solution, cream | keratoses certain skin cancers | blocks the growth of certain cells, causing cell death | *Adverse reactions:* burning, crusting, redness, pain, soreness, inflammation, or irritation of the skin |
| methotrexate | oral: tablets injection | certain cancers psoriasis that is not adequately responsive to other forms of therapy | blocks an enzyme needed for cell growth, which slows the growth of cancer cells and abnormal skin cells | *Adverse reactions:* dizziness headache loss of appetite mild hair loss nausea stomach pain or upset tiredness vomiting |

**Chapter Highlights**

- Drugs may be classified according to their primary action on the body. However, the primary use of a particular drug may have effects and actions on other systems of the body as well.

- Antibiotics are useful in treating a wide variety of bacterial infections. Some antibiotics work to kill bacteria, whereas others simply interrupt the way the bacteria reproduce.

- Many topical drugs are used to relieve itching and inflammation from various skin conditions. These drugs are thought to interfere with the body's inflammation response.

- Anti-inflammatory drugs are used to treat inflammation, swelling, and pain. They work in several ways, such as by inhibiting chemical processes that sense pain or interfering with cells that produce swelling, redness, and itching.

- Analgesics and antipyretics are used to treat pain and fever. It is thought that analgesics probably work on the CNS to prevent the pain response from occurring.

- Physicians may prescribe muscle relaxants for patients experiencing muscle stiffness, spasms, or spasticity. These drugs work in one of two ways: either by acting on the CNS or by acting directly on skeletal muscles.

- Cardiac drugs are used to treat a variety of conditions, such as hypertension, angina, and arrhythmias. These drugs are also used to lower cholesterol levels and to prevent the risk of blood clots. They work in many different ways, by dilating blood vessels, acting directly on the heart, acting on the liver, or by interfering with factors in the blood clotting process.

- Respiratory medications are used to treat TB, asthma, bronchitis, emphysema, cough, nasal congestion, and seasonal allergies. Antitubercular drugs work by killing or stopping the growth of TB bacteria. Other respiratory drugs act by dilating bronchial passages, acting on the cough center in the brain, breaking down mucus, reducing swelling in nasal passages, or blocking the action of histamines.

- Drugs that affect the digestive system are indicated for heartburn, nausea and vomiting, ulcers, irritable bowel syndrome, diarrhea, and constipation. Some digestive drugs work by decreasing stomach acid, some work in the brain or nervous system, and others act directly on the intestines.

- Urinary drugs are used to treat UTIs, to relieve pain and other symptoms associated with UTIs, and to relieve the symptoms of an overactive bladder. They work by relieving pain on the lining of the urinary tract or by killing the bacteria causing a UTI.

- Diuretic drugs are used to rid the body of excess fluid, which allows these drugs to play a major role in treating hypertension and other cardiovascular conditions. Diuretics work by helping the kidneys remove water and electrolytes from the body.

- Nervous system medications are used in treating various types of seizures as well as symptoms of Parkinson disease, such as muscle rigidity and tremors. These drugs work by affecting chemicals and nerve impulses in the brain.

- Drugs that affect the endocrine system are used for hormone replacement therapy as well as to treat conditions such as hypoglycemia, allergic reactions, skin conditions, and rheumatic disorders. These drugs work in one of several ways. They may mimic the effects of naturally occurring hormones, replace or supplement an underactive gland in the endocrine system, or influence or regulate functions such as the immune response and control of the anti-inflammatory response.

- Oncology medications are used to slow or stop the growth of various cancers. These drugs work by interfering, slowing, or preventing tumor cells from reproducing and/or repairing.

## Chapter 6

# SUPPLEMENTS AND IMMUNIZATIONS: WAYS TO PROTECT OUR HEALTH

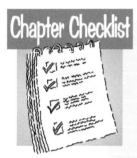

**Chapter Checklist**

- Differentiate between fat-soluble and water-soluble vitamins
- Explain the body's need for vitamins and natural sources
- Explain the body's need for minerals and natural sources
- List uses for commonly used herbal preparations
- Identify safety issues with complementary herbal therapy
- Describe the components of the National Childhood Vaccine Injury Act
- Identify the diseases for which common immunizations are administered
- Identify the most frequent adverse reactions of the vaccines usually given

**Chapter Competencies**

- Demonstrate knowledge of federal and state health care legislation and regulations (CAAHEP Competency 3.c.2.e.)
- Monitor legislation related to current health care issues and practices (ABHES Competency 5.g.)

The patients who come into a medical office are all different. Some are thorough when it comes to taking their medications as ordered. Others forget to take their medications, can't afford their prescriptions, or stop taking their medications for a variety of reasons. Some patients believe in self-medicating. Others trust traditional medicine to cure what ails them. The patients you'll meet may take vitamins, supplements, herbal preparations, and remedies of all kinds. As a clinical medical assistant, you'll need to be aware of what people put into their bodies so that you can document complete medical histories.

Patients will also visit the medical office for various immunizations. These include childhood immunizations, travel immunizations, and flu shots to protect patients' health. Immunizations are a frequent and important part of the care your medical office provides, so it's important for you to be familiar with them.

## Vitamins

**Vitamins** are organic compounds that we get mainly from plant sources and animal protein in our diet. Vitamins are officially classified as micronutrients because the body needs only small amounts of them to function normally. By comparison, macronutrients are the fats, carbohydrates, and proteins that form the bulk of the human diet. Our bodies break down these macronutrients to create energy and to build body tissue. Vitamins assist in that process and do other jobs as well.

## What Vitamins Do and Where They Come From

Vitamins help maintain normal body function such as formation of bone and tissue, production of white and red blood cells, and cell repair. Lack of vitamins can cause disease, poor eyesight, and other problems. Vitamins work with other vitamins and with enzymes produced by the body to help cells function correctly.

With two exceptions, the body does not make vitamins. It gets them from the food people eat.

- The first exception is vitamin D, which your skin makes when it's exposed to sunlight.
- Vitamin K is the other exception. It's made by bacteria in the intestines.

## Closer Look

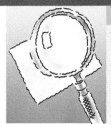

### MULTIVITAMINS—A SCAM OR THE SOLUTION?

Packages of multivitamins line the shelves of pharmacies, health food stores, and specialty stores. Americans have made multivitamins more than a billion-dollar industry. At the same time, many nutritionists say that a proper diet generally supplies all of the vitamins a person needs to stay healthy. So, what's the truth?

The truth is that, except for the special needs of pregnant women, the jury is out. The medical community is in disagreement about the value of multivitamins. For every study that finds a benefit, another study claims there's none. At the very least, they say, taking multivitamins may give people a false sense of security—that taking extra vitamins can make up for poor lifestyle and diet choices.

For the moment, listen to both sides with an open mind. If patients ask you what you think, tell them to ask the physician. The physician will take the patient's nutritional needs and lifestyle into consideration before making a recommendation. Meanwhile, be sure the physician is aware of any vitamins and multivitamins patients are taking on their own.

The U.S. Pharmacopeia recently established standards for vitamin supplements. These supplements have "USP" printed on the product label.

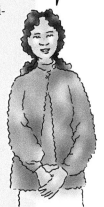

Vitamins can also be made synthetically, in the laboratory.

The body either stores vitamins intact, without breaking them down into other substances, or excretes them through the kidneys.

- **Fat-soluble vitamins** are stored in the body's fatty tissues for up to six months.
- **Water-soluble vitamins** pass through the bloodstream and leave the body when you urinate.

### FAT-SOLUBLE VITAMINS

Fat-soluble vitamins are stored in the body's fatty tissues for up to 6 months. If someone takes in too much of a fat-soluble vitamin, it gets stored in the liver and may cause health problems. In addition, rapid weight loss can cause swift release of stored fat-soluble vitamins, which can also cause toxicity. The following vitamins fall into this category:

- vitamin A
- vitamin D
- vitamin E
- vitamin K

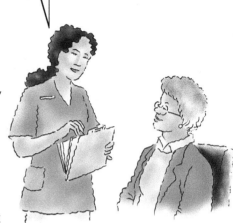

Because fat-soluble vitamins build up in body fat, you should not take them more often or in larger doses than the physician prescribes.

### Vitamin A

Vitamin A/retinol (Aquasol A, Palmitate-A, Solatene) is a fat-soluble vitamin that is found naturally in many sources, including liver, kidney, eggs, and dairy products. It is also found in dark or yellow vegetables and fruits. Vitamin A is included in most multivitamin preparations.

Vitamin A is necessary for maintaining vision. An early sign of vitamin A **deficiency**, or not enough vitamin A, is night blindness.

Vitamin A has important effects. It:

- helps prevent night blindness
- prevents chronic conjunctivitis ("pink eye")
- promotes growth of body cells
- is necessary for healthy hair and skin

Patients should avoid taking vitamin A at the same time they take mineral oil or cholestyramine (Questran), a cholesterol-reducing drug. Both slow down how fast vitamin A gets into the system.

---

## Closer Look | PRESCRIPTION-STRENGTH VITAMIN A

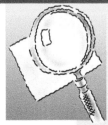

Physicians use prescription preparations that include vitamin A to treat acne. These include:

- tretinoin (Avita, Renova, Retina-A, Retin-A Micro)
- isotretinoin (Accutane)

Isotretinoin may cause severe adverse reactions, such as suicidal thoughts, and must never be used by a pregnant woman. It should be used only for severe, resistant acne that can't be cured with other medications.

## Vitamin D

Vitamin D (Calciferol, Calderol, Drisdol) is a fat-soluble vitamin that is found naturally in fish, eggs, fortified milk, cod liver oil, and other foods. Sunlight is another important source of vitamin D. Ten minutes a day in the sun is enough to prevent deficiencies. Vitamin D is included in most multivitamin preparations.

Vitamin D's job is to keep calcium and phosphorus in the blood at the right levels. It helps the body absorb calcium, which builds strong bones. Physicians use it to treat two diseases caused by a lack of vitamin D:

- rickets—a disease of infants and children marked by weak bones
- osteomalacia—a disease marked by fragile bones and muscular weakness, which in turn may lead to osteopenia or osteoporosis

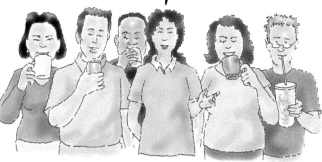

We have developed a habit of substituting coffee, tea, soft drinks, and water for milk as a daily beverage. But milk isn't just for young children—the vitamins in milk are important for everyone!

Patients who are taking vitamin D should avoid using mineral oil or taking magnesium-based antacids, such as Mylanta Liquid, Mylanta Tablets, Maalox Extra Strength Suspension, or Maalox Suspension.

## Vitamin E

Vitamin E/tocopherol (Aquasol E) is a fat-soluble vitamin with antioxidant properties. Antioxidants are found in fruits, vegetables, and whole grains.

Vitamin E's job is to help make red blood cells. It also protects essential fatty acids and plays a role in metabolism.

Vitamin E is used as a dietary supplement for people who lack enough vitamin E. This condition is rare. There are no proven medical uses for vitamin E beyond the minimum daily allowance needed for health.

High doses of vitamin E supplements may affect how well patients react to blood thinners such as warfarin (Coumadin), heparin, or aspirin (Bayer Aspirin, St. Joseph's Aspirin). Patients are usually instructed to stop taking vitamin E at least 1 to 2 weeks before surgery due to the effect on clotting.

### Vitamin K

Vitamin K (Aqua Mephyton, Mephyton) is a fat-soluble vitamin that is found naturally in green leafy vegetables, meat, and dairy products. We get most of the vitamin K we need from food. Bacteria in the intestines make a second form of vitamin K, called $K_2$, which we also need. Vitamin K is available in both oral and injectable forms.

The injectable form of vitamin K must be used only when the oral form can't be used. Injectable vitamin K can cause a rare but possibly fatal reaction even at the first injection.

Vitamin K is important for blood clotting. It works in the liver to create the chemicals called clotting factors that make blood clot properly. Liver failure or insufficient vitamin K can lead to clotting problems and excessive bleeding.

Lack of vitamin K is rare. But it can happen in people who suffer from chronic malnutrition, alcoholism, or liver problems. Vitamin K is routinely given to newborns to prevent bleeding problems from birth trauma or if surgery is planned.

## WATER-SOLUBLE VITAMINS

Water-soluble vitamins are not easily stored in the body. Because they are eliminated in the urine, they must be replenished every day. The following vitamins fall into this grouping:

- vitamin $B_1$/thiamin
- vitamin $B_2$/riboflavin
- vitamin $B_3$/niacin
- vitamin $B_6$/pyridoxine
- vitamin $B_9$/folic acid
- vitamin $B_{12}$/cyanocobalamin
- vitamin C/ascorbic acid

These vitamins are conveniently found in many foods. However, they are easily lost from some foods during cooking.

### Vitamin $B_1$/Thiamin

Vitamin $B_1$/thiamin (Betamine, Thiamilate) is a water-soluble vitamin that is found naturally in beef, brewer's yeast, beans, lentils, milk, nuts, oats, oranges, pork, rice, seeds, wheat, whole-grain cereals, and yeast.

Thiamin plays a role in many body functions, including the following:

- functioning of the nervous system
- normal digestion

- carbohydrate metabolism
- production of hydrochloric acid, which is necessary for digestion

Physicians use thiamin to prevent or treat stomach, heart, or nerve problems caused by thiamin deficiency. Severe thiamin deficiency is called beriberi.

Thiamin has few adverse reactions, even at high doses.

> Food products made from refined white flour usually have thiamin added because it is lost in the refining process.

## Vitamin B₂/Riboflavin

Vitamin $B_2$/riboflavin is a water-soluble vitamin that is found naturally in milk and other dairy products, eggs, enriched cereals and grains, meats, liver, and green vegetables such as asparagus or broccoli. The body's supply of riboflavin must be replenished daily.

Riboflavin is most commonly found in multivitamin and vitamin B-complex formulations.

Riboflavin is necessary for normal cell function, growth, and energy production. It breaks down carbohydrates, fats, and proteins for use by the body. It is also helpful for the following functions:

- keeping the skin, muscles, nerves, heart, and eyes healthy
- producing red blood cells and antibodies
- ensuring proper use of iron, folic acid, and vitamins $B_1$, $B_3$, and $B_6$ in the body
- producing hormones by the adrenal glands
- maintaining health of the mucous membranes in the digestive system
- promoting healthy development of the fetus

Vitamin $B_2$ deficiency is quite uncommon. It may occur in alcoholics, older adults with a poor diet, people who can't digest dairy products, and women who use oral contraceptives. The most common symptoms include visual problems, such as cataracts and extreme sensitivity to light. Drugs such as those used to treat Parkinson disease and other medications may affect how well the body can absorb riboflavin.

## Vitamin B₃/Niacin

Vitamin $B_3$ (Niacor, Niaspan, Slo-Niacin) is made up of niacin, or nicotinic acid, and niacinamide. It is found naturally in many foods, including meat, poultry, liver, fish, nuts, green vegetables, whole grains, and potatoes. Vitamin $B_3$ is often included in preparations with other B vitamins. These preparations are used to treat a lack of niacin. Niacin is also used in the following cases:

- to treat pellagra, a disease caused by niacin deficiency characterized by symptoms of diarrhea, dermatitis (skin rash), dementia, and, if left untreated, death
- to reduce bad cholesterol (LDL) levels in the blood and increase good cholesterol (HDL)

Taking niacin along with drugs that cause liver damage may make the damage worse. Niacin may also increase blood glucose levels in patients with diabetes. It appears in breast milk, so nursing mothers should stop taking niacin. This will keep large levels of it from building up in an infant's body.

## Vitamin B$_6$/Pyridoxine

Vitamin B$_6$/pyridoxine (Aminoxin, Pyri-500, Rodex, Vitabee 6) is a water-soluble vitamin that is found naturally in cereal grains, legumes, vegetables (carrots, spinach, peas), potatoes, milk, cheese, eggs, fish, liver, meat, and flour. It is not affected by cooking. The body needs only small amounts of it, and what you take in from food is usually enough. Vitamin B$_6$ is frequently included with other B vitamins in vitamin B-complex formulations.

The body needs vitamin B$_6$ for three very important reasons:

- to break down proteins, carbohydrates, and fats
- to make the neurotransmitters (brain chemicals) serotonin and norepinephrine
- to make myelin, an insulating material that surrounds the nerves

Many people are mildly lacking vitamin B$_6$. Vitamin B$_6$ deficiency can happen in people with uremia (kidney failure), alcoholism, cirrhosis, hyperthyroidism (overactive thyroid), congestive heart failure (CHF), and conditions that affect how drugs are absorbed. Some medications can also cause a mild deficiency of vitamin B$_6$. A lack of it may lead to anemia, nerve damage, seizures, skin problems, and sores in the mouth.

## Vitamin B$_9$/Folic Acid

Folic acid (FA-8) is the synthetic form of a water-soluble B vitamin called folate that is found in its natural form in many foods. Among these foods are leafy green vegetables (spinach, broccoli, lettuce), okra, asparagus, fruits (bananas, melons, lemons), legumes, yeast, mushrooms, organ meat (beef liver, kidney), orange juice, and tomato juice. It is also found in cereals and baked goods. Folic acid is frequently included with other B vitamins in vitamin B-complex formulations.

Folic acid helps the body form healthy cells, especially red blood cells. It causes few adverse reactions and rarely causes a severe allergic reaction. Physicians use folic acid to treat and prevent certain kinds of anemia, particularly those caused by the following conditions:

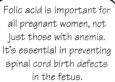

Folic acid is important for all pregnant women, not just those with anemia. It's essential in preventing spinal cord birth defects in the fetus.

- poor diet
- pregnancy
- alcoholism
- liver disease
- various stomach/intestinal problems
- kidney dialysis

Other important uses of folic acid include the following:

- relief from the tiredness and diarrhea caused by anemia
- prevention of birth defects in an infant's spinal cord

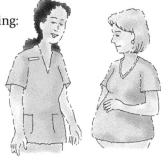

Pregnant women should be sure to have enough folic acid in their bodies by eating the right foods or taking supplements.

## Vitamin B$_{12}$/Cyanocobalamin

Vitamin B$_{12}$/cyanocobalamin (Cobolin-M, Cyanoject) is a water-soluble vitamin that is found naturally in a variety of foods such as fish, shellfish, meats, and dairy products. The body stores several years' supply of vitamin B$_{12}$, making it likely that most people will have enough of it in their systems. Exceptions are older adults, strict vegetarians, and people on macrobiotic diets (consumption of grains as a staple food).

Vitamin B$_{12}$ is frequently included with other B vitamins in vitamin B-complex formulations. It's also available by itself in oral tablet, sublingual tablet, or injectable form. Vitamin B$_{12}$ has an essential role in health. It is needed for the following functions:

- to keep nerve cells and red blood cells healthy
- to make DNA, the genetic material in our cells

Stomach acid releases the vitamin B$_{12}$ in food during digestion.

## Vitamin C/Ascorbic Acid

Vitamin C/ascorbic acid (Cecon, Ce-Vi-Sol, Vita-C) is a water-soluble vitamin that is found naturally in fruits and vegetables, especially citrus fruits such as oranges. Vitamin C is included in

## Closer Look   VITAMIN B₁₂ INJECTIONS

Patients with certain medical conditions can't absorb vitamin $B_{12}$ through the intestine. These patients may have one of the following conditions:

- pernicious anemia, a condition in which the body does not make enough intrinsic factor to absorb vitamin $B_{12}$ from food
- a diseased intestine (for example, Crohn disease, ulcerative colitis)
- a large part of the stomach or intestine removed (for example, from bariatric surgery)

These patients must receive $B_{12}$ by injection from a physician or other health care professional. Injections are intramuscular, or directly into the muscle. At the start, a patient may need an injection every day. Maintenance doses are given monthly.

Adverse reactions to a $B_{12}$ injection may include mild diarrhea, itching, and temporary warmth and pain at the injection site. Less likely but possible adverse reactions are trouble breathing, congestion, and tightness in the chest.

thousands of multivitamin formulations. Vitamin C is necessary to form collagen (the main fibrous protein) in bones, cartilage, muscle, and blood vessels. Vitamin C also helps the body absorb iron.

A severe lack of vitamin C causes a disease called scurvy. Scurvy is rare, but it can happen to the following people:

- people who are malnourished
- pregnant or breastfeeding women
- infants on unsupplemented milk diets

Symptoms of scurvy include liver spots on the skin, spongy gums, and bleeding from the mucous membranes. Severe scurvy can cause sudden death. Scurvy is treated with vitamin C administered under a physician's care.

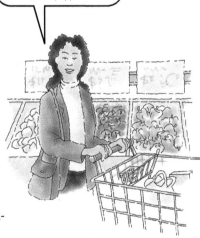

Vitamin C-rich fruits and vegetables include lemons, grapefruit, strawberries, tomatoes, tangerines, and green peppers.

**SMOOTH SAILING**

Sailors hundreds of years ago often came down with scurvy because they were away from shore and sources of fresh fruit for long periods of time. In the late 1800s, British sailors were given lime juice to prevent this disease. That's where the nickname "limey" comes from. It was originally "lime juicer."

Vitamin C is safe in the amounts people usually get from their normal diets. It is also present in breast milk. Taking high doses of vitamin C (over 1,000 mg each day) can cause many adverse reactions, including the following:

- kidney stones
- severe diarrhea
- nausea
- stomach inflammation (gastritis)

## IRON/FE

The mineral **iron** is a component of **hemoglobin,** which is a protein found in red blood cells. Iron (Femiron, Feosol, Fer-In-Sol) is also known by its generic names, ferrous sulfate and ferrous gluconate, and by its chemical name, Fe. Iron is found in meat, liver, kidney beans, oysters, dark green vegetables, carrots,

**Your Turn to Teach**    **VITAMIN C AND THE COMMON COLD**

Many patients that you see have probably heard that vitamin C can cure the common cold and respiratory infections. However, large clinical trials have shown that taking vitamin C does not reduce the risk of getting a cold. It also does not have any effect on the severity of the cold. For a small number of people, it reduces the length of a cold. So, what should you say to a patient who asks if it will help to start taking vitamin C after the cold starts? Break the news gently: the studies say no. Although it won't hurt the patient to drink some extra orange juice, it's not likely to have any effect on the patient's cold.

## Closer Look | MINERALS

In breakfast cereal commercials, the words *vitamins* and *minerals* seem to always go hand in hand. You've read about vitamins, but what are minerals exactly? **Minerals** are substances that miners dig out of the earth. However, small quantities of some minerals, like iron, are also in food. They help the body function properly and stay healthy.

The body can make two vitamins on its own—vitamin D and vitamin K. The rest of the essential vitamins and all essential minerals must be received from food. Furthermore, the body needs those dietary minerals to absorb vitamins.

Dietary minerals in different quantities are among the building blocks of bone, teeth, soft tissue, muscles, blood, and nerve cells. The body also uses minerals to make hormones and regulate the heartbeat.

Multivitamins usually contain small amounts of minerals. Mineral supplements are also available. However, in most cases, a diet rich in whole grains, seafood, fruits, and vegetables will provide all the minerals the body needs.

egg yolks, and other foods. It's also available in liquid, tablets, and capsules.

The body needs iron to bring oxygen to the cells. Although most people get enough iron in their diets, some people must take iron supplements to treat iron deficiency anemia. Iron deficiency anemia happens when there is not enough iron in the blood. If you're treating a patient with iron deficiency anemia, stress to the patient the importance of including iron-rich foods in his diet. If the physician recommends it, the patient may also take an iron supplement.

When it comes to iron supplements, what's in a name: ferrous sulfate or ferrous gluconate? What is the difference? Ferrous sulfate is actually harder on the stomach and harder to digest. People who get an upset stomach and constipation from ferrous sulfate may do better with ferrous gluconate. You should warn patients that iron supplements can cause constipation and make the stool dark. Therefore, it's important for the patient to increase fluid intake. It's also important to note that iron and

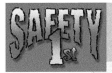

## IRON SUPPLEMENTS AND YOUNG CHILDREN

Although iron is a mineral purchased over the counter in vitamin supplements, it can be dangerous. It is the number one poison that kills children. Multivitamins taste sweet, and children sometimes watch caregivers taking vitamins and copy the behavior. It does not take a large overdose of iron to be fatal to a small child. Remind parents to keep all medications and supplements out of reach of children.

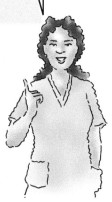

Because iron is found in several commonly eaten animal products, vegetarians must be particularly mindful that they are getting enough iron in their diets.

calcium supplements should be taken at least 1 hour apart since both compete for the same binding receptors.

## CALCIUM/CA

**Calcium** (Caltrate 600, Os-Cal 500) is an essential mineral in everyone's diet. It is also known by its generic name, calcium carbonate, and its chemical name, Ca. It is found in milk and milk products such as yogurt, cheese, and ice cream. But these foods are not the only possible source of calcium. Calcium is also found in dried beans and vegetables including broccoli and kale. Some foods, such as cereal, orange juice, and energy bars, have added calcium. Calcium supplements are available in liquid, tablet, or chewable tablet form.

What's in a name: calcium carbonate or calcium citrate? What is the difference? Most over-the-counter (OTC) calcium supplements are calcium carbonate. In order for the body to use this form, the stomach has to be functioning properly because carbonate needs hydrochloride to convert it to a usable form. Calcium citrate already has the acid molecule bound to it, so it releases better in a patient who underproduces acid or who does not have the body surface area to produce a sufficient amount of acid to convert the other form.

The body needs calcium for a number of important functions, including the following:

- formation of teeth and bones
- neuromuscular activity
- blood clotting
- cell wall permeability

## ZINC/ZN

**Zinc**/zinc gluconate is a mineral found in many supplemental drugs. Its chemical name is Zn. It helps the body's immune system function properly. Zinc is found naturally in seafood (especially oysters), meats, liver, eggs, and peanuts.

Zinc has a number of important roles in the body. It is needed for the following functions:

- building enzymes and insulin
- helping cells grow and divide and helping wounds heal
- developing the senses of smell and taste

Zinc is sold as lozenges to be used as a cold remedy for adults to shorten the length of a cold. However, zinc has not been proven to be effective for children with colds. Adverse reactions to zinc lozenges are not serious and include an unpleasant taste in the mouth and nausea. However, long-term effects have not been studied, so high doses of zinc supplements should not be taken over a long period of time.

## POTASSIUM/K

The mineral **potassium**/potassium chloride (K-Dur, K-Lor, Klotrix) is also known by its chemical name, K. Potassium aids with the functioning of the heart, kidneys, nerves, muscles, and the digestive system. You can get potassium from foods including bananas, oranges, and potatoes. Potassium supplements are sold as tablets, effervescent tablets, oral liquid, and soluble powder. Potassium is also available in the form of solution for IV injection.

Potassium aids the body with the following functions:

- muscle contractions
- conduction of nerve impulses
- balance of fluids and electrolytes

Most people get enough potassium in their diets. However, some medical conditions and the use of diuretics create low potassium levels in the body. Physicians may prescribe potassium therapy to these patients.

## FLUORIDE/FL

**Fluoride**/sodium fluoride (Fluor-A-Day, Karidium, Luride, Pediaflor) is a mineral that is essential for healthy teeth. Fluoride is also known as its chemical name, Fl.

Fluoride is added to the drinking water in most U.S. cities. However, it's sometimes prescribed as a liquid, tablet, or

## Your Turn to Teach

### TIPS FOR TAKING POTASSIUM SUPPLEMENTS

Suppose the physician has prescribed oral potassium therapy for a patient who has been diagnosed with **hypokalemia** (low blood potassium). During his next office visit, the patient says he has stopped taking the supplement because it made him nauseous. What should you tell the patient?

Gastrointestinal distress is a common adverse reaction to oral potassium. To avoid unpleasant reactions, the supplement must be taken exactly as directed on the prescription container. Oral potassium should be taken immediately after meals or with food and a full glass of water. Doses should not be increased, decreased, or omitted except on the advice of the prescribing physician. Other tips for taking various forms of oral potassium include:

- Do not chew or crush potassium tablets; these should be swallowed whole.
- If effervescent tablets have been prescribed, place the tablet in 4 to 8 ounces of cold water or juice. Wait until the fizzing stops before drinking. Sip the liquid during a period of 5 to 10 minutes.
- If the physician has prescribed an oral liquid or powder, measure the dose accurately and add it to 4 to 8 ounces of cold water or juice. Sip the mixture slowly during a period of 5 to 10 minutes.

Remind the patient to consult the physician about the use of nonprescription drugs or salt substitutes (many contain potassium). In addition, the patient should contact his health care provider if he experiences any of the following reactions:

- tingling of the hands and feet
- unusual tiredness or weakness
- a feeling of heaviness in the legs
- severe nausea
- vomiting
- abdominal pain
- black stools (GI bleeding)

chewable tablet for people who live in places where the water does not have added fluoride.

Fluoride has a number of health benefits and is used to do the following:

- prevent tooth decay
- help the teeth resist acid
- stop bacteria from forming cavities

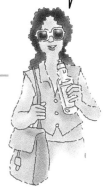

Bottled water is popular, but it may not contain the fluoride that you need for healthy teeth.

## Herbal Supplements

The FDA classifies vitamins, minerals, and herbal supplements as **dietary supplements.** As defined by law, these products contain ingredients that are meant to supplement, or add to, a person's regular diet.

Herbal medicine was humanity's first medicine. In the modern world, devotees call it **alternative medicine** or **traditional medicine.** Practitioners of herbal medicine still exist in many cultures. Indeed, modern pharmaceutical companies look to nature to find the chemicals to make tomorrow's cures.

The herbs used in medications and supplements are called *medicinal herbs.* Herbs used in cooking are called *culinary herbs.* Medicinal herbs often come from shrubs or woody plants. Culinary herbs are usually made from the leaves of nonwoody plants.

Herbal supplements have become very popular. But, sometimes, they can cause medical problems or interfere with prescription and over-the-counter medications.

### LACK OF REGULATION BY THE FEDERAL GOVERNMENT

The Food and Drug Administration (FDA) requires drug manufacturers to submit their products through a rigorous process of testing and approval before they can be sold on the market. There is no similar process for herbal supplements. The FDA does not have the authority to approve herbal supplements as safe and effective.

The Dietary Supplement Health and Education Act (DSHEA) of 1994 set the standards for the safety and labeling of dietary supplements. According to DSHEA, the maker alone is responsible for guaranteeing that the product is safe. The maker also must be sure that there is adequate evidence to back up any claims the seller makes about the health benefits of the product. However, the manufacturer does *not* have to submit any of this evidence to the FDA. The maker does not even have to register its products with the FDA before selling them to the public.

What happens if something goes wrong and a product causes unwanted adverse reactions? According to DSHEA, once a product is on the market, the FDA then becomes responsible for showing that a product is "unsafe." If the charge is proven, the product can be taken off the market or be restricted in its use.

## INTERACTIONS WITH OTHER MEDICATIONS

Some herbal medications do not mix well with over-the-counter and prescription medications that patients may be taking. If a patient is taking herbal medications, the medication may not work as well as it should.

Patients may experience serious adverse reactions if they take one of the following kinds of drugs along with herbal medications:

- antidepressants or antianxiety drugs

- anticonvulsant drugs

- blood thinners

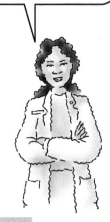

An herb called kava was being sold as a remedy for stress and anxiety. In 2002, the FDA issued a strong advisory against using it. Evidence was mounting that kava causes severe liver damage—including hepatitis, cirrhosis, and liver failure.

## Your Turn to Teach      BUYING HERBAL SUPPLEMENTS

Teach patients to follow these guidelines before purchasing herbal supplements:

- *Do your research.* Find out as much as you can about the products you're considering using.

- *Talk to your physician.* Let your physician know that you've been thinking about taking an herbal supplement. Ask if it's safe to take the supplement with other prescription and over-the-counter medications you're currently taking.

- *Read labels carefully.* Labels on products with more than one herb often do not tell how much of each herb is in the formula. That's why it's safer to buy single-herb products. The label should also show how much of the herb each dose contains.

- *Be very cautious about herbal supplements from other countries.* Some can contain ingredients with health risks.

- *Be wary of outrageous claims that sound too good to be true.* No single remedy can cure every possible ill.

- blood pressure medicines
- heart medicines
- diabetes drugs
- cancer drugs

## COMPLICATIONS DURING AND AFTER SURGERY

Herbal medicines can also interfere with surgery. If you're helping patients who are preparing for surgery, remind them to tell the physician what herbal preparations they are taking—even if they have taken those preparations for a long time without problem. The physician may want patients to stop taking supplements for as long as 3 weeks before surgery. This will ensure that nothing is left in their systems that may cause harm.

Here is a sampling of the problems that some herbs can cause for a patient in surgery.

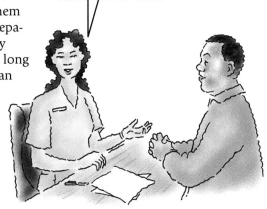

Everything you put into your body has some effect on it. Remind patients to tell the physician if they are using any kind of herbal supplement.

### Herbal Supplements and Possible Surgical Complications

| Supplement | Complications |
| --- | --- |
| echinacea | • may interfere with immune functioning<br>• may make the body more likely to reject a replacement organ after transplant surgery |
| garlic | • may cause bleeding<br>• may keep blood from clotting normally |
| ginkgo biloba | • may cause bleeding |
| St. John's wort | • may affect how some drugs work during and after surgery |
| valerian | • may interfere with anesthesia |

## COMMONLY USED HERBAL SUPPLEMENTS

Medical science is testing the usefulness of many herbal medications. Following are the findings about a selection of popular herbal supplements.

## Echinacea

Echinacea belongs to the aster family. Oral preparations made from the roots and above-ground parts of this species are popular in the United States and Europe for treating upper respiratory tract infections (URIs).

Human trials in Europe have found that taking echinacea when symptoms of a URI start to appear can shorten the infection and make it less severe. Clinical trials on adults in the United States, however, do not support the results of the European trials. Overall, the evidence leads to no clear conclusion, and better trials are needed.

In addition, studies have found the following:

- Human trials show that taking echinacea daily does not prevent URIs.
- No benefit to children ages 2 to 11 years has been reported.
- Preliminary studies of taking echinacea by mouth to treat genital herpes are inconclusive.
- No evidence supports suggestions that echinacea can help wounds heal or have an effect on *Candida albicans* infections.

## Lavender

Lavender flowers are used in aromatherapy. Manufacturers use lavender's fragrant oils to make candles, cosmetics, detergents, jellies, massage oils, perfumes, shampoos, soaps, teas, and many other products. English lavender is most commonly used.

Many people find lavender aromatherapy relaxing. There is some evidence to suggest that lavender can also reduce anxiety. However, until better studies are done, the evidence is still weak.

Lavender aromatherapy is also used as a hypnotic, or sleep aid. However, there isn't enough evidence to support this use.

## Ginkgo Biloba

People have used ginkgo biloba as a medicinal herb for thousands of years. Although not FDA approved, evidence shows that it's effective against the following conditions:

- leg pain caused by clogged arteries (claudication)
- dementia (decreasing brain function) due to multiple strokes or Alzheimer disease
- poor concentration and other problems that come from poor blood flow to the brain ("cerebral insufficiency")

It is no longer thought that ginkgo biloba offers any benefit to people suffering from tinnitus (ringing in the ears).

Ginkgo biloba may cause bleeding. Patients using blood thinners should use it with caution. They should also use it with caution before some surgical or dental procedures.

### Ginseng

The ginseng root has been a staple of Chinese traditional medicine for more than 2,000 years. Ginseng has been used to increase stamina and endurance and to increase mental and physical performance. Siberian ginseng, another species, has been used to build up resistance to colds and other mild infections.

Studies also report good (but not strong) scientific evidence for using ginseng to lower blood sugar in patients with type 2 diabetes. For this use, however, the long-term effects of ginseng are not clear. Patients should not use ginseng in place of standard diabetes treatments.

> As an employee of a medical office, it's important to know the physician's position on herbal remedies. Avoid offering patients your own opinions about herbal supplements and refer specific questions to the physician instead.

### Saw Palmetto

In Europe, saw palmetto is the most common herbal remedy for an enlarged prostate. Long ago in the Americas, the Mayan people used it as a tonic. The Seminole people used it as an expectorant and an antiseptic.

The following uses of saw palmetto have been tested scientifically:

- Strong scientific evidence suggests that saw palmetto improves nighttime urination problems and urine flow in men who have enlarged prostates.
- Unclear scientific evidence exists for using saw palmetto to treat male-pattern baldness and underactive bladders.
- A fair amount of evidence exists for *not* using saw palmetto to treat prostate infections or chronic pelvic pain.

### Ginger

Ginger has had an important role in Chinese, Japanese, and Indian medicine since the 1500s. There is little scientific evidence for many of its popular uses, such as curing upset stomach, nausea, and motion sickness. However, good (but not strong) scientific evidence exists for using ginger to control nausea and vomiting during pregnancy if it's used for less than 5 days.

Supplements containing ginger have often had harmful impurities and additives. Since the 1500s, ginger tea has been a common, safe way to deliver this herb.

## Cinnamon

Used often in cooking today, cinnamon was used historically for its medicinal properties. The Egyptians used cinnamon in embalming. During the bubonic plague in the Middle Ages, people placed cinnamon mixed with cloves and water in victims' bedrooms.

Some recent scientific studies have shown some results of interest:

- memory improvements
- help with urinary tract infections
- lowering blood sugar levels
- lowering blood cholesterol

The tests were generally limited in scope, however, and further study is needed.

## Lycopene

Lycopene is the pigment that makes tomatoes red. This water-soluble pigment (called a carotenoid) is found in human blood, the liver, the adrenal glands, the lungs, the prostate, the colon, and the skin.

Many studies indicate that eating large amounts of foods that contain lycopene may lower the risk of cancer, heart disease, and macular degeneration, a condition that can lead to blindness. However, these studies are based on eating tomatoes, not lycopene supplements. Because tomatoes also contain vitamin C, folate, and potassium, these studies do not offer clear proof that lycopene alone is the source of these benefits.

## Peppermint

Good (though not strong) scientific evidence exits for the use of peppermint to treat heartburn and symptoms of irritable bowel syndrome (IBS).

Unclear scientific evidence exists for using peppermint to treat coughs, nasal congestion, nausea, pain from herpes zoster, tension headaches, or urinary tract infections. Further research is needed.

Peppermint oil is available as enteric-coated capsules, soft gelatin capsules, and in liquid form. Liquid preparations may contain sugar or alcohol. Patients with diabetes and people who suffer from alcohol addiction should use the product with caution.

## SAFETY 1st

### USE CAUTION WITH SALVIA

Leaves from the sage plant (*Salvia officinalis*), a member of the mint family, have been used to treat excessive sweating, indigestion, and loss of appetite. Researchers have found no evidence for these claims. Laboratory tests of some supplements containing salvia have found possibly harmful additives or impurities in the sample.

Liquid preparations of salvia may contain sugar or alcohol. Patients with diabetes and people with alcohol dependence should use the product with caution and read the label carefully. The FDA has not yet reviewed salvia for safety or effectiveness.

Another member of the mint family, *Salvia divinorum*, is being sold on the Internet. This herb, also known as Diviner's Sage and Magic Mint, is an unregulated hallucinogen that's being marketed as an alternative to regulated plant hallucinogens. *S. divinorum* is used by shamans of the Mazatec people of southern Mexico to go on "spirit journeys."

### St. John's Wort

Extracts of St. John's wort (*Hypericum perforatum* L.) were used in the past to treat many medical conditions. Today, its most popular use is to treat depression. These are the important scientific findings:

- Many short-term studies report that St. John's wort is more effective than tricyclic antidepressants such as amitriptyline (Elavil) to treat mild to moderate major depression.

- Evidence for using St. John's wort to treat severe depression remains unclear.

A fair amount of scientific evidence exists against using St. John's wort to treat these conditions:

- human immunodeficiency virus (HIV)
- social phobia

Wort is an old name meaning "root plant." You'll find it in other traditional names for plants, too. Figwort, liverwort, moneywort, and spiderwort are some examples.

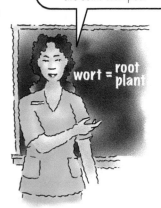

wort = root plant

## *Immunizations*

One of the most important jobs that you may have in a medical office is to assist with **immunizations.** It may be unpleasant to work with toddlers—and even adolescents—who would do anything to avoid getting an injection. However, despite a few seconds of discomfort, the benefits to the patient are immense. Children who are up-to-date with their immunizations will avoid the major diseases of childhood.

It's not just children who benefit from immunizations. During flu season, many adults will start asking when they can get their flu vaccine.

These are the immunizations you'll learn about:

- MMR (measles, mumps, and rubella)
- DTaP (diphtheria, whooping cough, and tetanus)
- varicella (chickenpox)
- hepatitis B virus (HBV)
- pneumococcal
- influenza

You'll also learn about other available immunizations for children under 18 and for travelers.

> Smallpox was the first disease for which scientists developed an effective vaccine. The last case of smallpox in the United States was in 1949. The last case in the world was in 1977, in Somalia.

## PURPOSE OF IMMUNIZATIONS

Before immunizations were available, people—especially children—died from a range of diseases that are easily prevented today. Those diseases caused disfigurement, deformity, and even death. Today, millions of people are spared the effects of these diseases thanks to immunization with **vaccines.**

What is a vaccine? It's a weakened or dead form of a disease or a related disease. When a physician or nurse injects a vaccine into someone, the vaccine puts the body's immune system to work. It creates disease-fighting antibodies that protect the body from the disease or that lessen the disease's effects.

## IMMUNIZATION SCHEDULES

If your medical office has many infants, children, and adolescents among its patients, your supervisor may ask you to use an immunization schedule to check dates. The CDC publish these schedules and update them each year. Downloadable versions are also available for keeping track of these dates electronically.

There are separate schedules for children from birth through age 6 and from ages 7 to 18. There is also a catch-up schedule for people whose immunizations were delayed. These immunization schedules are shown on pages 226–228.

## Legal Brief | NATIONAL VACCINATION ACT

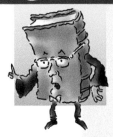

The full name of the 1986 National Vaccination Act is the National Childhood Vaccine Injury Act (NCVIA). This law protects vaccine manufacturers from lawsuits regarding injury from vaccine injections. The fear was that drug companies might be unable to prepare enough supplies of a vaccine in time if they also had to use their funds and resources to resolve lawsuits.

As a result of this law, physicians must take part in the Vaccine Adverse Event Reporting System (VAERS). VAERS is operated by the Centers for Disease Control and Prevention (CDC) and the FDA. This system allows the government to collect information about possible adverse reactions from immunizations. (A copy of the reporting form that VAERS uses is shown on page 225.)

Additionally, physicians must give a vaccine information statement (VIS) to each patient, her parent, or her legal guardian before receiving certain vaccines. You must use the official VIS forms your office has. A VIS is required for the following vaccines:

- diphtheria
- tetanus
- pertussis
- polio
- measles
- mumps
- rubella
- hepatitis B virus
- Hib (*Haemophilus influenzae* type b)
- varicella

Remember what you learned about charting vaccinations in Chapter 3. Your office will need the exact and accurate information you provide if a patient suffers from an adverse reaction.

WEBSITE: www.vaers.hhs.gov   E-MAIL: info@vaers.org    FAX: 1-877-721-0366

## VAERS

**VACCINE ADVERSE EVENT REPORTING SYSTEM**
24 Hour Toll-Free Information  1-800-822-7967
P.O. Box 1100, Rockville, MD 20849-1100
**PATIENT IDENTITY KEPT CONFIDENTIAL**

**For CDC/FDA Use Only**

VAERS Number _____

Date Received _____

Patient Name: _____

Last        First        M.I.

Address _____

City        State        Zip

Telephone no. (____) _____

Vaccine administered by (Name): _____

Responsible
Physician _____
Facility Name/Address _____

City        State        Zip

Telephone no. (____) _____

Form completed by (Name): _____

Relation    ☐ Vaccine Provider  ☐ Patient/Parent
to Patient  ☐ Manufacturer      ☐ Other
Address (*if different from patient or provider*)
_____

City        State        Zip

Telephone no. (____) _____

| 1. State | 2. County where administered | 3. Date of birth  mm / dd / yy | 4. Patient age | 5. Sex  ☐ M ☐ F | 6. Date form completed  mm / dd / yy |

7. Describe adverse events(s) (symptoms, signs, time course) and treatment, if any

8. Check all appropriate:
☐ Patient died       (date ___ / ___ / ___ )
                              mm   dd   yy
☐ Life threatening illness
☐ Required emergency room/doctor visit
☐ Required hospitalization (_____days)
☐ Resulted in prolongation of hospitalization
☐ Resulted in permanent disability
☐ None of the above

9. Patient recovered    ☐ YES  ☐ NO  ☐ UNKNOWN

12. Relevant diagnostic tests/laboratory data

10. Date of vaccination
mm / dd / yy
Time _____ AM PM

11. Adverse event onset
mm / dd / yy
Time _____ AM PM

13. Enter all vaccines given on date listed in no. 10

|  | Vaccine (type) | Manufacturer | Lot number | Route/Site | No. Previous Doses |
|---|---|---|---|---|---|
| a. | | | | | |
| b. | | | | | |
| c. | | | | | |
| d. | | | | | |

14. Any other vaccinations within 4 weeks prior to the date listed in no. 10

|  | Vaccine (type) | Manufacturer | Lot number | Route/Site | No. Previous doses | Date given |
|---|---|---|---|---|---|---|
| a. | | | | | | |
| b. | | | | | | |

15. Vaccinated at:
☐ Private doctor's office/hospital    ☐ Military clinic/hospital
☐ Public health clinic/hospital       ☐ Other/unknown

16. Vaccine purchased with:
☐ Private funds  ☐ Military funds
☐ Public funds   ☐ Other/unknown

17. Other medications

18. Illness at time of vaccination (specify)

19. Pre-existing physician-diagnosed allergies, birth defects, medical conditions (specify)

20. Have you reported this adverse event previously?
☐ No      ☐ To health department
☐ To doctor   ☐ To manufacturer

**Only for children 5 and under**

22. Birth weight _____ lb. _____ oz.

23. No. of brothers and sisters

21. Adverse event following prior vaccination (check all applicable, specify)

|  | Adverse Event | Onset Age | Type Vaccine | Dose no. in series |
|---|---|---|---|---|
| ☐ In patient | | | | |
| ☐ In brother or sister | | | | |

**Only for reports submitted by manufacturer/immunization project**

24. Mfr./imm. proj. report no.

25. Date received by mfr./imm.proj.

26. 15 day report?    ☐ Yes   ☐ No

27. Report type    ☐ Initial   ☐ Follow-Up

Health care providers and manufacturers are required by law (42 USC 300aa-25) to report reactions to vaccines listed in the Table of Reportable Events Following Immunization.
Reports for reactions to other vaccines are voluntary except when required as a condition of immunization grant awards.

Form VAERS-1(FDA)

DEPARTMENT OF HEALTH AND HUMAN SERVICES • CENTERS FOR DISEASE CONTROL AND PREVENTION

# Recommended Immunization Schedule for Persons Aged 0–6 Years—UNITED STATES • 2007

| Vaccine ▼     Age ▶ | Birth | 1 month | 2 months | 4 months | 6 months | 12 months | 15 months | 18 months | 19–23 months | 2–3 years | 4–6 years |
|---|---|---|---|---|---|---|---|---|---|---|---|
| **Hepatitis B**[1] | HepB | HepB | *see footnote 1* | | HepB | | | | | HepB Series | |
| **Rotavirus**[2] | | | Rota | Rota | Rota | | | | | | |
| **Diphtheria, Tetanus, Pertussis**[3] | | | DTaP | DTaP | DTaP | | DTaP | | | | DTaP |
| ***Haemophilus influenzae* type b**[4] | | | Hib | Hib | *Hib*[4] | Hib | | Hib | | | |
| **Pneumococcal**[5] | | | PCV | PCV | PCV | PCV | | | | PCV PPV | |
| **Inactivated Poliovirus** | | | IPV | IPV | | IPV | | | | | IPV |
| **Influenza**[6] | | | | | | Influenza (Yearly) | | | | | |
| **Measles, Mumps, Rubella**[7] | | | | | | MMR | | | | | MMR |
| **Varicella**[8] | | | | | | Varicella | | | | | Varicella |
| **Hepatitis A**[9] | | | | | | HepA (2 doses) | | | | HepA Series | |
| **Meningococcal**[10] | | | | | | | | | | MPSV4 | |

Range of recommended ages

Catch-up immunization

Certain high-risk groups

This schedule indicates the recommended ages for routine administration of currently licensed childhood vaccines, as of December 1, 2006, for children aged 0–6 years. Additional information is available at http://www.cdc.gov/nip/recs/child-schedule.htm. Any dose not administered at the recommended age should be administered at any subsequent visit, when indicated and feasible. Additional vaccines may be licensed and recommended during the year. Licensed combination vaccines may be used whenever any components of the combination are indicated and other components of the vaccine are not contraindicated and if approved by the Food and Drug Administration for that dose of the series. Providers should consult the respective Advisory Committee on Immunization Practices statement for detailed recommendations. Clinically significant adverse events that follow immunization should be reported to the Vaccine Adverse Event Reporting System (VAERS). Guidance about how to obtain and complete a VAERS form is available at http://www.vaers.hhs.gov or by telephone, 800-822-7967.

**1. Hepatitis B vaccine (HepB).** *(Minimum age: birth)*
**At birth:**
- Administer monovalent HepB to all newborns before hospital discharge.
- If mother is hepatitis surface antigen (HBsAg)-positive, administer HepB and 0.5 mL of hepatitis B immune globulin (HBIG) within 12 hours of birth.
- If mother's HBsAg status is unknown, administer HepB within 12 hours of birth. Determine the HBsAg status as soon as possible and if HBsAg-positive, administer HBIG (no later than age 1 week).
- If mother is HBsAg-negative, the birth dose can only be delayed with physician's order and mother's negative HBsAg laboratory report documented in the infant's medical record.
**After the birth dose:**
- The HepB series should be completed with either monovalent HepB or a combination vaccine containing HepB. The second dose should be administered at age 1–2 months. The final dose should be administered at age ≥24 weeks. Infants born to HBsAg-positive mothers should be tested for HBsAg and antibody to HBsAg after completion of ≥3 doses of a licensed HepB series, at age 9–18 months (generally at the next well-child visit).
**4-month dose:**
- It is permissible to administer 4 doses of HepB when combination vaccines are administered after the birth dose. If monovalent HepB is used for doses after the birth dose, a dose at age 4 months is not needed.

**2. Rotavirus vaccine (Rota).** *(Minimum age: 6 weeks)*
- Administer the first dose at age 6–12 weeks. Do not start the series later than age 12 weeks.
- Administer the final dose in the series by age 32 weeks. Do not administer a dose later than age 32 weeks.
- Data on safety and efficacy outside of these age ranges are insufficient.

**3. Diphtheria and tetanus toxoids and acellular pertussis vaccine (DTaP).** *(Minimum age: 6 weeks)*
- The fourth dose of DTaP may be administered as early as age 12 months, provided 6 months have elapsed since the third dose.
- Administer the final dose in the series at age 4–6 years.

**4. *Haemophilus influenzae* type b conjugate vaccine (Hib).**
*(Minimum age: 6 weeks)*
- If PRP-OMP (PedvaxHIB® or ComVax® [Merck]) is administered at ages 2 and 4 months, a dose at age 6 months is not required.
- TriHiBit® (DTaP/Hib) combination products should not be used for primary immunization but can be used as boosters following any Hib vaccine in children aged ≥12 months.

**5. Pneumococcal vaccine.** *(Minimum age: 6 weeks for pneumococcal conjugate vaccine [PCV]; 2 years for pneumococcal polysaccharide vaccine [PPV])*
- Administer PCV at ages 24–59 months in certain high-risk groups. Administer PPV to children aged ≥2 years in certain high-risk groups. See *MMWR* 2000;49(No. RR-9):1–35.

**6. Influenza vaccine.** *(Minimum age: 6 months for trivalent inactivated influenza vaccine [TIV]; 5 years for live, attenuated influenza vaccine [LAIV])*
- All children aged 6–59 months and close contacts of all children aged 0–59 months are recommended to receive influenza vaccine.
- Influenza vaccine is recommended annually for children aged ≥59 months with certain risk factors, health-care workers, and other persons (including household members) in close contact with persons in groups at high risk. See *MMWR* 2006;55(No. RR-10):1–41.
- For healthy persons aged 5–49 years, LAIV may be used as an alternative to TIV.
- Children receiving TIV should receive 0.25 mL if aged 6–35 months or 0.5 mL if aged ≥3 years.
- Children aged <9 years who are receiving influenza vaccine for the first time should receive 2 doses (separated by ≥4 weeks for TIV and ≥6 weeks for LAIV).

**7. Measles, mumps, and rubella vaccine (MMR).** *(Minimum age: 12 months)*
- Administer the second dose of MMR at age 4–6 years. MMR may be administered before age 4–6 years, provided ≥4 weeks have elapsed since the first dose and both doses are administered at age ≥12 months.

**8. Varicella vaccine.** *(Minimum age: 12 months)*
- Administer the second dose of varicella vaccine at age 4–6 years. Varicella vaccine may be administered before age 4–6 years, provided that ≥3 months have elapsed since the first dose and both doses are administered at age ≥12 months. If second dose was administered ≥28 days following the first dose, the second dose does not need to be repeated.

**9. Hepatitis A vaccine (HepA).** *(Minimum age: 12 months)*
- HepA is recommended for all children aged 1 year (i.e., aged 12–23 months). The 2 doses in the series should be administered at least 6 months apart.
- Children not fully vaccinated by age 2 years can be vaccinated at subsequent visits.
- HepA is recommended for certain other groups of children, including in areas where vaccination programs target older children. See *MMWR* 2006;55(No. RR-7):1–23.

**10. Meningococcal polysaccharide vaccine (MPSV4).** *(Minimum age: 2 years)*
- Administer MPSV4 to children aged 2–10 years with terminal complement deficiencies or anatomic or functional asplenia and certain other high-risk groups. See *MMWR* 2005;54(No. RR-7):1–21.

The Recommended Immunization Schedules for Persons Aged 0–18 Years are approved by the Advisory Committee on Immunization Practices (http://www.cdc.gov/nip/acip), the American Academy of Pediatrics (http://www.aap.org), and the American Academy of Family Physicians (http://www.aafp.org).

SAFER • HEALTHIER • PEOPLE™

DEPARTMENT OF HEALTH AND HUMAN SERVICES • CENTERS FOR DISEASE CONTROL AND PREVENTION

# Recommended Immunization Schedule for Persons Aged 7–18 Years—UNITED STATES • 2007

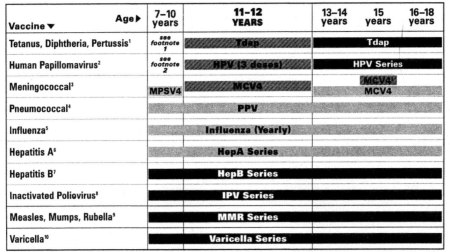

| Vaccine ▼ / Age ▶ | 7–10 years | 11–12 YEARS | 13–14 years | 15 years | 16–18 years |
|---|---|---|---|---|---|
| Tetanus, Diphtheria, Pertussis[1] | see footnote 1 | Tdap | Tdap | | |
| Human Papillomavirus[2] | see footnote 2 | HPV (3 doses) | HPV Series | | |
| Meningococcal[3] | MPSV4 | MCV4 | MCV4 / MCV4 | | |
| Pneumococcal[4] | | PPV | | | |
| Influenza[5] | | Influenza (Yearly) | | | |
| Hepatitis A[6] | | HepA Series | | | |
| Hepatitis B[7] | | HepB Series | | | |
| Inactivated Poliovirus[8] | | IPV Series | | | |
| Measles, Mumps, Rubella[9] | | MMR Series | | | |
| Varicella[10] | | Varicella Series | | | |

Legend:
- Range of recommended ages
- Catch-up immunization
- Certain high-risk groups

This schedule indicates the recommended ages for routine administration of currently licensed childhood vaccines, as of December 1, 2006, for children aged 7–18 years. Additional information is available at http://www.cdc.gov/nip/recs/child-schedule.htm. Any dose not administered at the recommended age should be administered at any subsequent visit, when indicated and feasible. Additional vaccines may be licensed and recommended during the year. Licensed combination vaccines may be used whenever any components of the combination are indicated and other components of the vaccine are not contraindicated and if approved by the Food and Drug Administration for that dose of the series. Providers should consult the respective Advisory Committee on Immunization Practices statement for detailed recommendations. Clinically significant adverse events that follow immunization should be reported to the Vaccine Adverse Event Reporting System (VAERS). Guidance about how to obtain and complete a VAERS form is available at http://www.vaers.hhs.gov or by telephone, 800-822-7967.

1. **Tetanus and diphtheria toxoids and acellular pertussis vaccine (Tdap).** *(Minimum age: 10 years for BOOSTRIX® and 11 years for ADACEL™)*
   - Administer at age 11–12 years for those who have completed the recommended childhood DTP/DTaP vaccination series and have not received a tetanus and diphtheria toxoids vaccine (Td) booster dose.
   - Adolescents aged 13–18 years who missed the 11–12 year Td/Tdap booster dose should also receive a single dose of Tdap if they have completed the recommended childhood DTP/DTaP vaccination series.

2. **Human papillomavirus vaccine (HPV).** *(Minimum age: 9 years)*
   - Administer the first dose of the HPV vaccine series to females at age 11–12 years.
   - Administer the second dose 2 months after the first dose and the third dose 6 months after the first dose.
   - Administer the HPV vaccine series to females at age 13–18 years if not previously vaccinated.

3. **Meningococcal vaccine.** *(Minimum age: 11 years for meningococcal conjugate vaccine [MCV4]; 2 years for meningococcal polysaccharide vaccine [MPSV4])*
   - Administer MCV4 at age 11–12 years and to previously unvaccinated adolescents at high school entry (at approximately age 15 years).
   - Administer MCV4 to previously unvaccinated college freshmen living in dormitories; MPSV4 is an acceptable alternative.
   - Vaccination against invasive meningococcal disease is recommended for children and adolescents aged ≥2 years with terminal complement deficiencies or anatomic or functional asplenia and certain other high-risk groups. See *MMWR* 2005;54(No. RR-7):1–21. Use MPSV4 for children aged 2–10 years and MCV4 or MPSV4 for older children.

4. **Pneumococcal polysaccharide vaccine (PPV).** *(Minimum age: 2 years)*
   - Administer for certain high-risk groups. See *MMWR* 1997;46(No. RR-8):1–24, and *MMWR* 2000;49(No. RR-9):1–35.

5. **Influenza vaccine.** *(Minimum age: 6 months for trivalent inactivated influenza vaccine [TIV]; 5 years for live, attenuated influenza vaccine [LAIV])*
   - Influenza vaccine is recommended annually for persons with certain risk factors, health-care workers, and other persons (including household members) in close contact with persons in groups at high risk. See *MMWR* 2006;55 (No. RR-10):1–41.
   - For healthy persons aged 5–49 years, LAIV may be used as an alternative to TIV.
   - Children aged <9 years who are receiving influenza vaccine for the first time should receive 2 doses (separated by ≥4 weeks for TIV and ≥6 weeks for LAIV).

6. **Hepatitis A vaccine (HepA).** *(Minimum age: 12 months)*
   - The 2 doses in the series should be administered at least 6 months apart.
   - HepA is recommended for certain other groups of children, including in areas where vaccination programs target older children. See *MMWR* 2006;55 (No. RR-7):1–23.

7. **Hepatitis B vaccine (HepB).** *(Minimum age: birth)*
   - Administer the 3-dose series to those who were not previously vaccinated.
   - A 2-dose series of Recombivax HB® is licensed for children aged 11–15 years.

8. **Inactivated poliovirus vaccine (IPV).** *(Minimum age: 6 weeks)*
   - For children who received an all-IPV or all-oral poliovirus (OPV) series, a fourth dose is not necessary if the third dose was administered at age ≥4 years.
   - If both OPV and IPV were administered as part of a series, a total of 4 doses should be administered, regardless of the child's current age.

9. **Measles, mumps, and rubella vaccine (MMR).** *(Minimum age: 12 months)*
   - If not previously vaccinated, administer 2 doses of MMR during any visit, with ≥4 weeks between the doses.

10. **Varicella vaccine.** *(Minimum age: 12 months)*
    - Administer 2 doses of varicella vaccine to persons without evidence of immunity.
    - Administer 2 doses of varicella vaccine to persons aged <13 years at least 3 months apart. Do not repeat the second dose, if administered ≥28 days after the first dose.
    - Administer 2 doses of varicella vaccine to persons aged ≥13 years at least 4 weeks apart.

The Recommended Immunization Schedules for Persons Aged 0–18 Years are approved by the Advisory Committee on Immunization Practices (http://www.cdc.gov/nip/acip), the American Academy of Pediatrics (http://www.aap.org), and the American Academy of Family Physicians (http://www.aafp.org).

SAFER • HEALTHIER • PEOPLE™

# Catch-up Immunization Schedule
## for Persons Aged 4 Months–18 Years Who Start Late or Who Are More Than 1 Month Behind

**UNITED STATES • 2007**

The table below provides catch-up schedules and minimum intervals between doses for children whose vaccinations have been delayed. A vaccine series does not need to be restarted, regardless of the time that has elapsed between doses. Use the section appropriate for the child's age.

### CATCH-UP SCHEDULE FOR PERSONS AGED 4 MONTHS–6 YEARS

| Vaccine | Minimum Age for Dose 1 | Minimum Interval Between Doses | | | |
|---|---|---|---|---|---|
| | | Dose 1 to Dose 2 | Dose 2 to Dose 3 | Dose 3 to Dose 4 | Dose 4 to Dose 5 |
| Hepatitis B[1] | Birth | 4 weeks | 8 weeks (and 16 weeks after first dose) | | |
| Rotavirus[2] | 6 wks | 4 weeks | 4 weeks | | |
| Diphtheria, Tetanus, Pertussis[3] | 6 wks | 4 weeks | 4 weeks | 6 months | 6 months[3] |
| Haemophilus influenzae type b[4] | 6 wks | 4 weeks if first dose administered at age <12 months / 8 weeks (as final dose) if first dose administered at age 12-14 months / No further doses needed if first dose administered at age ≥15 months | 4 weeks[4] if current age <12 months / 8 weeks (as final dose)[4] if current age ≥12 months and second dose administered at age <15 months / No further doses needed if previous dose administered at age ≥15months | 8 weeks (as final dose) This dose only necessary for children aged 12 months–5 years who received 3 doses before age 12 months | |
| Pneumococcal[5] | 6 wks | 4 weeks if first dose administered at age <12 months and current age <24 months / 8 weeks (as final dose) if first dose administered at age ≥12 months or current age 24–59 months / No further doses needed for healthy children if first dose administered at age ≥24 months | 4 weeks if current age <12 months / 8 weeks (as final dose) if current age ≥12 months / No further doses needed for healthy children if previous dose administered at age ≥24 months | 8 weeks (as final dose) This dose only necessary for children aged 12 months–5 years who received 3 doses before age 12 months | |
| Inactivated Poliovirus[6] | 6 wks | 4 weeks | 4 weeks | 4 weeks[6] | |
| Measles, Mumps, Rubella[7] | 12 mos | 4 weeks | | | |
| Varicella[8] | 12 mos | 3 months | | | |
| Hepatitis A[9] | 12 mos | 6 months | | | |

### CATCH-UP SCHEDULE FOR PERSONS AGED 7–18 YEARS

| Vaccine | Minimum Age for Dose 1 | Dose 1 to Dose 2 | Dose 2 to Dose 3 | Dose 3 to Dose 4 | |
|---|---|---|---|---|---|
| Tetanus, Diphtheria/ Tetanus, Diphtheria, Pertussis[10] | 7 yrs[10] | 4 weeks | 8 weeks if first dose administered at age <12 months / 6 months if first dose administered at age ≥12 months | 6 months if first dose administered at age <12 months | |
| Human Papillomavirus[11] | 9 yrs | 4 weeks | 12 weeks | | |
| Hepatitis A[9] | 12 mos | 6 months | | | |
| Hepatitis B[1] | Birth | 4 weeks | 8 weeks (and 16 weeks after first dose) | | |
| Inactivated Poliovirus[6] | 6 wks | 4 weeks | 4 weeks | 4 weeks[6] | |
| Measles, Mumps, Rubella[7] | 12 mos | 4 weeks | | | |
| Varicella[8] | 12 mos | 4 weeks if first dose administered at age ≥13 years / 3 months if first dose administered at age <13 years | | | |

1. **Hepatitis B vaccine (HepB).** *(Minimum age: birth)*
   - Administer the 3-dose series to those who were not previously vaccinated.
   - A 2-dose series of Recombivax HB® is licensed for children aged 11–15 years.

2. **Rotavirus vaccine (Rota).** *(Minimum age: 6 weeks)*
   - Do not start the series later than age 12 weeks.
   - Administer the final dose in the series by age 32 weeks. Do not administer a dose later than age 32 weeks.
   - Data on safety and efficacy outside of these age ranges are insufficient.

3. **Diphtheria and tetanus toxoids and acellular pertussis vaccine (DTaP).** *(Minimum age: 6 weeks)*
   - The fifth dose is not necessary if the fourth dose was administered at age ≥4 years.
   - DTaP is not indicated for persons aged ≥7 years.

4. **Haemophilus influenzae type b conjugate vaccine (Hib).** *(Minimum age: 6 weeks)*
   - Vaccine is not generally recommended for children aged ≥5 years.
   - If current age <12 months and the first 2 doses were PRP-OMP [PedvaxHIB® or ComVax® (Merck)], the third (and final) dose should be administered at age 12– 15 months and at least 8 weeks after the second dose.
   - If first dose was administered at age 7–11 months, administer 2 doses separated by 4 weeks plus a booster at age 12–15 months.

5. **Pneumococcal conjugate vaccine (PCV).** *(Minimum age: 6 weeks)*
   - Vaccine is not generally recommended for children aged ≥5 years.

6. **Inactivated poliovirus vaccine (IPV).** *(Minimum age: 6 weeks)*
   - For children who received an all-IPV or all-oral poliovirus (OPV) series, a fourth dose is not necessary if third dose was administered at age ≥4 years.
   - If both OPV and IPV were administered as part of a series, a total of 4 doses should be administered, regardless of the child's current age.

7. **Measles, mumps, and rubella vaccine (MMR).** *(Minimum age: 12 months)*
   - The second dose of MMR is recommended routinely at age 4–6 years but may be administered earlier if desired.
   - If not previously vaccinated, administer 2 doses of MMR during any visit with ≥4 weeks between the doses.

8. **Varicella vaccine.** *(Minimum age: 12 months)*
   - The second dose of varicella vaccine is recommended routinely at age 4–6 years but may be administered earlier if desired.
   - Do not repeat the second dose in persons aged <13 years if administered ≥28 days after the first dose.

9. **Hepatitis A vaccine (HepA).** *(Minimum age: 12 months)*
   - HepA is recommended for certain groups of children, including in areas where vaccination programs target older children. See *MMWR* 2006;55(No. RR-7):1–23.

10. **Tetanus and diphtheria toxoids vaccine (Td) and tetanus and diphtheria toxoids and acellular pertussis vaccine (Tdap).** *(Minimum ages: 7 years for Td, 10 years for BOOSTRIX®, and 11 years for ADACEL™)*
    - Tdap should be substituted for a single dose of Td in the primary catch-up series or as a booster if age appropriate; use Td for other doses.
    - A 5-year interval from the last Td dose is encouraged when Tdap is used as a booster dose. A booster (fourth) dose is needed if any of the previous doses were administered at age <12 months. Refer to ACIP recommendations for further information. See *MMWR* 2006;55(No. RR-3).

11. **Human papillomavirus vaccine (HPV).** *(Minimum age: 9 years)*
    - Administer the HPV vaccine series to females at age 13–18 years if not previously vaccinated.

Information about reporting reactions after immunization is available online at **http://www.vaers.hhs.gov** or by telephone via the 24-hour national toll-free information line 800-822-7967. Suspected cases of vaccine-preventable diseases should be reported to the state or local health department. Additional information, including precautions and contraindications for immunization, is available from the National Center for Immunization and Respiratory Diseases at **http://www.cdc.gov/nip/default.htm** or telephone, **800-CDC-INFO (800-232-4636).**

**DEPARTMENT OF HEALTH AND HUMAN SERVICES • CENTERS FOR DISEASE CONTROL AND PREVENTION • SAFER • HEALTHIER • PEOPLE**

## MMR IMMUNIZATION

The letters *MMR* are short for measles, mumps, and rubella. These are the three viral diseases against which the MMR vaccine provides immunity.

> Be sure to become familiar with the names and uses of the vaccines the medical professionals in your office use.

### MMR Immunization

| Disease | Symptoms | Can lead to . . . |
|---------|----------|-------------------|
| measles | rash, cough, runny nose, eye irritation, and fever | pneumonia, seizures, brain damage, and death |
| mumps | fever, headache, and swollen glands | deafness, meningitis, swollen testicles or ovaries, and death |
| rubella (German measles) | mild rash | serious birth defects in the child of a woman who gets rubella while pregnant |

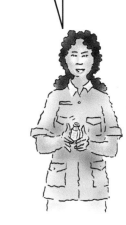

### Use

MMR is a "three in one" vaccine that offers lifetime immunity against the three target diseases. It is usually given subcutaneously (SubQ) according to the following schedule:

- first injection—at ages 12 months to 15 months
- second injection—at ages 4 to 6 years (before starting school)

> You should be familiar with your state's laws regarding MMR vaccination for school-aged children.

The second vaccination can actually be given at any time after age 6. It is administered to guarantee protection in case full immunity did not result from the first vaccination.

Most schools require proof that a child was immunized before she can start school. Some states mandate a second MMR specifically at the start of kindergarten.

### Effects on the Body

For most people, the MMR vaccine causes few or no problems. The most common complaint is soreness and redness where the injection was given. One in six children may get a fever. One in 20 patients may develop a rash. Swollen glands or seizures are uncommon or rare.

However, women who are pregnant or who may become pregnant within 28 days after vaccination should not be immunized. Significant fetal deformities, including blindness and death of the fetus, may occur if a pregnant woman is exposed to the measles vaccine or disease.

> Many adults born before 1956 are immune—they had measles and mumps when they were kids. Adults born after 1956 should consider getting an MMR if they aren't sure whether they were vaccinated as children.

### Tips

If a child is ill the day the vaccine is to be administered, make sure you tell the physician. If the child has anything more serious than a cold, the physician might want the child to come back when he is healthy.

Be sure the physician also knows if an older child had any problems when he got his first MMR as an infant. The vaccine should not be given to pregnant women or to patients with immune system problems.

## DTAP IMMUNIZATION

Diphtheria, tetanus, and pertussis are serious bacterial infections. The DTaP immunization protects from all three and is highly recommended for all children.

### DTaP Immunization

| Disease | Symptoms | Can lead to . . . |
|---------|----------|-------------------|
| diphtheria | bad sore throat, swollen glands, fever, and chills | paralysis, heart failure |
| tetanus (lockjaw) | painful tightening of muscles in the jaw or all over the body | death by suffocation |
| pertussis (whooping cough) | a cough with a "whooping" sound on the in-breath | • difficulty eating, drinking, or breathing |
| | choking spells, coughing so hard that vomiting may result | • very dangerous in infants |

The DTaP vaccine is a safer form of the older vaccine called DPT, which is no longer used in the United States. However, you may hear some health care professionals still use the older name from habit.

The DTaP immunization is for children under age 7. It is not meant for older children or adults. Physicians use

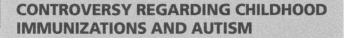

## Ask the Professional

## CONTROVERSY REGARDING CHILDHOOD IMMUNIZATIONS AND AUTISM

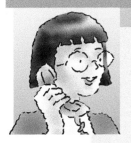

**Q:** *I've heard that there may be a link between the MMR vaccination and autism in children. Is this true?*

**A: Autism** is a collection of developmental disabilities that first start to appear before a child is 3 years old. Children and adults with autism have difficulty expressing themselves or knowing how to interact with others in social situations. This brain disorder has a different effect on every person who has it. People who are only mildly autistic can cope well in most situations. The most severely autistic individuals have great difficulty communicating and can appear nonresponsive and withdrawn.

According to the CDC, 1 child in 150 births has some form of autism, and the numbers are growing. The cause of autism is not clear. At present, there is no cure.

However, almost every significant research study shows that there is no causal connection between the MMR vaccine and autism. The rumors of a connection between the two resulted from a great deal of media attention to a handful of flawed research studies. In 2004, 10 of the 13 authors of the study retracted their findings. They now say that there are not enough data to make the connection.

If a parent asks if the MMR vaccination can cause autism, though, be sure to refer the parent to the physician. If the physician hasn't already provided preprinted material responding to concerns, he or she will handle the situation by answering the parent's questions.

Tetanus bacteria live in soil, manure, and saliva. They get into the body through a cut. People of any age can be exposed to tetanus.

vaccines without the pertussis component for these older age groups.

**Use**

The specific vaccine a patient gets depends on the patient's age.

### For Young Children

Two vaccines are available for children under the age of 7 years.

- **DTaP vaccine**—a three-in-one vaccine that protects against all three diseases: diphtheria, tetanus, and pertussis.

- **DT vaccine**—a two-in-one vaccine that does not contain a pertussis component.

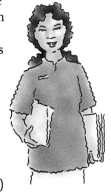

It's safe to give the DTaP vaccine at the same time as other vaccines.

Unless there is a medical reason against it, physicians usually administer the DTaP vaccine. If you're helping to administer the DTaP immunization, check the child's medical records for any allergic reactions the child may have had to an earlier immunization. Warn the nurse or physician if you find such a notation.

The DTaP and the DT vaccines are usually given as a series of five doses by injection into the arm or thigh. One dose is given at each of the following ages:

- 2 months
- 4 months
- 6 months
- 15 to 18 months
- 4 to 6 years of age, before starting school (booster shot)

### For Older Children and Adults

Unlike the MMR immunization, immunization against diphtheria and tetanus does not last forever. Older children and adults should get booster shots of an age-appropriate vaccine.

Two vaccines are available for children over age 7 and for adults.

- *Td vaccine.* A booster shot containing tetanus and diphtheria vaccine should be given to children at age 11 to 12 years and every 10 years thereafter.

- *T vaccine.* A "tetanus shot" can be given to any older child or adult with a serious cut or puncture would, such as from stepping on a nail. You may be asked to give a tetanus shot if the wound is dirty and if the patient hasn't had a Td booster shot in 5 years.

## Effects on the Body

Mild reactions to DTaP immunization are common. One in four children may get a slight fever or have soreness and redness where the shot was given. One in three recipients may become fussy. One in ten may feel tired or lose appetite.

Serious reactions are much less common. For instance, swelling of the whole arm or leg where the shot was given happens to 1 in 30 patients. High fever or seizures may happen to 1 in 14,000 or more patients.

## Closer Look   COMBINATION VACCINES

The National Network for Immunization Information points out that children can get up to 20 vaccinations in their first 2 years of life. A child could receive as many as five different injections during a single office visit. That's a lot of tears and crying!

Drug companies are developing combination vaccines that protect against two to five different diseases with a single infection. Two of them have been used for many years. You probably received them yourself when you were an infant:

- MMR—against measles, mumps, and rubella
- DTaP—against diphtheria, tetanus, and pertussis (whooping cough)

Newer formulas add additional protections:

- Pediarix—DTaP plus hepatitis B and polio vaccines
- Comvax—hepatitis B and Hib (*H. influenzae* type b)
- TriHIBit—DTaP and Hib

However, according to some reports, children are more likely to run a fever after getting a "five-in-one" vaccine at the same time as other inoculations.

## VARICELLA IMMUNIZATION

Varicella is the medical name for **chicken-pox,** an infectious disease caused by the varicella virus. Chickenpox usually affects children under age 15. However, older children and even adults can get chickenpox, too. These cases tend to be more severe.

Chickenpox is an uncomfortable blister-like rash, itching, fatigue, and fever. It usually appears on the face, scalp, or upper body, although it can spread over the entire body. It's relatively mild in children and goes away in five to ten days. Chickenpox tends to be more serious when an adult or older child gets it.

It's possible to get chickenpox more than once. However, most people who have had it once will never get it again.

> More than 20 states require children who are going to school or day care to be immunized against chickenpox. Be sure that you know the law in your state.

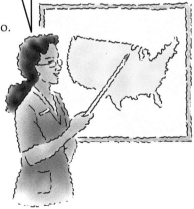

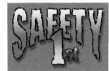

## AVOID ASPIRIN WITH CHICKENPOX

Children who are given aspirin when they have chicken-pox are at risk of developing **Reye syndrome** (RS). RS causes swelling in the brain and also affects the liver.

Reye syndrome can strike children who already have a viral infection like the flu or chickenpox. Physicians do not know yet what causes RS, and there is no cure for it. However, some evidence points to a connection between taking aspirin and developing RS in these circumstances. It's best to be safe and advise patients to avoid aspirin without the physician's specific approval. When you're seeing a child with chickenpox, be sure that the physician reminds parents to avoid giving aspirin to the child.

### Use

The varicella vaccine is 85% effective against chickenpox. It is usually given subcutaneously in the upper arm according to the following schedule:

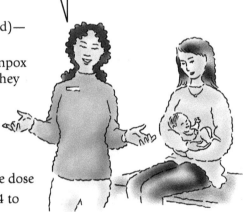

Certain specialty practices, such as oncology practices and OB-GYN offices, may require employees to submit proof of varicella vaccination or varicella titer. This precaution is in place to protect patients with compromised immune systems and unborn babies from exposure to the virus.

- first dose—at age 12 months to 15 months
- second dose (newly recommended)— at age 4 to 6 years

Children who have already had chickenpox do not need to be vaccinated because they develop their own immunity.

Children who have *not* already had chickenpox should be vac-cinated according to the following schedule:

- age 19 months to age 12—a single dose
- people 12 and older—two doses 4 to 8 weeks apart

### Effects on the Body

There are some common adverse reactions for this vaccine. The most common ones are burning, stinging, pain, or redness where the injection was given, mild fever, and skin rash.

## Closer Look    ZOSTAVAX

In 2006, the FDA approved the vaccine Zostavax to prevent shingles in older adults. Shingles is caused by the varicella-zoster virus (which also causes chickenpox). People who develop shingles experience a blister-like rash accompanied by severe pain. The pain can last for weeks, months, or even years.

People who have had chickenpox are at risk for developing shingles later in life when their immune systems are weakened. This is because the chickenpox virus remains dormant in the body after the initial infection disappears. As people get older, the virus may reappear and cause shingles. The FDA estimates that shingles affects approximately 20% of people at some point in their lifetime.

The shingles vaccine may be administered to patients aged 60 years and older. It is given in the form of an injection and may cause the following adverse reactions:

- swelling at the injection site
- redness, pain, and tenderness
- itching
- headache

## HEPATITIS B IMMUNIZATION

**Hepatitis B** is one kind of hepatitis, which is liver disease. Hepatitis B is caused by the hepatitis B virus (HBV). It's spread by contact with blood, semen, or other body fluids from a person who has HBV. An infant can get it at birth from her mother.

HBV is rare in the United States. However, chronic hepatitis is a major public health problem in many other parts of the world, especially in developing countries.

Use

Hepatitis B immunization is part of the immunization schedule for children. It is given according to the following schedule:

- first dose—at birth, before leaving the hospital
- second dose—at ages 1 to 2 months
- third dose—at ages 6 to 18 months

If the child's mother tested positive for HBV when the child was born, the child should be tested for the virus after the third dose, at the next well-child office visit.

Adults at risk of contracting hepatitis B are given a different vaccine than the one used for children. The hepatitis B vaccine is strongly recommended by OSHA for all health care workers. After the first dose has been administered, the adult vaccine follows this schedule:

- second dose—given 30 days after the first dose

- third dose—given 5 to 7 months after the second dose

- fourth dose—given 6 months after the third dose (only administered if the patient's blood test results reveal that he is not yet immune to the virus)

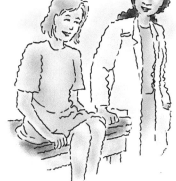

Hepatitis B is a major public heath problem. If you know that a patient is going to travel to a developing country, remind her to ask the physician about getting a hepatitis B injection.

### More About HBV Infections

If a person has contracted hepatitis B, it will show up on a blood test. Sometimes HBV has no symptoms, and people can have it without knowing it. In other cases, people with HBV think they have the flu. The disease usually improves by itself after a few months. If it does not, however, it can become a chronic infection. Chronic hepatitis can damage the liver and cause liver failure or liver cancer.

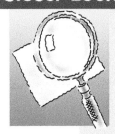

## Closer Look ADULTS WITH HEPATITIS B

Younger people are generally well protected because hepatitis B immunization is part of the childhood vaccination program. Most children and about 60 percent of adolescents ages 13 to 15 have been immunized.

Among adults, about 95% of pregnant women have been tested. But the following segments of the adult population are still at risk:

- heterosexuals with multiple sex partners

- IV drug users

- homosexual males who are sexually active

- sex partners of persons with chronic HBV

- persons from Asian Pacific countries

### Effects on the Body

The most common adverse reactions to hepatitis B immunization are a result of the injection itself. They include irritation, redness, itching, bruising, or swelling at the injection site. Most patients report no adverse reactions at all.

A few patients may experience headache, fatigue, sore throat, fever, nausea, dizziness, flu-like symptoms, or body discomfort. If patients have any other symptoms after the injection, remind them to tell the physician.

## PNEUMOCOCCAL IMMUNIZATION

Pneumococcal disease is a very dangerous bacterial infection that's carried in the bloodstream. It can cause the following:

- **pneumonia**—a serious infection of the lungs
- **bacteremia**—a serious infection of the blood
- **meningitis**—a serious infection of the covering of the brain

In the past, penicillin was used to treat these infections. However, the pneumococcus bacterium has become resistant to penicillin. Now physicians try to prevent these infections by immunizing people against them.

### Use

Two pneumococcal vaccines are in use. The pneumococcal conjugate vaccine (PCV), also known as PCV7, is part of the recommended immunization schedule for healthy children ages 6 weeks to 5 years old. This vaccine is administered as an injection into the muscle or fatty tissue of the arm or leg. Doses are given at 2, 4, 6, and 12 to 15 months of age.

Another vaccine, the pneumococcal polysaccharide vaccine (PPV), or PPV23, is formulated for patients ages 65 and over. It is also given by IM injection to anyone over the age of 2 years who has certain long-term health problems, such as heart disease or sickle cell anemia, or a disease that lowers resistance to infection, such as Hodgkin disease, leukemia, HIV, or AIDS. This vaccine protects against 23 strains of pneumococci.

### Effects on the Body

Both the PCV and the PPV vaccines are very safe. Like other vaccinations, there may be some mild adverse reactions.

- One in five children who receives a PCV injection may develop redness, tenderness, or swelling where the shot was given. One in 10 patients may develop a fever.

- Up to 50% of the people who get a PPV injection may have a mild reaction where the shot was given. One in 100 people may get a fever, muscle aches, or more severe reactions at the injection site.

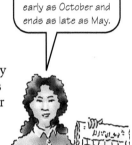

Flu season begins as early as October and ends as late as May.

## INFLUENZA IMMUNIZATION

Influenza—or the flu—usually spreads from person to person by means of coughing or sneezing. There are many different strains of the flu. So, each year, particular strains of the flu are selected for the vaccine that will be made for that year.

People who have been immunized can still get the flu if they come into contact with another strain of flu. They can also get other viral infections and experience flu-like symptoms.

The best time to get vaccinated is in October or November. But physicians may still give the flu vaccine in December, or even later.

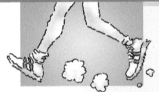

## Running Smoothly    WHO SHOULD GET A FLU SHOT?

*What if a patient asks if he needs a flu shot?*

As of 2007, the flu vaccine is one of the recommended immunizations for everyone under age 18. Patients under 18 years old should get immunized each year.

Children under the age of nine who are receiving a flu shot for the first time should get two injections 4 to 6 weeks apart. The timing depends on the vaccine the physician uses.

The following people should also get the flu vaccine each year:

- men and women over age 50
- workers in nursing homes and other health care facilities and institutions
- adults with a chronic disease
- children and adolescents ages 6 months to 18 years who are taking aspirin therapy. They are in danger of developing Reye syndrome (swelling of the brain) if they get the flu.

## Use

Two forms of flu vaccine are available.

- In a standard "flu shot," the vaccine is made from dead viruses. It is injected by needle into the arm. It's approved for everyone older than 6 months of age.

- In a nasal-spray flu vaccine (LAIV), the vaccine is made from live but weakened viruses. It's approved for healthy people between ages 5 and 49 years.

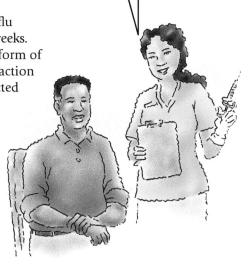

Some patients worry that they will get the flu from the flu shot. Remind these concerned patients that they can't get the flu from the flu vaccine because the viruses within are dead!

## Effects on the Body

Antibodies that protect against the flu develop in the body after about 2 weeks.

Very few people who get either form of the flu vaccine experience a bad reaction to it. Adverse reactions to the injected form of the virus are soreness or redness where the needle entered the skin, low-grade fever, and body aches.

When children receive the nasal spray vaccine, they may develop a runny nose, headache, muscle aches, or fever. Adults using the spray may get a runny nose, headache, sore throat, or a cough.

## Tips

People should *not* get the flu vaccine if any of the following apply to them:

- if they are allergic to eggs
- if they are still sick from an acute illness
- if they are in the first trimester of pregnancy, although it's safe to get a flu vaccine during the second and third trimesters of pregnancy

In some years, the flu vaccine is in short supply. When that happens, the CDC instruct physicians to give the vaccine to patients over 65 and other specified groups first before administering the vaccine to otherwise healthy patients.

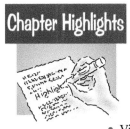
**Chapter Highlights**

- Fat-soluble vitamins are stored intact in the body's fatty tissues for up to 6 months. The body does not break them down into other substances. Vitamins A, D, E, and K are the fat-soluble vitamins.

- Water-soluble vitamins pass through the bloodstream and leave the body through the kidneys. Vitamin $B_1$, $B_2$, $B_3$, $B_6$, $B_9$, $B_{12}$, and C are the water-soluble vitamins.

- Vitamins help maintain normal body functions such as formation of bone and tissue, production of white and red blood cells, and cell repair. Lack of vitamins can cause disease, poor eyesight, and other problems.

- Dietary minerals in different quantities are among the building blocks of bone, teeth, soft tissue, muscles, blood, and nerve cells. The body also uses minerals to make hormones and regulate the heartbeat.

- Multivitamins usually contain small amounts of minerals. Mineral supplements are also available. However, a diet rich in whole grains, seafood, fruits, and vegetables provides all the minerals needed.

- Commonly used herbal supplements are echinacea, lavender, ginkgo biloba, ginseng, saw palmetto, ginger, cinnamon, lycopene, salvia, peppermint, and St. John's wort. Except for ginkgo biloba and St. John's wort, these herbal supplements have inconclusive evidence to support their use.

- Ginkgo biloba improves concentration and helps patients who have had multiple strokes. St. John's wort is more effective than tricyclic antidepressants, such as amitriptyline, to treat mild to moderate major depression and may be as effective as the SSRI antidepressants fluoxetine hydrochloride or sertraline hydrochloride.

- Patients may experience serious adverse reactions if they take herbal medications with antidepressants, antianxiety drugs, anticonvulsant drugs, blood thinners, blood pressure medicine or heart medicines, diabetes drugs, or cancer drugs.

- Herbal medicines can also interfere with surgery. The doctor may want such patients to stop taking supplements for as early as three weeks before an operation.

- The FDA encourages pregnant women to talk to their doctors before taking herbal supplements. Some herbs can cause miscarriage, premature birth, uterine contractions, and harm to the fetus.

- A vaccine is a weakened or dead form of a disease or a related disease. A vaccine causes the immune system to create antibodies that protect the body from the target disease or that lessen its effects.

- The National Childhood Vaccine Injury Act (NCVIA) of 1986 requires medical offices to take part in the Vaccine Adverse Event Reporting System (VAERS). It also requires physicians to provide a vaccine information statement (VIS) to each patient, her parent, or her legal guardian before certain vaccines may be given.

- The MMR vaccine offers lifetime immunity against measles, mumps, and rubella.

- The DTaP immunization protects against diphtheria, tetanus, and pertussis (whooping cough). DTaP immunization is for children under age 7. Vaccines without the pertussis component or the diphtheria component are used for older age groups.

- Varicella immunization protects against chickenpox.

- Hepatitis B immunization protects against the strain of hepatitis caused by the hepatitis B virus (HBV). HBV is now rare in the United States because of the immunization program. However, certain groups in the adult population, such as IV drug users, are still at risk.

- Pneumococcal immunization protects against pneumococcal disease, which can cause pneumonia, bacteremia, and meningitis.

- Influenza immunization protects against the strains of the flu selected for that year's vaccine.

- Other available immunizations include vaccines to prevent *H. influenzae* type b (Hib), hepatitis A, human papillomavirus (HPV), polio, meningococcal meningitis, and rotavirus.

- Common adverse reactions for vaccines include pain, stinging, itching, or burning at the injection site, mild fever, and skin rash.

## Chapter 7

# ABUSE AND MISUSE OF SUBSTANCES

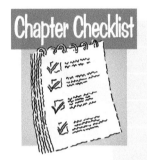

## Chapter Checklist

- List the various costs of substance abuse.

- Identify the signs and symptoms of abuse.

- Explain how prescription drugs can be abused.

- Describe the special problems of abuse in older adults.

- Describe the special problems of abuse in health care workers.

- Explain how legal substances such as caffeine, nicotine, and alcohol can be addictive.

- State the dangers of secondhand smoke.

- Identify problems and symptoms related to the use of marijuana, cocaine, opiates, hallucinogens, and club drugs.

- Describe the symptoms and abuse of household substances.

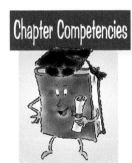

## Chapter Competencies

- Identify community resources (CAAHEP Competency 3.c.3.d.)

Substance abuse is the use of natural and synthetic substances to alter mood or behavior in a manner that differs from their generally accepted use. It cuts across racial, economic, social, and generational lines.

In this chapter, you'll learn how to recognize the signs and symptoms of substance abuse within and outside the medical office.

## Recognizing Substance Abuse

The signs of abuse are different for each substance. Sometimes, it's obvious that a patient has slurred speech, an unsteady gait, or the smell of alcohol on his breath. For many substances, there are some general behavior changes:

- sudden problems with relationships, job, school, or health
- legal problems
- keeping a hidden supply of a substance
- increased tolerance to a substance and the need to take more to achieve the same effect

People come up with many convincing arguments to "prove" that they do not have a problem. Some of these include:

- "I'm not an alcoholic. I only drink hard on weekends."
- "I'm not hooked. I just need another pill for the pain."

Many people rationalize their use of drugs or alcohol. They may say things like:

- "It's only beer."
- "No one really understands how bad my pain is."

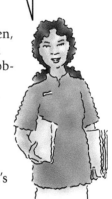

Patient information is CONFIDENTIAL. Do not discuss it in the hallway with coworkers or with friends or strangers outside the office.

### BEHAVIORS SEEN IN A MEDICAL PRACTICE

In your medical office, you may treat mostly young children, older adults, or the severely injured. Or maybe you'll see a broad mix of patients. It is likely that some will have a problem with substance abuse. Be on the lookout for telltale signs of substance abuse, such as alcohol on the breath or dilated pupils.

You have the opportunity to notice many possible problems—and an ethical obligation to let the physician know about them. Just remember to discuss any concerns with the physician in private. As a health care professional, it's your duty to maintain patient confidentiality at all times.

## REASONS FOR SUBSTANCE ABUSE

But why do people abuse substances such as alcohol, drugs, or nicotine? Several reasons include:

- self-medication
- peer pressure
- curiosity
- relief from stress
- dependence on prescription drugs

Regardless of the reason for substance abuse, the personal and social costs are enormous.

## COSTS OF SUBSTANCE ABUSE

According to researchers at the Johns Hopkins School of Medicine, alcohol, tobacco, and illicit drug use is responsible for one in four deaths in the United States each year. Substance abuse touches every corner of American life.

### In the Workplace

The federal government estimates that productivity losses caused by substance abuse rose from $77.4 billion in 1992 to $128.6 billion in 2002. Lateness, absences, and work-related accidents all contributed to these numbers. According to the National Institute on Drug Abuse (NIDA), medical claims and workers' compensation claims from drug abusers cost their employers more than twice as much as claims from drug-free employees.

### In the Family

It's not just teens and young adults who are abusing drugs and alcohol. Researchers at the Johns Hopkins School of Medicine provide the following facts:

- Among women age 60 and above, substance abuse is at epidemic levels. Cigarettes, alcohol, and psychoactive prescription drugs are the main substances of abuse.
- Of older adult patients in emergency rooms, 14% show symptoms of alcoholism.
- Seventy-five percent of domestic violence victims report that their abuser was drunk or high at the time.
- Children of smokers are more likely to develop ear infections and asthma and miss approximately 33% more school days than children of nonsmokers.

- Children of substance abusers are more likely to skip school, get low grades, and have emotional problems than children from families that do not experience substance abuse.

## In Society

Alarming facts continue to accumulate.

- Smoking-related illnesses, including lung cancer, cost the nation one dollar of every 14 dollars spent on health care.
- Thirty-three million Americans engage in binge drinking, or consuming five or more drinks at a single sitting.
- The use of cocaine and crack cocaine is growing. In seven urban areas studied in 2002, 40% of people admitted to the hospital for illicit drug use were there because of cocaine use.
- Heroin use is a major problem in Boston, Chicago, Detroit, Newark, Philadelphia, San Francisco, and other U.S. cities.

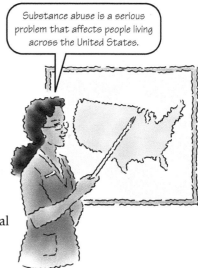

Substance abuse is a serious problem that affects people living across the United States.

- Increases are reported in the misuse of prescription opiates such as the combination drug hydrocodone and acetaminophen (Vicodin).
- Marijuana use continues to rise among adolescents and young adults.
- Methamphetamine use also continues to rise.
- Use of "club drugs," such as Ecstasy, is spreading beyond dance clubs and into high school parties.
- Scandals over steroids haunt professional sports. Use of these performance-enhancing drugs is spreading to amateur and school athletes, too.

## In the Individual

There are several physical costs to the individual drinker, drug user, or smoker. Tobacco users face increased risk of lung cancer, throat cancer, mouth cancer, high blood pressure, vascular disease, and impotence. Chronic alcoholics can develop cirrhosis of the liver, pancreatitis, and esophageal varices (varicose veins in the esophagus that can burst, causing the person to vomit blood). Intravenous drug users can contract hepatitis, HIV infections, STDs, tuberculosis, and other infections from sharing needles.

In the short term, drugs and alcohol become central to the abuser's life. Habitual users can't stop drinking or getting high once they start. A decision to quit lasts only days or even hours until the user needs to drink or get high again. Users find themselves needing a drink or drugs just to start the day. They feel guilty. They lie about their habit. Some steal to support it. They blank out or can't remember what they did while under the influence. Violence toward themselves and others is very common. Without treatment and rehabilitation, their lives can lose all direction.

# How Problems with Substances Occur

Substance abuse has become a worldwide problem. The terms *substance abuse* and *drug abuse* are often used to mean the same thing. That's because some of the substances, like tobacco, have chemicals in them that "hook" users. As family members and friends will tell you, it's hard to stop smoking once you've started. Other substances, like alcohol, have a potential for abuse—even though many people who take an occasional social drink will never become alcoholics.

## PRESCRIPTION DRUGS

The substances that people abuse are the ones that alter a person's mood or behavior. The prescription drugs that fit this description are usually painkillers. For example, a physician may prescribe morphine for severe pain, which is the intended therapeutic use of the drug. The drug is not intended to give the patient a high, or euphoria, but that may be the reason why he continues taking morphine. This is a misuse or abuse of the drug, as is using more of it to avoid withdrawal symptoms. Prescription drug abuse is one of the reasons why it's important to keep blank prescription forms in a locked cabinet.

## ILLEGAL DRUGS

Street drugs are another story. Heroin, crack cocaine, methamphetamine, and similar drugs are illegal to make, buy, or use. These are also mood- and behavior-altering drugs. Many of these drugs cause the brain's pleasure center to release the chemical dopamine, producing temporary feelings of euphoria. People use illegal drugs for various reasons.

- Some people use these drugs to achieve a high.
- Others begin using illegal drugs in response to pressure from peers.

- People whose pain isn't relieved by prescription drugs may turn to illegal drugs to relieve the pain.

## What Does "Substance Abuse" Really Mean?

**Substance abuse** is a pattern of excessive or harmful use of substances we put into our bodies. Most people use the term to refer to illegal drugs, but it's broader than that. Substance abuse includes a whole range of items that do not fit into neat categories, but may still cause problems, such as:

- mood-altering substances, such as coffee, tobacco, alcohol, inhalants, street drugs, club drugs, prescription painkillers, and similar products
- other problem-causing substances, such as anabolic steroids

Sometimes, the line between reasonable use and abuse is not clearly drawn. Alcohol is a good example. According to some medical studies, moderate consumption of red wine seems to be good for the heart and circulatory system. However, a lifetime of heavy drinking causes irreparable harm to the body.

## What Does Addiction Mean?

Drug **addiction** is the compulsive dependence on a legal or illegal drug, despite any possible consequences. These are some of the things an addict experiences:

- an overpowering desire or need to keep taking the drug
- a need to get the drug by any means possible
- a tendency to increase the dose of the drug
- a mental and physical dependence on the effects of the drug

### Physical Dependency

People who are physically dependent on a drug need their substance to "feel normal." Imagine needing an alcoholic beverage in the morning to settle your stomach before being able to eat breakfast or needing a drink to stop your hands from shaking. Needing an "eye-opener" is a sign of dependence. It results in the addicted person needing to plan to use his substance and having a hidden supply.

### Psychological Dependency

People who are psychologically dependent on a drug have a compulsive need to take the drug because of how good the drug makes them feel. They crave the effect that the drug has on them.

### Tolerance

After taking a drug for a while, the person usually builds up a tolerance to it. The same dose no longer has the same effect. The person needs to take more of it to get the original high.

### Withdrawal Symptoms

An addict usually experiences withdrawal symptoms when the substance is no longer available. When cigarette smokers stop using nicotine, they will likely become grumpy and irritable. Withdrawal symptoms from substances such as heroin are far more severe. Depression, anxiety, tremors, and other symptoms of withdrawal can be frightening and uncomfortable. Alcohol and benzodiazepine withdrawal can result in delirium tremens ("the DTs"), hallucinations, serious deviations in vital signs, and even death. Alcohol and benzodiazepine withdrawal should be monitored by a physician.

## SPECIAL ISSUES WITH OLDER ADULTS

Older people living in retirement communities often develop alcoholism, especially if social get-togethers are frequent. Problem drinking is also found among nursing home patients. Drinking can be a particular problem because alcohol can mask pain or change how the body reacts to narcotic painkillers and medications that treat depression.

## SPECIAL ISSUES WITH TEENS

Some young people start experimenting with drugs, alcohol, and tobacco during middle school. Many children will know a classmate who drinks, smokes, or does drugs. This is why many schools in the United States have drug education programs for their students.

Teens have many risk factors for drug abuse. Many are impulsive or sensation seekers. They think many of their friends are using drugs, even if they are not. Lacking experience, many teens do not yet understand how harmful drugs, alcohol, and tobacco can be.

## SPECIAL ISSUES WITH HEALTH CARE WORKERS

Health care workers can be at risk because they have easy access to prescription drugs in the medical office. Remember what you learned in Chapter 3 about reporting the disappearance of controlled substances from the medical office. (See page 78.)

## *Caffeine*

What did you drink with breakfast this morning? Chances are, it had caffeine in it.

### MOST COMMONLY USED DRUG IN THE UNITED STATES

Caffeine is the most commonly used drug in the United States. According to the Center for Science in the Public Interest (CSPI), four out of five Americans drink some form of caffeine each day. The average amount is what you'd get from two 8-ounce cups of coffee—about 200 mg. Drinking a 20-ounce coffee from your local coffee shop will put about 480 mg of caffeine in your body. The same sized cup of decaffeinated coffee drops the hit to only 20 mg of caffeine.

### SOURCES

Caffeine is a stimulant, so you'll find in it in many beverages and products that people use to give themselves an energy boost. These foods and beverages include:

- coffee
- tea
- energy drinks
- cola drinks and other soft drinks
- chocolate
- some pain-relief medications, such as Excedrin, which contains aspirin, acetaminophen, and caffeine

### EFFECTS ON THE HUMAN BODY

Because of its effect on the brain, caffeine temporarily heightens concentration and keeps you from feeling fatigued. It also increases the effect of painkillers, which is why it's included in some aspirin-based products.

A cup of coffee takes effect within 30 to 60 minutes and takes 4 to 6 hours to wear off. Smoking lessens the effect of caffeine, so smokers often drink more coffee to compensate.

What happens if you consume excessive amounts of caffeine? The following symptoms may occur:

- anxiety
- excitability
- tachycardia

- stimulated appetite
- restlessness
- dizziness
- irritability
- inability to concentrate
- gastrointestinal (GI) aches
- headaches that do not seem to go away
- trouble with sleeping

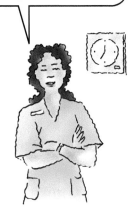

Remember the myth that coffee can sober you up if you've had too much to drink? Well, it's not true. It might wake you up, but it won't sober you up! Only time will do that.

Caffeine withdrawal makes you feel overtired and sleepy. You may have difficulty concentrating, too, so how can you stop? Unless you want a severe headache, the best way to stop drinking large amounts of caffeine is to cut back gradually.

## Alcohol

Alcohol is a natural product made by fermenting grains, fruits, or vegetables. Different forms of alcohol are used as cleaners, fuels, antiseptics, and sedatives. Alcohol is even an ingredient in some medications.

### A HIGH RATE OF CONSUMPTION

After caffeine, alcohol is the most commonly abused substance in the United States. According to the Centers for Disease Control and Prevention (CDC), 61% of adult Americans drank alcohol at least once in 2004. At least once that year, 32% of them had more than five drinks at one sitting.

This practice, called "binge drinking," isn't just an adult thing. In 2005, 10% of eighth graders, 21% of tenth graders, and 28% of twelfth graders admitted to binge drinking at least once. Binge drinking is exceptionally dangerous and can lead to death. Binge drinkers can pass out, vomit, aspirate (inhale into the lungs) their own vomit, and die. Celebration of special events may tempt people to binge on alcohol, but it's very risky behavior.

### DRUGS THAT INTERACT WITH ALCOHOL

Few medicines can be taken safely while a person is drinking alcohol. Many prescription medications and over-the-counter products have special warnings on the label that warn patients not to use them while drinking. Here are some examples:

## The Effects of Alcohol on Certain Drugs

| Drug | Alcohol's Effect |
| --- | --- |
| warfarin (Coumadin, Jantoven) and other blood thinners | lowers the drug's ability to keep blood from clotting |
| amitriptyline hydrochloride (Elavil) and other tricyclic antidepressants | increases the sedative effects |
| metronidazole (Flagyl) and other antibiotics | may cause nausea, vomiting, headache, and convulsions |
| diphenhydramine hydrochloride (Benadryl, Benylin Cough) and other antihistamines | may intensify the drowsiness these drugs cause |
| chlorpromazine (Thorazine) and other anti-psychotic drugs | increases the sedative (calming) effects; may cause fatal breathing problems |
| methyldopa (Aldomet) and other blood pressure drugs | reduces the effect of the drug |
| meperidine (Demerol) and other narcotic pain relievers | increases the sedative (calming) effect of both drugs |
| diazepam (Valium) and many benzodiazepines | may cause severe drowsiness when used with alcohol |
| lorazepam (Ativan), a benzodiazepine | dangerously lowers heartbeat and breathing |

## HOW ALCOHOL AFFECTS THE BODY

Alcohol depresses the central nervous system. The effects depend on how much alcohol is in a person's brain and body tissues. Alcohol affects a person's:

- judgment
- behavior
- coordination
- consciousness

Alcohol is absorbed into the bloodstream very quickly. Carbonated beverages get absorbed faster than noncarbonated drinks. Foods high in carbohydrates and fats slow down the rate that alcohol gets into the blood. The effects of alcohol start to appear as it reaches the brain, within 10 minutes.

Alcohol stays in the bloodstream until the liver breaks it down. A person's blood alcohol level rises if he takes in alcohol faster than his body can get rid of it.

Ethanol, or drinking alcohol, is toxic to the liver. After years of heavy drinking, people may develop alcoholic liver disease, including cirrhosis and hepatitis. Binge drinking can also lead to acute alcoholic hepatitis. Genetics and gender also play a role. Some people are more prone to liver disease than others, and women may be more susceptible to chronic liver disease than men are.

## SPECIAL CONCERNS

Alcohol affects pregnant women, older adults, and teenagers in different ways than it affects other adults.

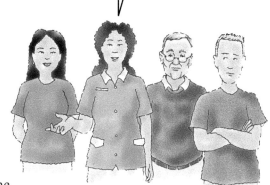

Alcohol affects different people in different ways.

### Pregnant Women

Many medical experts agree that even moderate drinking during pregnancy can lead to various problems for the unborn child. Every alcoholic drink the mother consumes is also consumed by the developing fetus, but the fetus does not have the mother's tolerance for alcohol. The fetus does not get enough oxygen and may be malnourished. As a result, the baby may be born with either of the following:

- **fetal alcohol syndrome (FAS)**—a group of problems that includes low birth weight, developmental delays, behavior problems, and possible mental retardation
- **fetal alcohol effects (FAE)**—a lesser but similar group of problems

### Older Adults

The National Institute on Alcohol Abuse and Alcoholism (NIAAA) has reported that alcoholism among Americans age 65 and older is on the rise. The NIAAA also studied hospital admissions for patients in that age group. Researchers found that 6% to 11% of hospitalized patients and 14% of emergency room patients show symptoms of alcohol abuse.

Among other NIAA findings are:

- Older adults who drink are more likely to fracture a hip in a fall. Alcohol affects bone density.
- Age plus alcohol slows the reaction time of older adults who drink. Thus, they are more likely to be injured or die in car crashes than nondrinkers.
- The average number of medications that older adult patients take (seven) makes it more likely that alcohol will interact with one of the medications.
- Depression is common among older adults, and this often leads to misuse of alcohol.

## Teens

Adolescence is a confusing time for many young people. It is also a time for risk-taking as teens try to define themselves. Teenagers experiment with alcohol for many of the same reasons that they experiment with other drugs. Some are curious. Some want to feel older; some feel pressured by friends to drink. Some want to reduce stress.

Teens who are at risk for developing problems with alcohol and drugs include those who:

- have a family history of substance abuse
- are depressed
- have low self-esteem
- feel that they do not fit in

Alcohol affects a teenager's brain in different ways than it affects an adult's brain. A great deal of functional brain development happens during adolescence. A 2004 Duke University study compared how alcohol affects teens and adults. The authors report that, compared to adults, teens who drink:

- are more likely to have problems with learning and memory
- are less likely to feel sleepy or drowsy
- have fewer problems with motor coordination, including walking without stumbling

## Closer Look — A DRUG THAT HELPS CHRONIC ALCOHOLICS

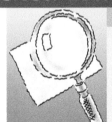

As part of long-term treatment, physicians sometimes prescribe disulfiram (Antabuse) to patients with chronic alcoholism. This drug has no effect when it's taken by itself. However, if it's taken with alcohol—even a small amount—it causes nausea, vomiting, and diarrhea.

Patients must be aware of the drug's effect and give their informed consent before they can take disulfiram.

Alcoholics often abuse other drugs as well as alcohol. Treatment with disulfiram may just cause them to shift their dependence to sedatives. Be sure to listen for and watch for signs of this shift, so that the physician can offer help.

## *Nicotine*

Tobacco smoke has two components that cause medical problems:

- **nicotine**—an addictive stimulant. Nicotine from a cigarette enters the bloodstream and rapidly reaches the brain. Its half-life in the body is about 2 hours.

- **tar**—cancer-causing particles from partly burned tobacco, marijuana, or other plant products. Over time, these particles damage the smoker's lungs.

Nicotine is in all of the tobacco products your local store sells—cigars, cigarettes, pipe tobacco, and chewing tobacco, which is sometimes called "smokeless tobacco," "chew," or "dip." Tobacco users get a stronger dose of nicotine from chewing tobacco than from smoking because some of the nicotine is lost in the smoke.

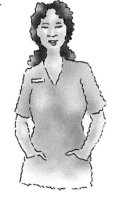

The tar from tobacco is not the same tar that workers use in road work and repair. Tar is the yellowish-brown residue you see inside the filter of a cigarette or when you blow tobacco smoke through a handkerchief.

### HOW NICOTINE AFFECTS THE BODY

Nicotine is highly addictive. When tobacco is smoked, the lungs absorb the nicotine in the smoke and move it into the bloodstream. It reaches the brain within 7 or 8 seconds of being inhaled. Nicotine can also enter the body though the skin or the mucous membranes of the mouth and nose. Once in the body, nicotine:

- changes the heart rate
- raises blood pressure
- acts on the nerves that control breathing
- stimulates the areas of the brain that produce feelings of pleasure and reward
- releases dopamine, the same brain chemical that narcotics also release

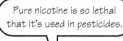

Pure nicotine is so lethal that it's used in pesticides.

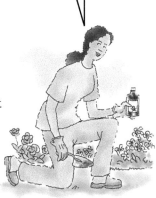

The side effects of nicotine become chronic problems for many smokers, who may experience:

- a breathless feeling
- chronic cough and phlegm
- paralysis of the cilia, which usually sweep foreign particles out of the lungs
- chronic bronchitis
- emphysema, a chronic "out of breath" condition that keeps many people from running or even walking around

When smokers stop smoking, they also suffer withdrawal symptoms, such as:

- constipation
- irritability
- slowing of the pulse
- hunger
- weight gain
- craving for tobacco

The craving can last for a few days or months. For some smokers, the craving lasts for years.

## OPTIONS FOR QUITTING

When it comes to quitting, many experts stress the importance of a patient's will and determination to stop. One way, if the patient can stand the initial discomforts of withdrawal, is just to quit—go "cold turkey." Other patients prefer a more gradual approach. Beyond this, there are psychological and medical ways to quit.

### Behavior Modification

Smokers often go back to smoking within 6 to 12 months of stopping. Behavior therapy tries to help smokers learn self-control by such positive activities as:

- removing things like ashtrays that remind them of smoking
- identifying the pleasurable or stressful times when they feel the urge to smoke
- substituting one behavior for another; for example, nibbling on carrot sticks when you feel the need to smoke
- focusing on the personal and social rewards, such as new clothes or the praise of friends

Hypnosis also works to help some people "recondition" themselves against smoking.

Nicotine lozenges are not ordinary candy, and nicotine gum is not ordinary chewing gum. Tell patients to keep them out of the reach of children.

### Decreasing Nicotine Through Patches and Gums

Nicotine patches, gums, and similar products are more properly called nicotine replacement therapy. They are best used along with behavior modification therapy. The table on page 256 gives several examples of the kinds of products that are available.

## Nicotine Replacement Therapy

| Method | What to Know |
|---|---|
| nicotine patch (Nicoderm CQ, Nicotrol) | • releases a constant amount of nicotine into the body through the skin<br>• must be worn all day<br>• usually changed every 24 hours<br>• comes in three different "steps," or strengths, to gradually reduce the symptoms of smoking withdrawal<br>• possible side effects: skin irritation, dizziness, racing heartbeat, headache, nausea, vomiting<br>• available over the counter, but also available by prescription |
| nicotine gum (Nicorette) | • works faster than the patch to deliver nicotine, but still takes a few minutes to reach the brain<br>• designed to be kept in the mouth, not chewed like ordinary gum<br>• beverages can affect how well it works<br>• possible side effects: may make teeth and gums sore, cause indigestion, or irritate the throat<br>• available over the counter |
| nicotine lozenge (Commit, NiQuitin CQ) | • slowly releases nicotine as it dissolves in the mouth<br>• maximum dose: 20 lozenges per day<br>• possible side effects: may make teeth and gums sore, cause indigestion, or irritate the throat<br>• available over the counter |
| nicotine nasal spray (Nicotrol NS) | • rapidly absorbed through the nasal membranes to relieve cravings<br>• useful for highly dependent smokers<br>• common side effects: nose and throat irritation<br>• available by prescription only |
| nicotine inhaler (Nicotrol Inhaler) | • shaped like a cigarette<br>• delivers nicotine by puffs into the mouth, not the lungs<br>• one cartridge = two cigarettes<br>• maximum dose: 16 cartridges per day<br>• common side effects: mouth and throat irritation<br>• available by prescription only |

### Bupropion

Bupropion (Zyban) has no nicotine in it at all. Bupropion is an antidepressant that is sold under the trade name Zyban to help people stop smoking. For use as an antidepressant, it's sold under the name Wellbutrin. Like nicotine, the drug stimulates the pleasure center of the brain to release the chemical dopamine. This:

- decreases the craving for a cigarette
- reduces the symptoms of nicotine withdrawal

Treatment with bupropion tablets begins a week before the smoker's official "quit date." Treatment continues for 7 to 12 weeks, depending on the patient. If the patient does not stop smoking within this time period, the physician should take him off the drug.

Bupropion can interact with many prescription medications, so it's important to take an accurate medication history for the physician. Because the drug is an antidepressant, it can have some uncommon but serious side effects. These include seizures, hallucinations, irrational fears, irregular heartbeat, and hives.

### Exciting New Options on the Horizon

Varenicline tartrate (Chantrix) is the newest antismoking medication approved by the FDA. Patients who are taking varenicline tartrate will probably find a cigarette less pleasurable to smoke, so they'll be likely to smoke less. This drug does two things.

- It reduces the symptoms of nicotine withdrawal (like bupropion does).
- It blocks the brain from taking in nicotine.

Like bupropion, treatment with varenicline tartrate lasts 12 weeks. The most common side effects of varenicline tartrate include nausea, headache, vomiting, gas, insomnia, abnormal dreams, and a change in the sense of taste.

## Ask the Professional    SMOKING AND PREGNANCY

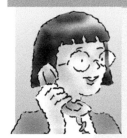

**Q:** *I know that pregnant women shouldn't drink because alcohol can affect the fetus. But what about smoking?*

**A:** That's an important question for any medical assistant who may work with pregnant patients. Empathize with them. Agree that it's difficult to stop smoking. But let them know about some of the risks.

A woman who smokes throughout her pregnancy increases her risk of some serious problems:

- ectopic pregnancy (pregnancy outside the uterus)
- problems with the placement of the placenta (placenta previa)
- premature rupture of the membranes
- premature birth
- low birth weight
- stillborn infant
- birth defects
- possible physical or mental damage to the child

## SECONDHAND SMOKE AND RESPIRATORY ILLNESS IN CHILDREN

Secondhand smoke is tobacco smoke that nonsmokers breathe in from the smokers around them. Second-hand smoke affects everyone and causes health problems. A 2006 report from the sur-geon general states that secondhand smoke contains over 250 chemicals, including form-aldehyde, benzene, vinyl chloride, arsenic, ammonia, and hydrogen cyanide.

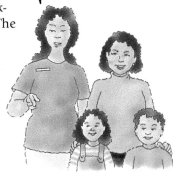

Urge the parents of children not to smoke. If they must smoke, make certain it isn't around the kids!

The surgeon general compared children of smok-ers and children from a smoke-free environment. The conclusion? Children who breathe in secondhand smoke are more likely to:

- develop pneumonia, bronchitis, and other lung diseases
- develop asthma
- have more asthma attacks if the child already has asthma
- have more ear infections

## Marijuana

Public policy experts consider marijuana a "gateway drug." This means that people who smoke marijuana are more likely to try harder drugs such as cocaine and heroin. Other experts think that marijuana is a "starter drug" only because it's more avail-able. They think that genetic and social reasons explain why some people are more likely to do drugs than others.

As a medical assistant, you need to know the medical implica-tions of marijuana use. You'll also need to be aware of the user's attitudes toward drug use and where those attitudes may lead—from occasional recreational use to dependence and addiction.

### SOURCES

Marijuana comes from the leaves and flowering tops of the hemp plant *(Cannabis sativa)*, which grows in many areas of the world. The chemical in marijuana that causes the drug's mind-altering effects is THC, which is short for delta-9-tetrahydrocannabinol.

THC is also in hashish, or hash, which is a resin collected from the same parts of the plant. Because it's concentrated, hashish has five to ten times more THC than marijuana does.

## Closer Look   DIFFERING LEVELS OF THC

It's not just hashish that's stronger. Marijuana itself is also getting stronger. A research group at the University of Mississippi has been tracking the potency of marijuana since the 1980s. In 2007, the group reported that the amount of THC in recent samples is twice as high as in samples from the mid-1980s. In other words, even recreational use may carry more risks than it once did.

### SHORT-TERM EFFECTS OF MARIJUANA

The THC from smoking marijuana reaches the brain the same way nicotine from a cigarette does—through the lungs and into the bloodstream. THC goes to the parts of the brain that influence pleasure, memory, thought, concentration, and coordination. It makes the heart beat faster. It also changes how fast a person thinks time is passing and may intensify the sense of smell, taste, sight, sound, or touch.

The short-term effects of marijuana can include:

- problems with memory and learning
- distorted perception
- difficulty in thinking and problem-solving
- loss of coordination
- increased heart rate
- hallucinations (in some users)

Outwardly, marijuana affects coordination and reflexes. Tasks such as driving or using heavy machinery become more difficult, and the chance of an accident increases.

### LONG-TERM EFFECTS OF MARIJUANA

Long-term users of marijuana may become psychologically dependent on the drug. Some long-term users may become paranoid or psychotic.

Respiratory problems can also occur. Users hold the inhaled smoke in the lungs longer than tobacco smoke. Thus, long-term users may also experience lung damage from the cancer-causing "tars" in the unfiltered smoke.

THC decreases the motility of sperm and may affect male fertility. It also weakens the immune system. Long-term users tend to take more sick days than nonusers. Additionally, THC makes it more difficult to learn or remember information. *Amotivational syndrome* may occur, in which the marijuana user loses initiative and desire for success. Mellow and content with life as it is, the user does not aspire to be promoted at a job or attend classes to receive a diploma.

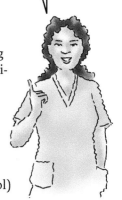

Tell young mothers not to smoke marijuana during pregnancy. THC passes right through the placenta. Tell them, "What you smoke your unborn baby smokes."

## MEDICAL USE OF MARIJUANA

The possible medical use of marijuana is a public policy issue. The real focus of attention, however, is on smoking marijuana as part of therapy, not on manufacturing medications derived from marijuana.

The debate pits those who favor medical use against those who oppose decriminalization of any illegal drug.

### Dronabinol

The FDA has approved a drug called dronabinol (Marinol) for two purposes:

- to treat nausea and vomiting in patients who are in chemotherapy for cancer. It is used only when other medications do not work.
- to increase appetite in AIDS patients who are losing weight

Dronabinol is a synthetic, or man-made, version of THC, the active ingredient in marijuana. Product information from the drug company clearly states that the product "is not marijuana" and does not contain chemicals from the cannabis plant that are in marijuana.

Common side effects are very much like marijuana's and include:

- clumsiness or unsteadiness
- dizziness
- drowsiness
- false sense of well-being
- trouble thinking

### Treating Other Diseases

Other possible medical uses for marijuana include treatments for:

- glaucoma
- Parkinson disease
- severe nausea from chemotherapy

# Cocaine

Cocaine is a very addictive drug that stimulates the central nervous system. It is the most potent natural stimulant available. It has caused death, even in small doses. Cocaine use is a serious substance abuse problem in the United States.

> Cocaine has a number of street names, including blow, flake, snow, sneeze, dust, and nose candy. Crack cocaine is sometimes called rock.

## MEDICAL USE OF COCAINE

In medicine, cocaine is used for local anesthesia of mucous membranes and for children. It is applied topically to avoid the use of injections.

## ILLEGAL USE OF COCAINE

Users have found a number of ways to ingest cocaine.

- They snort, or inhale through the nose, the powder form of cocaine. This is referred to as "snorting a line."
- They dissolve it and inject it by needle into the bloodstream.
- They mix it with heroin and inject a "speed ball."
- They smoke a freebase form of cocaine. It gets to the brain much faster than by snorting.
- They smoke a purified form of the drug called crack. They put it in a pipe and smoke it. Users may also mix crack with marijuana or tobacco.

Smoking crack produces a fast, intense high followed by a deep low. It is inexpensive and the quickest way to become addicted.

## SHORT-TERM EFFECTS OF COCAINE

Cocaine stimulates the central nervous system. The short-term effects of using cocaine are:

- raised temperature, heart rate, and blood pressure
- constricted blood vessels
- dilated pupils
- feelings of restlessness, irritability, and anxiety

Users may also have an irregular heartbeat, have difficulty breathing, or stop breathing. Some users have seizures or become violent.

## LONG-TERM EFFECTS OF COCAINE

Cocaine use results in physical dependence on the drug. Some users become dependent after only one or two uses. The long-term effects of using cocaine are:

- irregular heartbeat
- high blood pressure
- chronic cough
- chest congestion
- chronic runny nose
- inflammation around the heart (myocarditis)
- memory problems
- personality and behavior changes
- ulcers (sores) on the nasal passages
- perforated septum (the cartilage between the nostrils) from inhaling cocaine
- burns on the face, fingertips, or eyebrows of crack smokers
- needle tracks on the skin of those who inject the drug intravenously
- weight loss
- loss of contact with reality (psychosis)
- hallucinations

During withdrawal, cocaine abusers often feel depressed, psychotic, and restless. They feel an intense craving for the drug. They are irritable and unable to concentrate.

## Closer Look    COCAINE AND PREGNANCY

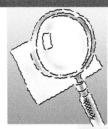

Cocaine, like other illicit drugs, can cause problems during pregnancy and after the child is born. These include:

- The mother can have a miscarriage, give birth early, or experience problems during delivery.
- The fetus can have a stroke and suffer brain damage or die.
- The newborn may not do well on the tests of reflexes and responsiveness done immediately after birth.
- The newborn may be easily startled or hard to comfort, or he may cry at even a gentle touch or sound.

## *Narcotic Analgesics (Opiates)*

Analgesics are painkillers. The strongest analgesics are opiates, or narcotics, which you can get only by prescription. They give relief to patients who suffer from severe, disabling pain after surgery, major injuries, or accidents. These drugs are also often abused. Some abusers started innocently enough with a legitimate prescription and then developed a craving for the drug. Other abusers take them from a family member's medicine cabinet or buy them illegally on the street.

### OPIATES USED TO TREAT PAIN

These opium-derived drugs are commonly used to treat pain:

- codeine
- morphine
- meperidine (Demerol)
- hydromorphone (Dilaudid)
- methadone
- oxycodone (OxyContin)
- paregoric—used to treat diarrhea

The drug naltrexone (ReVia, Vivitrol) is used to prevent relapse in patients who have been treated for opioid addiction. It comes in the form of tablets and as an extended-release injection.

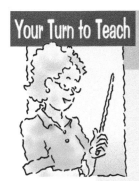

**Your Turn to Teach**

### HOW ELSE IS METHADONE USED— AND WHY?

Methadone is a man-made drug that is similar to morphine, from which heroin is made. As a painkiller, methadone relieves moderate to severe pain. It is also used in drug treatment programs.

Methadone effectively suppresses the effects of withdrawal from heroin, morphine, and other opiates. It is also a narcotic, but it does not give the euphoric rush that heroin gives. For this reason, methadone is sometimes given to those addicts who can't quit or be detoxified. Instead of turning to crime and violence to obtain their drug of choice, drug users may receive treatment at methadone clinics. However, because methadone is a controlled substance, only certain clinics and hospitals can dispense methadone for this purpose with the DEA's blessing.

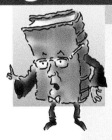

## Legal Brief — MISLEADING CLAIMS FOR OXYCONTIN BRING FINES

In May 2007, Purdue Pharma was fined $600 million for giving false or misleading information about oxycodone (OxyContin) to physicians and the public.

The drug manufacturer asserted that OxyContin users were less likely to abuse the drug or become addicted to it than to fast-acting narcotic painkillers such as oxycodone with acetaminophen (Percocet). OxyContin's time-release formula was the reason.

However, according to evidence given in federal court, the product did not live up to these claims. Recreational users soon discovered that they could get an immediate heroin-like high from OxyContin. All they had to do was break the tablets open and then swallow, snort, or inject the drug. Inside was pure, powerful oxycodone.

## TOLERANCE AND ADDICTION TO PRESCRIPTION DRUGS

People who use narcotic pain relievers build up a tolerance to the drug very quickly. Depending on the size of the dose and how often they get it, they can become physically dependent on the drug.

Narcotic painkillers produce a feeling of euphoria. Depending on the particular narcotic, the high can be very intense. Eventually, the user takes the drug to prevent withdrawal symptoms rather than to get high.

## WHO HAS AN ADDICTION?

It's no longer shocking news that some famous person has confessed to a drug problem or has gone into rehab. Drug addiction cuts across all segments of society and all age groups—from movie stars to politicians, from the famous to the unknown.

## TODAY'S WAR ON HEROIN

Most heroin in the United States today is smuggled into the country from Mexico, Canada, China, Colombia, the Dominican Republic, Burma, Thailand, and Laos. In the second half of

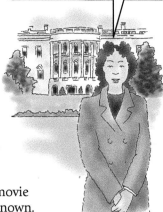

Betty Ford, wife of President Gerald Ford, was first lady from 1974 to 1977. She became addicted to painkillers and, later, to alcohol. In 1982, she founded the Betty Ford Center in Rancho Mirage, California, to treat people suffering from chemical dependency.

the 1990s, Afghanistan became the world's largest supplier of heroin.

## HEROIN'S EFFECT ON THE BODY

Heroin affects the body quickly. Symptoms include the following:

- surge ("rush") of euphoria
- flushing of the skin
- dry mouth
- pinpoint pupils
- a feeling of heaviness in the limbs
- alternating wakeful and sleepy states
- clouded mental functioning

Long-term use of heroin can cause the following medical problems:

- collapsed veins
- needle marks and tracks (scarring) along arteries and veins
- infection of the heart lining and valves
- abscesses
- cellulitis (bacterial skin infection)
- pneumonia

Heroin and other narcotics cross the placental barrier. This means that the drugs enter the fetus' bloodstream. A child born to a mother who is addicted to heroin is also addicted to heroin. At birth, the baby can have the same symptoms of addiction as an older user.

## SYMPTOMS OF HEROIN WITHDRAWAL

Withdrawal symptoms start 8 to 12 hours after the last dose. They can last 2 to 3 days. Mild withdrawal symptoms include:

- watery eyes
- runny nose
- yawning
- goosebumps
- sweating

As withdrawal continues, the following symptoms may appear:

- extreme agitation
- restless activity
- anxiety

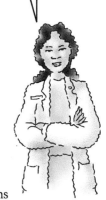

Street names for heroin include skag, horse, H, dope, smack, and junk. Other names are "brand names" of specific types, such as Body Bag, Homicide, and Pink Panther.

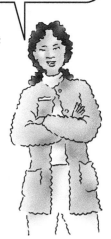

Injecting heroin can also lead to HIV, hepatitis, and blood poisoning (septicemia).

- irritability
- nausea and vomiting
- chills and fever
- allover body aches
- tremors and muscle spasms
- high blood pressure
- increased heart rate

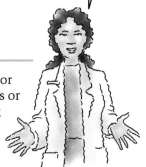

The symptoms of heroin withdrawal are often grouped together and described as a terrible case of the flu with aches, vomiting, headache, and diarrhea.

## Hallucinogens

Certain drugs cause changes in the way people perceive, or are aware of, reality. These drugs are called hallucinogens or psychedelics. People who take such drugs report hearing sounds, seeing images, and feeling sensations that are not actually real.

### TYPES OF HALLUCINOGENS

One type of hallucinogen is "shrooms" or "magic mushrooms." They're natural hallucinogens because the active chemicals in them occur in nature: psilocin and psilocybin. Other mushrooms, such as the *Amanita muscaria* (fly agaric), have similar properties but a different chemical makeup.

Below are two other natural hallucinogenic drugs. These, as well as psilocybin, can also be manufactured in the lab:

Whether natural or made in the lab, all these drugs are Schedule I controlled substances. They're all illegal.

- mescaline—from the peyote cactus
- DMT (dimethyltryptamine)—found in many plant species

Many of the other hallucinogenic drugs are known by their initials because they are only made in the lab. These drugs are:

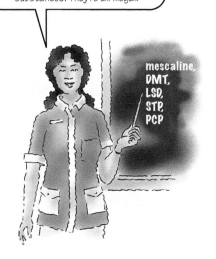

mescaline, DMT, LSD, STP, PCP

- LSD (acid)—lysergic acid diethylamide
- STP (DOM)—2,5-dimethoxy-4-methyl-amphetamine
- PCP (angel dust)—phencyclidine

### SHORT-TERM EFFECTS OF LSD

LSD is 100 times more powerful than the psilocybin in magic mushrooms and 4,000 times more powerful than mescaline. A typical "trip" starts 30 to 90 minutes after taking the drug and lasts for about 12 hours. These are the physical effects:

- dilated pupils
- higher body temperature
- fast heart rate
- high blood pressure
- sweating
- loss of appetite
- sleeplessness
- dry mouth
- tremors

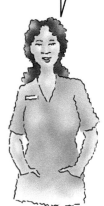

LSD is unpredictable. How people react to LSD depends on their personalities, how they're feeling, where they are, and what they expect will happen.

LSD has a dramatic effect on the senses. Everything is intensified. Some even say that they can "hear" colors and "see" sounds. Often, though, one experiences a "bad trip" that is unpleasant and as frightening as a terrible nightmare.

### LONG-TERM CONCERNS ABOUT LSD

LSD users quickly develop tolerance to the drug and need larger doses each time they use it. They also develop tolerance for other hallucinogenic drugs. However, this tolerance lasts only a few days. There are no reports of people experiencing physical withdrawal symptoms after chronic use.

In some users, LSD produces flashbacks even years after they stop taking the drug. Flashbacks are sometimes hallucinations, but in many other cases, they're a spontaneous return to the original experience—along with whatever distortions the person felt back then. Physicians call these flashbacks HPPD—hallucinogen persisting perception disorder. A single dose can be enough to cause them.

LSD can also cause long-term psychosis, or loss of contact with reality. Symptoms include dramatic mood swings, visual disturbances, and hallucinations. These symptoms can last for years even in people who have no history of psychological problems.

## Club Drugs

Club drugs, also called designer drugs, are increasingly popular among teens and young adults. The drugs are often sold, exchanged, or used at all-night dances called raves and in after-hours dance clubs. One of these drugs, Ecstasy, has become an icon of alternative culture.

## SOURCES OF CLUB DRUGS

Many club drugs are "homemade," meaning commercial laboratories do not produce them. The strength and exact chemicals can be different from batch to batch, and impurities may be present. Club drugs are often taken in combination with other illegal drugs or with alcohol, a practice that makes them even more potent and dangerous.

> Anterograde amnesia means you can't remember what happened after taking the drug. Events never go from short-term memory to long-term memory.

## TYPICAL CLUB DRUGS AND THEIR EFFECTS

As a medical assistant, you need to know about the club drugs that patients who visit the physician might be using. The chart below gives information about five typical club drugs.

## Club Drugs and Their Effects

| Drug Name | Street Names | Type/Effects | Adverse Effects |
|---|---|---|---|
| MDMA (methylenedioxy-methamphetamine) | • Ecstasy<br>• X<br>• XTC<br>• Adam<br>• Eve<br>• E | MDMA is a stimulant/hallucinogen that causes:<br>• too much energy<br>• increased sense of alertness<br>• higher heart rate, blood pressure, and body temperature | • lasts 4 to 6 hours<br>• builds up in the body to harmful levels after repeated use over a short time<br>• can cause depression, sleep problems, and anxiety for days to weeks after a dose<br>• can cause dehydration, forcing the user to drink too much water |
| GHB (gamma-hydroxybutyrate) | • Liquid Ecstasy<br>• Liquid X<br>• Liquid E<br>• Grievous Bodily Harm<br>• Georgia Home Boy<br>• Easy Lay<br>• Vita-G | GHB is a central nervous system depressant that causes:<br>• intoxicating effects similar to alcohol but more intense<br>• feelings of euphoria | • lasts up to four hours<br>• causes impaired motor skills and confusion<br>• sleep, coma, or death from higher doses<br>• hard to detect; clears from the body quickly<br>• also releases human growth hormones<br>• can be lethal when combined with alcohol |
| flunitrazepam (Rohypnol) | • Roofies<br>• Rophies<br>• Forget-Me Pill | Rohypnol is a central nervous system depressant that causes the user to become drowsy and fall asleep. | • profound loss of memory (anterograde amnesia)<br>• decreased blood pressure<br>• drowsiness |

## Club Drugs and Their Effects (continued)

| Drug Name | Street Names | Type/Effects | Adverse Effects |
|---|---|---|---|
| | | | • visual disturbances<br>• dizziness<br>• confusion<br>• upset stomach<br>• urinary retention |
| ketamine | • K<br>• Special K<br>• Vitamin K<br>• Super K | Ketamine is a dissociative anesthetic that is sold legally for veterinary use.<br>*Low doses:*<br>• feeling of floating<br>• disconnection from the body<br>*Large doses:*<br>• dreamlike states<br>• altered consciousness<br>• hallucinations | *Low doses:*<br>• impaired attention<br>• impaired learning ability<br>• impaired memory<br>*Higher doses:*<br>• delirium<br>• memory loss (amnesia)<br>• impaired motor function<br>• high blood pressure<br>• depression<br>• breathing problems |
| methamphetamine | • Meth<br>• Crystal<br>• Crystal Meth<br>• Crank<br>• Tweak<br>• Go-fast<br>• Ice<br>• Tina | Methamphetamine is a stimulant that causes:<br>• agitation<br>• excited speech<br>• decreased appetite<br>• increased physical activity levels | • memory loss<br>• aggression<br>• violence<br>• psychotic behavior<br>• damage to the heart and nervous system |

## ILLEGAL ACTS AND CLUB DRUGS

According to a 2005 survey, methamphetamine, or "meth," use is the biggest drug problem facing many counties in the United States. The report links meth users to increases in domestic violence, robbery, and theft. The drug is made with household ingredients such as cold medicine, and it's made in basements and garages.

Meth has harmful effects on the body. For example, this drug may increase heart rate and blood pressure, cause arrhythmias, and speed up respiration. High doses of the drug can raise body temperatures to unsafe levels. Under the influence, users may become irritable, confused, anxious, and aggressive.

Two club drugs are well-known date rape drugs. Rohypnol, or "roofies," acts as a sedative and leaves victims unable to remember what happened to them while under the influence of the drug. It's odorless, tasteless, and dissolves easily in carbonated drinks.

Until 1992, GHB, or Liquid Ecstasy, was being sold legally in heath food stores to body builders. It has also been linked to sexual assaults. It can cause its victims to lose consciousness.

## Inhalants

Young people, aged 8 to 17 years old, are the age group most likely to inhale chemical vapors from common household products and similar items to get high. The street name for this practice is "huffing."

### TYPICAL SUBSTANCES INHALED

Inhalant abusers use any of several different kinds of substances. Most are legal and can be bought by anyone for their originally intended purpose.

- volatile solvents—"volatile" because they turn to vapor at room temperature, such as paint thinner, gasoline, nail polish remover, rubber cement, and felt-tip markers
- aerosol sprays—spray paints, hair sprays, deodorant sprays, fabric protectors, and cooking sprays
- household gases—propane, butane from lighters, whipped cream aerosols, and refrigerant gases
- medical gases—ether, chloroform, nitrous oxide ("laughing gas")

### SIGNS THAT HUFFING HAS OCCURRED

Using inhalants has these effects:

- lightheadedness
- euphoria
- excitation
- hallucinations
- suicidal feelings (in some users)

If the person is sniffing paint or lacquer from a spray can, there may be paint residue on the nose, mouth, or hands.

### EFFECTS ON THE BODY

The effects of an inhalant last only about 30 minutes. So, the user may be tempted to repeat the experience. Users do not become physically dependent on inhalants, but they may become psychologically dependent.

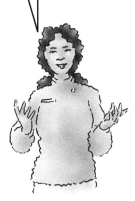

Thefts of cold medicines containing pseudoephedrine to make meth is the reason why drug stores must now sell these remedies from behind the counter and in small quantities. This is why in many states an OTC decongestant such as Sudafed is kept behind the counter and you have to show proof of identification to purchase it.

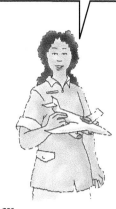

Model airplane glue was one of the items that huffers often used to use. Many communities no longer allow stores to sell it to minors.

Overdoses can have the following effects:

- irregular heartbeat (arrhythmia)
- low blood pressure (hypotension)
- delirium or coma
- violent behavior
- respiratory failure

Prolonged use can damage the lungs, heart, liver, kidneys, and central nervous system. Users may also suffer permanent brain damage.

## Treatment Options

Drug addiction is a chronic recurring illness. Many addicts compulsively fall back to their old behaviors despite the damage it does to themselves and their loved ones. Chronic addicts often need repeated treatments between relapses until they can finally recover and function without drugs.

No single method of treatment works for everyone. In addition, an effective treatment plan focuses on the whole person, not just the person's drug use. A whole array of other problems might contribute to the addiction. Medical, emotional, legal, family-related, and school- or job-related issues may all play a part.

Organizations such as NIDA are involved in researching treatment methods. For example, several medication options are now available and have been proven successful with some people. Other options include behavioral therapies, such as long-term residential programs, and support groups. Following are some of the options for drug addiction treatment in the United States.

## Closer Look    TREATING DRUG ADDICTION

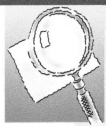

In 2004, more than 22 million Americans ages 12 and over needed treatment for alcohol or substance abuse. Fewer than four million of them received it. As a medical assistant, you should know as much as you can about the kinds of treatment that are available.

A good place to start is by visiting the NIDA website at www.drugabuse.gov/NIDAHome.html.

## Drug and Alcohol Addiction Treatment Options

| Treatment Option | Description |
| --- | --- |
| Detoxification | • often the first step in treating an addiction<br>• treats the physical effects of withdrawal<br>• done on an inpatient or outpatient basis |
| Drug maintenance programs | • usually done on an outpatient basis<br>• for addicts to heroin, morphine, and other opiates<br>• purpose: to prevent withdrawal, block the effects of the illegal drug, and decrease the craving for it<br>• drugs used: methadone, LAAM (levo-alpha-acetyl-methadol) |
| Treatment with naltrexone or buprenorphine (Subutex) | • usually done on an outpatient basis<br>• for addicts to alcohol or narcotics<br>• purpose: to block the effects of alcohol or narcotics and reduce the craving |
| Long-term residential programs | • 24-hour care<br>• for addicts to alcohol and illegal drugs<br>• usually not in a hospital setting<br>• often follows a "therapeutic community" approach |
| Outpatient drug-free treatment | • can be low intensity or as intensive as residential programs<br>• for addicts to alcohol and illegal drugs<br>• good for people with jobs or strong support structures in their lives<br>• may provide only drug information and counseling |

## TREATMENT ORGANIZATIONS AND GROUPS

Many organizations and groups give alcohol and drug addicts the support they need to stay sober and addiction free. The federal government is also very active in providing medical professionals and the public with information about these addictions.

### Alcoholics Anonymous

Alcoholics Anonymous, or AA, is an organization run by and for alcoholics. It has been successful in helping many people who have not been helped by other means. It follows a 12-step recovery program to reach sobriety.

A 12-step program encourages abusers to admit they have an uncontrollable problem and follow a specified series of steps to overcome it.

Alcoholics Anonymous describes itself as "a fellowship of men and women who share their experience, strength, and hope with each other that they may solve their common problem and help others to recover from alcoholism. The only requirement for membership is a desire to stop drinking."

AA was founded in 1935. There are meetings in almost every community in the United States.

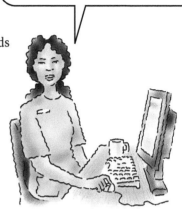

Encourage alcohol and drug abusers to look online and in the phone book for the locations of meetings. Tell them that no last names are used, so their identities will remain secret.

## Al-Anon and Alateen

This 50-year-old organization describes itself as "a fellowship of relatives and friends of alcoholics who share their experience, strength, and hope in order to solve their common problems." The purpose of the group is to give support to the families of alcoholics. Alateen groups are specifically for teenagers whose parents are alcoholics. There are Al-Anon and Alateen meetings in most communities. The group was founded in 1951, with guidance from AA's founder to create a support structure for family members of alcoholics in AA.

## Cocaine Anonymous

Cocaine Anonymous is a 12-step recovery program for cocaine abusers that is modeled on Alcoholics Anonymous. It welcomes crack abusers as well as abusers of all other mind-altering substances. Like AA, it's not affiliated with any religion, religious organization, or institution. Cocaine Anonymous was founded in Los Angeles in 1982. It has about 2,500 chapters worldwide.

## Marijuana Anonymous

Marijuana Anonymous is a 12-step recovery program for marijuana abusers. Like Cocaine Anonymous, it's modeled on AA. The organization was founded in 1989 and has more than 50 groups worldwide.

## Narcotics Anonymous

Narcotics Anonymous is a 12-step recovery program for drug abusers. It, too, is modeled on AA and is organized in a similar way. The group was founded in 1953. More than 33,500 meetings a week are conducted in 115 countries.

## National Clearinghouse for Alcohol and Drug Information

The National Clearinghouse for Alcohol and Drug Information is a comprehensive source of information about illegal drugs. The federal agencies that sponsor the clearinghouse are the U.S.

Department of Health and Human Services and SAMHSA (Substance Abuse and Mental Health Services Administration).

## National Institute on Drug Abuse

The National Institute on Drug Abuse has two functions. The first is to support and conduct research into drug addiction. The second is to put that research into the hands of medical professionals, schools, and families.

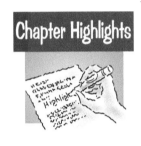

**Chapter Highlights**

- Substance abuse has personal costs that include problems with family, friends, job, school, health, money, or relationships. It also has societal costs. Substance abuse causes one in four deaths in the United States each year. Productivity losses to business have reached major levels.

- The signs and symptoms of abuse are different for each substance. For example, slurred speech and an unsteady gait are two physical signs that someone has been drinking to excess. A cocaine abuser may feel "high," "wired," restless, euphoric, and full of energy until the drug wears off.

- People who are physically dependent on a drug have a compulsive need to take the drug again and again to avoid withdrawal symptoms. People who are psychologically dependent on a drug have a compulsive need to take the drug because of how good the drug makes them feel.

- Older people living in retirement communities and nursing homes are often at risk for substance abuse. Drinking can be a particular problem because alcohol can mask pain or change how the body reacts to narcotic painkillers and medications that treat depression.

- Health care workers are at risk for drug abuse because many have easy access to drugs at work.

- Caffeine is the most commonly used drug in the United States. This stimulant is found in beverages and products that offer an energy boost, such as coffee, soft drinks, some pain-relief medications, and caffeine tablets. Caffeine withdrawal can cause fatigue, headaches, and difficulty concentrating.

- Alcohol is another commonly abused substance. One third of those who consume alcohol "binge drink," consuming more than five drinks at one sitting.

- Nicotine in tobacco is highly addictive. Once in the body, it changes the heart rate and blood pressure, stimulates feelings of pleasure and reward in the brain, and, like narcotics, releases dopamine.

- Secondhand smoke contains over 250 chemicals. Children and adults who breathe in secondhand smoke are more likely to develop pneumonia, bronchitis, and other lung diseases.

- The short-term effects of marijuana can include problems with memory and learning; distorted perception; difficulty in thinking and problem-solving; loss of coordination; and increased heart rate. Some users experience hallucinations. Long-term marijuana users may develop psychological dependence.

- Cocaine use results in physical dependence on the drug. Some long-term effects of using cocaine are personality and behavior changes, ulcers on the nasal passages, perforated septum, weight loss, loss of contact with reality (psychosis), and hallucinations.

- People who use narcotic pain relievers build up a tolerance to and dependence on the drug very quickly. Narcotic painkillers produce a feeling of euphoria. Depending on the particular narcotic, the high can be very intense. Eventually, the user takes the drug to prevent withdrawal symptoms rather than to get high.

- Hallucinogens cause changes in the way people perceive, or are aware of, reality. Users report hearing sounds, seeing images, and feeling sensations that are not real. Some hallucinogens can cause lingering effects. For example, LSD produces flashbacks in some users days, months, or even years after they last took the drug. LSD can also cause long-term psychosis, or loss of contact with reality.

- Club drugs include the stimulants MDMA (Ecstasy) and methamphetamine; the depressants GBH and Rohypnol, which are both known as "date-rape" drugs; and the dissociative anesthetic ketamine (Special K). Club drugs are often taken in combination with other illegal drugs or with alcohol, a practice that makes them even more potent and dangerous.

- Using inhalants causes lightheadedness, euphoria, excitation, and hallucinations. Users do not become physically dependent on inhalants, but they may become psychologically dependent. Prolonged use can damage the lungs, heart, liver, kidneys, and central nervous system. Users may also suffer permanent brain damage.

## Chapter 8

# ADMINISTRATION OF MEDICATIONS

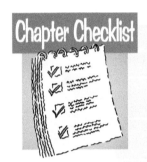

**Chapter Checklist**

- Locate important information on a medication label.

- Recall the steps to safely administer an oral medication.

- Describe how to select a site and administer a subcutaneous injection.

- Explain how to select a site and administer an intradermal injection.

- Describe how to select a site and give an intramuscular injection to an adult and a child.

- Explain the criteria in the selection of a needle gauge and length.

- Describe reconstitution of a powder to an injectable liquid.

- List steps in removing medication from a vial and an ampule.

- Compare the use of transdermal and topical medications.

- Describe the intravenous route of medication administration.

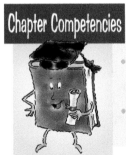

**Chapter Competencies**

- Apply principles of aseptic technique and infection control (ABHES Competency 4.c.)

- Prepare and administer oral and parenteral medications as directed by physician (ABHES Competency 4.m.; CAAHEP Competency 3.b.4.g.)

- Practice standard precautions (ABHES Competency 4.r.; CAAHEP Competency 3.b.1.e.)

In this chapter, you'll learn more about the clinical aspects of interpreting medication orders and administering medications to patients. You'll learn the correct procedures for administering oral, topical, and transdermal medications. You'll also learn the procedures for delivering medications by injection and inhaler, and how medication can be delivered by the intravenous route.

Remember two important restrictions as you start this chapter. The first is that only some states allow clinical medical assistants to administer drugs. Be sure that you know what the laws of your state allow you to do. The second is that medical assistants may only administer drugs under the direction of a physician or other licensed health care professional.

## Medication Orders

When a physician tells you orally or in writing to give a medication to a patient, the physician is giving a medication order.

### PARTS OF A MEDICATION ORDER

A medication order provides four important pieces of information:
- the name of the drug
- the strength of the dose
- the route of administration
- when or how often to administer the drug

For example, the physician might write the following in a patient's medication record: *ranitidine 150 mg PO twice a day.* This entry means that the physician would like the patient to take 150 mg of ranitidine (Zantac) by mouth twice a day.

### TYPES OF MEDICATION ORDERS

As you learned in Chapter 3, you'll most likely encounter only two different types of medication orders in the medical office. Many drug orders administered in a medical office are *single orders*. For example, you may help administer a patient's annual flu shot. Medications that must be administered immediately in emergency situations are referred to as *STAT single orders.*

## Reading the Medication Label

Before you can administer or help administer a drug, your most important task is to check the drug label against the medication order. You need to be sure you have the correct drug and the

## Closer Look — ONCE-PER-WEEK DRUGS

Some drugs are now available in once-per-week, twice-per-month, and even once-per-month forms. These drugs replace older formulations that were meant to be taken daily. For example, in 2001, the FDA approved two new strengths of the osteoporosis drug alendronate (Fosamax). Both strengths were designed to be given on a weekly basis to prevent or treat postmenopausal osteoporosis.

In 2005, the FDA approved a new, once-per-month version of ibandronate (Boniva), which is also used to treat and prevent postmenopausal osteoporosis. Women are instructed to take this 150-mg oral tablet on the same date each month.

correct dosage in your hand. Safe drug administration requires you to compare the physician's order as written on the medication order form against the drug label *three times.*

Many drugs, especially oral medications, are available in a number of strengths or concentrations. The drug label gives you exact information about the drug, including the name, the dose strength, and the expiration date.

## DRUG NAME

The labels on both prescription drugs and over-the-counter drugs generally give two names. The generic name is written in lowercase letters and appears, sometimes in parentheses, after the manufacturer's trade name. Physicians often order medications by their generic names, such as acetaminophen or ibuprofen. The trade name is often printed in large letters on the medication label and is often followed by the ™ or ® symbol.

### What's in a Name?

Generic drugs can be sold under more than one trade name. For example, the generic drug ibuprofen is sold under the trade names Advil, Motrin, and Nuprin, among others. Because drug formulations may differ, the physician may specify a trade name rather than a generic name in the medication order.

However, certain drugs are so widely used and so well known by their generic names that some manufacturers choose to avoid marketing under trade names. One example is lidocaine.

## Combination Drugs

Some medications are called combination drugs because they contain two or more medications together. In these cases, the drug label will list both generic names and will indicate how much of each drug is in the combination dose. These drugs are ordered by the trade name and the number of capsules or tablets or the volume of elixir to be given. For example, the drug order *Septra 1 tsp q12hr* indicates that the patient should receive one teaspoon of Septra every 12 hours.

### Closer Look  ANATOMY OF A DRUG LABEL

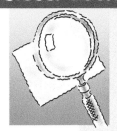

Take a quick look at this drug label. The label shows that this particular prescription-only antibacterial medication contains two different generic drugs. The small print on the left side tells how much of each generic drug is in a teaspoon (5 mL) of the elixir: 40 mg trimethoprim and 200 mg sulfamethoxazole. The medication order will state how many teaspoons of Septra to give the patient.

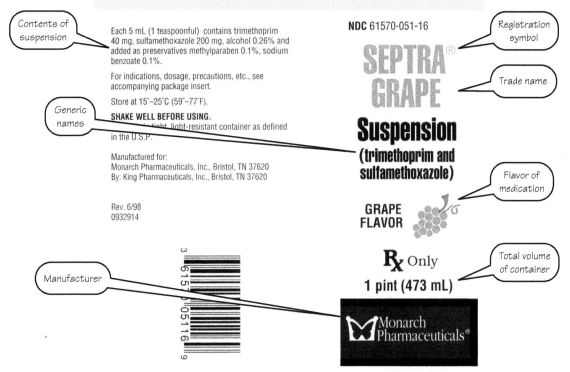

Contents of suspension

Each 5 mL (1 teaspoonful) contains trimethoprim 40 mg, sulfamethoxazole 200 mg, alcohol 0.26% and added as preservatives methylparaben 0.1%, sodium benzoate 0.1%.

For indications, dosage, precautions, etc., see accompanying package insert.

Store at 15°–25°C (59°–77°F).

SHAKE WELL BEFORE USING.

Generic names

light, light-resistant container as defined in the U.S.P.

Manufactured for:
Monarch Pharmaceuticals, Inc., Bristol, TN 37620
By: King Pharmaceuticals, Inc., Bristol, TN 37620

Rev. 6/98
0932914

Manufacturer

NDC 61570-051-16

Registration symbol

SEPTRA®
GRAPE

Trade name

Suspension
(trimethoprim and sulfamethoxazole)

Flavor of medication

GRAPE FLAVOR

Rx Only

Total volume of container

1 pint (473 mL)

Monarch Pharmaceuticals®

## Seal of Approval

The letters *USP* or *NF* may also appear on a drug label. These letters stand for *United States Pharmacopeia* and *National Formulary*. These initials mean that the drug has met standards of purity, potency (strength), and storage. The Food and Drug Administration enforces these standards.

> The letters *USP* or *NF* on a drug label indicate that the drug has been given the United States Pharmacopeia and National Formulary's seal of approval.

## DOSE STRENGTH

After checking the drug name, look for the dose strength on the label. Pay close attention: the labels and containers for different concentrations of the same drug may look exactly alike except for the numbers that tell the strength of the contents. Strengths can be given in metric measurements, units, or percentages. Be sure that the numbers on the package match the numbers on the medication order.

Insulin, heparin, and penicillin G are among the drugs most commonly measured in units. The unit system is an international standard of drug potency; it is not based on weight. The number of units appears on the drug label. (See the illustration below for an example.)

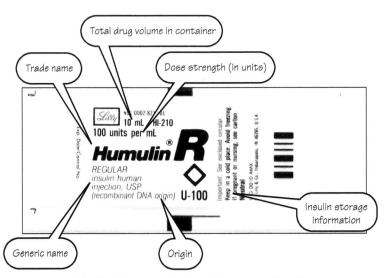

The label of an injectable drug that's measured in units includes the information shown here.

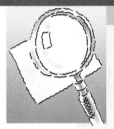

## Closer Look

## CAN YOU TELL THE DIFFERENCE BETWEEN THESE LABELS?

The oral solution labels below are examples of look-alike labels that you're likely to encounter. Reading labels carefully can help you avoid medication errors.

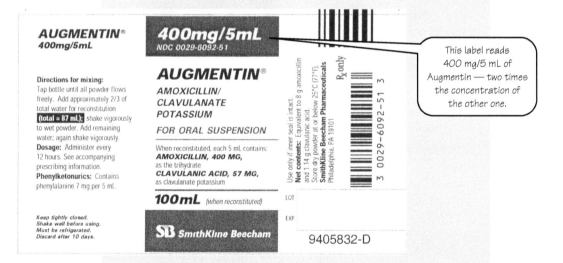

**AUGMENTIN®**
**200mg/5mL**
NDC 0029-6087-51

**AUGMENTIN®**
200mg/5mL

**Directions for mixing:**
Tap bottle until all powder flows freely. Add approximately 2/3 of total water for reconstitution **(total ≈ 91 mL);** shake vigorously to wet powder. Add remaining water; again shake vigorously.
**Dosage:** Administer every 12 hours. See accompanying prescribing information.
**Phenylketonurics:** Contains phenylalanine 7 mg per 5 mL.

Keep tightly closed.
Shake well before using.
Must be refrigerated.
Discard after 10 days.

**AUGMENTIN®**
AMOXICILLIN/
CLAVULANATE
POTASSIUM

FOR ORAL SUSPENSION

When reconstituted, each 5 mL contains:
**AMOXICILLIN, 200 MG,**
as the trihydrate
**CLAVULANIC ACID, 28.5 MG,**
as clavulanate potassium

**100mL** (when reconstituted)

**SB** SmithKline Beecham

Use only if inner seal is intact.
**Net contents:** Equivalent to 4 g amoxicillin and 0.57 g clavulanic acid.
Store dry powder at or below 25°C (77°F).
SmithKline Beecham Pharmaceuticals
Philadelphia, PA 19101

Rx only

3 0029-6087-51 9

LOT
EXP

9405728-D

This one is
Augmentin 200 mg/5 mL

**AUGMENTIN®**
**400mg/5mL**
NDC 0029-6092-51

**AUGMENTIN®**
400mg/5mL

**Directions for mixing:**
Tap bottle until all powder flows freely. Add approximately 2/3 of total water for reconstitution **(total ≈ 87 mL);** shake vigorously to wet powder. Add remaining water; again shake vigorously.
**Dosage:** Administer every 12 hours. See accompanying prescribing information.
**Phenylketonurics:** Contains phenylalanine 7 mg per 5 mL.

Keep tightly closed.
Shake well before using.
Must be refrigerated.
Discard after 10 days.

**AUGMENTIN®**
AMOXICILLIN/
CLAVULANATE
POTASSIUM

FOR ORAL SUSPENSION

When reconstituted, each 5 mL contains:
**AMOXICILLIN, 400 MG,**
as the trihydrate
**CLAVULANIC ACID, 57 MG,**
as clavulanate potassium

**100mL** (when reconstituted)

**SB** SmithKline Beecham

Use only if inner seal is intact.
**Net contents:** Equivalent to 8 g amoxicillin and 1.14 g clavulanic acid.
Store dry powder at or below 25°C (77°F).
SmithKline Beecham Pharmaceuticals
Philadelphia, PA 19101

Rx only

3 0029-6092-51 3

LOT
EXP

9405832-D

This label reads
400 mg/5 mL of
Augmentin — two times
the concentration of
the other one.

## EXPIRATION DATE

The final thing to check on the package or the container is the expiration date. The expiration date may be printed on the package label or stamped on the container. Expired drugs may have lost their strength or become chemically unstable. Be sure to dispose of expired drugs properly.

# Administering Oral Medications

As a medical assistant, you may often be asked to help administer pills, tablets, capsules, and liquids for patients to take by mouth. The oral route is the most frequent route of drug administration and rarely causes physical discomfort in patients. Administration of oral drugs is relatively easy for patients who are alert and can swallow.

Hands On Procedure 8-1 on page 300 outlines the exact steps to follow when you administer oral medications. Right now, let's put those steps in context and understand what makes them important.

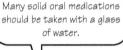

Many solid oral medications should be taken with a glass of water.

### WASHING YOUR HANDS

Observe proper hand hygiene. Do not let a hectic day keep you from washing your hands before administering any drug in any form. Some medical offices may prefer that you use soap and water. Others allow the use of alcohol-based hand rubs or gels.

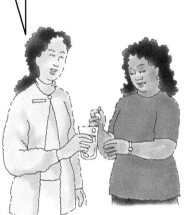

### GETTING ORGANIZED

To administer solid medications you'll need:

- a disposable calibrated cup to hold oral liquid, tablets, or capsules
- a glass of water for the patient

Some patients may have difficulty swallowing certain tablets or capsules. Do not crush medications or break them open unless directed to do so by the physician. Some drugs will affect the body in a different way if they are not taken as directed on the package.

When you fill the disposable cup with a liquid medication, take care to measure out the correct amount. Hold the cup at eye level. Use your thumbnail to identify how far up to fill the

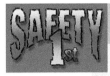

## RIGHT PATIENT, RIGHT DRUG, RIGHT DOSE

When you administer drugs, you can never be too careful. Giving the wrong drug or too strong a dose can cause serious harm to a patient. Do not assume anything. Get in the habit of checking your every move.

- If you're working with more than one patient at a time, be sure that the patient and the medication order match up. Remember to be conscious of trade names and generic names.

- If the supply cabinet contains different strengths of a medication, check that you've chosen the strength the physician prescribes.

- If you have more than one medication in front of you when you're with a patient, check that you've picked up the right one each time. Put the lid back on any medication you have finished using. Never have two medications open at one time.

Remember, when you've removed a drug from its container, you should ensure that it's the correct drug by carefully comparing the medication order with the package label for drug and dosage information.

cup with liquid. Pour only up to that level. The surface of the liquid may appear curved when observing from the side of the cup; this phenomenon is known as the **meniscus**. Be sure to measure the liquid from the lowest part of this curve.

## CALCULATING A DOSE

If a medication order calls for 500 mg of the antibiotic cefaclor (Ceclor) and the package you have contains 250-mg tablets, then you must calculate the dose. Review what you learned in Chapter 2 about calculating doses. If necessary, use a calculator to do the math.

- If you're unsure that you have made the correct calculation, ask your supervisor to check your results.

- If you discover you have given too little or too much of a medication, tell your supervisor immediately. The safety of patients must always come before any other consideration.

## AVOIDING CONTAMINATING THE MEDICATION

Many times you'll be administering solid drugs from a container of loose tablets or capsules. Liquids are also dispensed from multiple-dose containers. Here's how to avoid contaminating the contents:

- When you open a container, always place the open end of the lid so it faces up. This way, no bacteria from the surface on which you place the lid will contaminate it.

- Drop solid medications into the bottle cap. If more than one tablet or capsule drops into the bottle cap, pour them back into the container and start again. Do not stick your fingers into the container or touch the capsules or tablets with your fingers.

- If a tablet is in a unit-dose package, hold the dose over the disposable calibrated cup. Push the tablet into the cup by pressing on the backing. Adjust this technique to work with other packaging formats.

## GIVING THE MEDICATION

Tell the patient to place the pill or capsule on the back of the tongue. Have him or her tilt her head back to swallow a tablet or slightly forward to swallow a capsule. Encourage him or her to take a few sips of water to move the tablet or capsule down the esophagus and into the stomach. Then ask the patient to finish drinking the glass of water.

## AFTER GIVING THE MEDICATION

Be sure that the patient swallows the full dose that the physician has prescribed. Note any discrepancies in the patient's records. Have the patient remain in the office for 20 to 30 minutes, especially if a new medication is administered, so that he may be observed for any adverse reactions. Some drugs, such as antibiotics, may cause a severe allergic reaction that would require immediate care. If a reaction occurs, notify the physician immediately.

# Administering Medications by Injection

In some states, medical assistants are allowed to administer medications by injection. You'll hear this form of administration called the parenteral route (that is, the route that does not go through the gastrointestinal system).

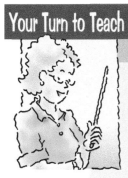

**Your Turn to Teach**

## USING PILL BOXES, PILL CUTTERS, AND PILL CRUSHERS

Once patients leave the medical office, it's often difficult for them to self-administer medications and keep their various medications organized. As a medical assistant, it may be your job to teach patients practical ways of managing their medications. Inform patients of the following resources:

- *Pill boxes.* Instruct patients to divide their medications into daily doses and store them in a weekly pill box. This is especially helpful for patients who have difficulty remembering to take their pills each day. Pill boxes are available at most drug and grocery stores and are often sold with large symbols or letters.

- *Pill cutters.* Inform patients about pill cutters, which easily divide oddly shaped pills. Some pill cutters come with a built-in magnifying glass and a storage compartment. Pill cutters are safer and easier to use than knives, especially for patients with unsteady hands or impaired vision. However, it's important to remind patients that pill cutters should not be used unless the pill is scored.

- *Pill crushers.* Advise patients to purchase a pill crusher if their medications must be dissolved in food. Crushers are easy and safe to use. Most models prevent cross-contamination when more than one pill must be crushed.

Hands On Procedure 8-2 on page 303 describes how to prepare injections, and Hands On Procedures 8-3 through 8-6 provide step-by-step instructions for administering injections. First, however, you need to learn about syringes, safety procedures, drug packaging, injection sites, and other useful facts.

### GETTING ORGANIZED

To administer an injection, you'll need these supplies:

- sterile gloves
- a syringe and needle of the right size for the injection site, the medication, and the age and size of the patient
- an ampule or vial of the correct medication at the strength specified in the medication order

- antiseptic wipes to clean the skin before the injection
- a small gauze pad to cover the injection site after the injection
- an adhesive bandage (or paper tape if the patient is allergic to adhesive bandages) to secure the gauze pad

## THE PARTS OF A SYRINGE AND NEEDLE

The illustration below gives the names for the parts of a **syringe** and needle. The **barrel** holds the medication. The **plunger** forces the medicine out of the barrel and into the patient's body.

A syringe has ruler-like markings on the side of the barrel to show the amount of the drug inside. It is measured in cubic centimeters or milliliters. Markings between numbers show fractions of a cubic centimeter or milliliter, so that you can measure out the exact quantity the medication order calls for.

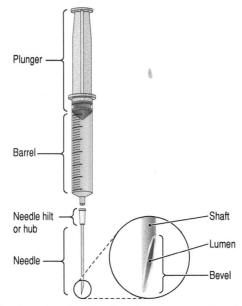

The plunger, barrel, and needle make up the parts of a syringe.

## SAFETY PROCEDURES AND STANDARD PRECAUTIONS

There are several safety procedures that you must follow when administering injections. These include:

- wearing gloves
- applying an antiseptic to the patient's skin
- properly disposing of used needles and other sharps

## Wearing Gloves

Gloves will protect you from potential blood spills when you administer medications by injection. The Centers for Disease Control and Prevention (CDC) recommend wearing gloves whenever you may have contact with blood, body tissues, mucous membranes, or broken skin.

Boxes of gloves are in most examining rooms. Read the label on the box before you use them. If your office uses standard latex gloves, ask patients if they're allergic to latex. Ask your supervisor where the nonlatex gloves are kept.

*Wearing gloves isn't just for your safety—it's for the patient's safety, too!*

## Applying Antiseptics

The skin is covered with bacteria. To clean the skin at the injection site, use an alcohol swab or other skin cleaner that your office specifies. Work methodically. Clean the skin with a circular motion, starting at an inner point and moving outward. Using this procedure will keep you from contaminating the injection site.

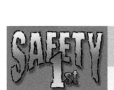

### GUIDELINES FOR WEARING GLOVES

The CDC guidelines include the following statement about wearing gloves:

The use of gloves does not eliminate the need for hand hygiene. Likewise, the use of hand hygiene does not eliminate the need for gloves. Gloves reduce hand contamination by 70% to 80%, prevent cross-contamination, and protect patients and health care personnel from infection. Hand rubs should be used before and after each patient, just as gloves should be changed before and after each patient.

For additional information about CDC hand hygiene guidelines, visit the website www.cdc.gov.

### Disposing of Used Needles and Syringes

Used needles need to be disposed of properly. Discarded carelessly in the office, they are a danger to patients and your fellow health care workers.

Needles and syringes should be disposed of in clearly marked sharps containers. Do not recap used syringes. Just drop them carefully into the appropriate waste container. If, by accident, you drop a ring or some other important personal item into the sharps container, do not reach in to get it.

OSHA recommends that all medical offices use a needle designed to prevent accidental needle sticks. This needle has a plastic guard that slips over the needle as it's withdrawn from the injection site. The guard locks in place, giving you a greater margin of safety. Dispose of this needle in the sharps box in the standard manner.

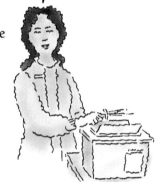

Dispose of used needles and syringes in the appropriate sharps container.

## HOW INJECTABLE MEDICATIONS ARE STORED

Injectable medications are stored in vials, ampules, or prefilled cartridges. When retrieving an injectable medication, observe these standard precautions:

- Check the expiration date on an ampule or vial.

- Check that the medicine is safe to give. Look for crystals or lumps. There should be none. Do not use the medicine if crystals or lumps are present.

- Check for the right color. Tell the physician if you think the medicine has become discolored.

## Containers for Injectable Medications

| Container | What You Need to Know |
|---|---|
| Prefilled cartridges | • Prefilled cartridges provide measured doses of a medicine in one-time-use syringes.<br>• A special syringe might be needed depending on the type of cartridge. However, some medications come in prefilled syringes with plastic plungers that must be screwed in.<br>• The entire unit should be discarded after use. |
| Ampules | • An ampule is a small glass bottle with a narrow neck and a long, hollow top. It holds a single dose of a drug.<br>• The ampule may be colored or clear. It may be scored to make breaking off the top easier.<br>• Sterile gauze or an ampule breaker should be used to break the ampule.<br>• Medicine sometimes gets lodged in the neck of the ampule. Flick the neck with your finger until the medicine flows down. If you do not, you'll not have the full dose to inject.<br>• Because glass fragments may be inside, a filter needle should be used to draw up the medication. Do not take medicine from the top of the ampule after you break it open. |
| Vials | • A vial is a small bottle with a plastic or metal top. In the middle is a rubber stopper.<br>• The vial may have a single dose inside or enough for several doses.<br>• If the vial holds more than one dose, write a note on the label. Give the date on which you first used the medication. |

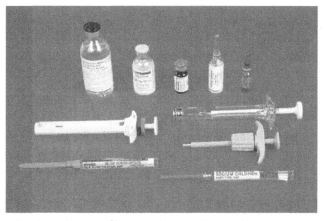

Ampules, vials, and prefilled cartridges contain injectable medications.

## Closer Look

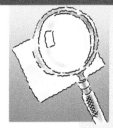

### RECONSTITUTING DRY MEDICATIONS

The contents of vials may be in the form of a solution or powder. Powders must be reconstituted—mixed with a specific amount and type of diluting agent. The **diluent**, or diluting agent, is usually sterile water or saline. Certain drugs, such as phenytoin (Dilantin) require a special diluent supplied by the manufacturer.

When a powdered drug is reconstituted in a multiple-dose vial, you must write some information on the label:

- date of reconstitution
- initials of the person who reconstituted the drug
- diluent used
- strength of the medicine that was produced

To reconstitute dry medication in a vial, follow these steps:

1. Check the vial label or manufacturer's instructions to find out how much diluent to add to the powder.

2. Wipe the top of the vial containing the diluent with an alcohol pad before inserting the needle. Inject the air from the needle into the vial, and then withdraw the correct amount of diluent using aseptic technique.

3. Add the diluent to the vial containing the powder. Wipe the top of the vial with an alcohol pad before inserting the needle.

4. Roll the vial between your palms until the powder is dissolved.

The concentration of the mixture will depend on how the medication will be given. The instructions from the drug's manufacturer usually tell how much diluent to add to the powder if the medication is to be given by IV, IM, or SubQ injection.

You must be sure that the concentration of the mixture is right for the method of administration. A dosage that's too strong for the way it's given may harm the patient's tissues. If the dose is too weak for the method of administration, the medicine may not have the proper effect.

## TYPES OF INJECTIONS

As you learned in Chapter 1, there are several different types of injections. You'll need to know how to administer the following:

- **Subcutaneous** (SubQ) injections—just under the skin
- intradermal injections—between the layers of the skin
- **intramuscular** (IM) injections—into a muscle

### Subcutaneous Injections

A SubQ injection places the drug into the tissues between the skin and the muscle. Drugs administered by this route are absorbed more slowly than IM injections. Heparin and insulin are two common examples of drugs given by SubQ injection.

A small volume of 0.5 to 1 mL is used for SubQ injections. Volumes larger than 1 mL are best given as IM injections.

Recommended sites for SubQ injections include:

- the upper arm
- the front of the thigh
- the upper abdomen

When a drug is given by the SubQ route, the needle is generally inserted at a 45-degree angle. The needle length and angle of insertion depend on the patient's body weight.

### Intradermal Medications

The intradermal route is usually used for sensitivity tests, such as the tuberculin test or allergy skin tests. Absorption is slow from this route, providing good results when testing for allergies or administering local anesthetics. Common injection sites are the inner part of the forearm and the upper back.

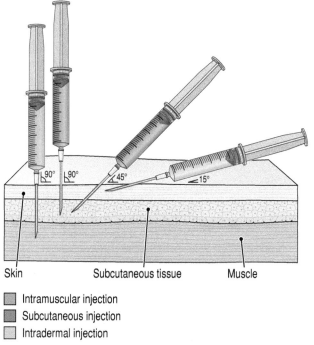

The angle of insertion varies depending on the type of injection being administered.

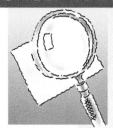

# Closer Look | CHOOSING THE RIGHT NEEDLE

Factors such as the type of injection and size of the patient require different needle lengths and gauges. Needle lengths vary from 0.375 inch to 1.5 inches for standard injections. The **gauge** of the needle refers to the diameter of the needle **lumen** (hole). Needle gauge varies from 18 (large) to 30 (small). As a general rule, remember that the higher the number, the smaller the gauge.

For IM injections, needle length varies from one to three inches depending on the site of injection and the type of medication being administered. The size of the patient and the fat-to-muscle ratio are also factors in determining the size of needle needed. For example, a deep IM injection in the buttocks of an adult female might require a 3-inch needle, whereas an IM injection in the deltoid muscle of an older adult patient might only require a 1-inch needle.

The needle gauge varies from 20 to 25 depending on the thickness of the medication to be administered. A small-gauge needle, such as 25 or 27, would make it difficult to draw thick medications into a syringe or inject them into a patient. Examples of thick medications are penicillins and hormones.

SubQ injections, however, are generally given using a short, small-gauge needle, such as 25 gauge (0.625 inch) or 23 gauge (0.5 inch).

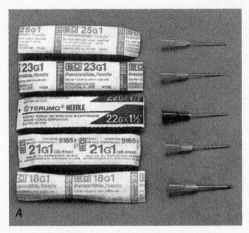

A) Medical supply companies package needles separately in color-coded packages. The sizes are written on the package.

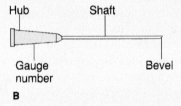

(B) The parts of a needle include the hub, shaft, and bevel.

When selecting an injection site, choose a hairless area of skin, away from moles, scars, or pigmented areas. Small volumes (less than 0.1 mL) are usually used for this type of injection. The needle should be inserted at a 15-degree angle between the upper layers of the skin. The injection produces a small raised area, or **wheal**, on the outer surface of the skin. If no wheal appears, you may have injected the drug into the subcutaneous layer. This would cause test results to be inaccurate.

## Intramuscular Injections

As you learned in Chapter 1, an IM injection is the administration of a drug into a muscle. Drugs that are irritating to subcutaneous tissue can be given by IM injection. Because of the rich blood supply of the muscle, drugs given intramuscularly are absorbed more rapidly than drugs given by the subcutaneous route of administration. Additionally, a larger volume (1–3 mL) of the drug can be given at one site. However, with a large drug volume, the drug must be divided and given as two separate injections. Volumes larger than 3 mL will not be absorbed properly at a single injection site.

**Selecting a Site**

The table on page 294 helps you identify the most common sites for IM injections. These sites include:

- the deltoid muscle
- the ventrogluteal site
- the dorsogluteal site
- the vastus lateralis

The thigh, or vastus lateralis site, is often used for infants' and children's injections, especially for children under the age of three years. In younger children, the vastus lateralis is more developed than the gluteal or deltoid sites, which are common injection sites for adults.

When using the deltoid site in adults, no more than 1 mL of medication should be injected into the muscle. Also in adults, no more than 3 mL of a drug should be injected into the ventrogluteal or vastus lateralis sites.

The rectus femoris, located on the anterior of the thigh, is only used when other sites are contraindicated. Often, drug manufacturers recommend sites for injecting specific drugs to assist in determining the best possible location for an injection.

**Administering the Injection**

After you've selected an appropriate site for an IM injection, cleanse the skin thoroughly with alcohol. Then, stretch the skin taut and insert the needle at a 90-degree angle to the skin.

The Z-track method of IM injection may be used to administer a drug that is highly irritating to subcutaneous tissues or one that may permanently stain the skin (see Hands On Procedure 8-6 on page 317).

## Intramuscular Injection Sites

| Muscle | Location | How to Find It | What It Looks Like |
|---|---|---|---|
| Deltoid | the upper arm | • *Patient position*: sitting or lying down<br>• Visualize a triangle on the patient's upper arm. Feel for a bone (called the acromion process) across the top of the upper arm. Use it as the base of the triangle. The point of the triangle is right below it, at about armpit level.<br>• Give the injection in the middle of the triangle, one to two inches below the base. | |
| Ventrogluteal | the hip | • *Patient position*: lying on the side, toes pointing inward<br>• Place your open hand on the patient's hip. The heel of your hand should be on the hip bone. The thumb should point at the groin. Form a "V" with your pointer and third fingers.<br>• With your little finger and ring finger, feel for the edge of a bone. Give the injection in the middle of the "V." | |

## Intramuscular Injection Sites (continued)

| Muscle | Location | How to Find It | What It Looks Like |
|---|---|---|---|
| Dorsogluteal | the upper buttocks | • *Patient position*: lying on the side, toes pointing inward<br>• Imagine a line from the top of the cleft of the buttocks to the side of the body. In the middle of that line, imagine a second line that forms a cross. The cross starts about three inches above the first line and goes halfway down the middle of the buttock.<br>• Feel for a curved bone in the upper outer square. Administer the injection below the curved bone. | Injection site — Posterior superior iliac spine — Greater trochanter — Sciatic nerve — |
| Vastus lateralis | the top of the thigh | • *Patient position*: reclining or lying down<br>• Divide the thigh into thirds horizontally and vertically. The injection goes into the outer middle third of the thigh. | Greater trochanter of femur — Femoral artery and vein — Sciatic nerve — Deep femoral artery — Vastus lateralis (Outer middle third) — Vastus lateralis — Lateral femoral condyle — |

### Other Things to Know About Intramuscular Injections

When you learn to give IM injections, you'll be told to aspirate for blood. This means to pull up on the plunger of the needle to see if you draw any blood up into the barrel. If blood appears, you've unintentionally injected the needle into a blood vessel, not into muscle. If you draw blood, discard the syringe and begin again. Do not reinject the now-contaminated medication. With SubQ or intradermal injections, however, aspirating is not necessary.

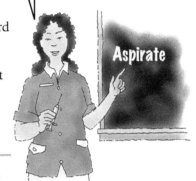

*Aspirate means "to take out by suction." You might be told to use a needle to aspirate the medication from a vial. This means to draw it into the syringe.*

**Aspirate**

## Administering Inhalant Medications

Asthma sufferers and patients with other breathing difficulties often receive medications as sprays or mists that they inhale into their lungs. The drugs given this way fall into three categories.

- bronchodilators, which open the breathing passages in the lungs
- mucolytics, which help patients bring up mucus from the lungs
- certain anti-inflammatory drugs

These drugs primarily have a local effect on the lungs.

### BEFORE YOU BEGIN

These drugs enter the bloodstream through the mucous membranes of the respiratory system. The patient breathes in the drug through a face mask, a nebulizer, or a positive-pressure breathing machine. A nebulizer turns liquid medication into a mist or vapor by pumping air or oxygen through it. The patient inhales the vapor through a tubelike mouthpiece and receives the drug in the process. Face masks are sometimes used with children and older adult patients.

If you're working with patients who need inhalant medications, you'll need to help them understand how to take these medications correctly. For example, many patients with asthma use an inhaler to make breathing easier. Each time they press the inhaler, it releases a **metered dose** of the medication inside. However, if patients do not use their inhalers correctly, they can deposit much of the drug on their tongues rather than taking it into their lungs. They won't get enough medication into their systems and will therefore lose the benefit of the therapy.

## TWO KINDS OF INHALERS

Metered-dose inhalers (MDIs) are meant to be placed in the mouth between the lips. Inhaled steroids are often delivered in pressurized inhalers (pMDIs). Pressurized inhalers are different because they use water vapors or mist to carry the medication into the lungs. These inhalers are meant to be sprayed at a distance of 1 to 2 inches from the mouth.

With both metered-dose and pressurized inhalers, the physician may advise the patient to use a spacer device that can be placed directly in the mouth. The spacer slows down the droplets and allows them to enter the airways more easily. Common spacers that you'll most likely encounter are the Aerochamber or E-Z Spacer.

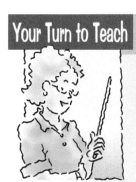

## Your Turn to Teach — USING A METERED-DOSE INHALER

As a medical assistant, you may be asked to instruct patients on the proper way to use a metered-dose inhaler. Teach patients to follow these steps:

1. Shake the inhaler immediately before using it.
2. Remove the cap covering the mouthpiece.
3. Hold the inhaler with the mouthpiece down.
4. Slowly exhale, letting all the air out of your lungs.
5. Place the mouthpiece between your lips and close them around it.
6. Firmly press the bottom of the inhaler down to produce the spray. Slowly breathe in deeply while pressing.
7. Hold your breath for 5 to 10 seconds while the medication takes effect. You may cough; this is natural.
8. If your prescription calls for a second dose, wait 1 to 2 minutes. Then repeat steps 4 through 7.
9. Replace the cap.
10. Rinse out your mouth with water.

# Administering Topical and Transdermal Medications

As you read in Chapter 1, topical medications include creams, lotions, ointments, and sprays. You administer them directly onto the skin. These medications produce local effects.

Transdermal medications, however, are usually administered using a patch placed on the skin. They produce systemic effects, or effects throughout the body. Medication administered transdermally is absorbed into the body through the skin. Transdermal patches deliver a slow, steady, stable level of medication to the body. Steps for applying transdermal medications are outlined in Hands On Procedure 8-7 on page 319.

## TOPICAL MEDICATIONS

Topical drugs act on the skin, but they are not absorbed into it. They're mainly used to soften, disinfect, or lubricate the skin. A few topical medications contain enzymes that help remove dead skin or cleanse skin ulcers. Others are used to treat minor skin infections.

The physician may sometimes tell the patient to apply the drug in a thin, even layer or to cover the area after applying the drug. The drug manufacturer may also have special instructions, such as applying the drug to a clean, hairless area of the body. Be sure that patients know and follow any special directions because the action of the drug may be affected.

## TRANSDERMAL PATCHES

Transdermal patches may be placed in several locations on the body, including:

- the chest
- the back
- the upper arm
- behind the ear

Drugs that are often given this way include nitroglycerin, which is used to treat cardiac problems, and scopolamine, which is effective in preventing nausea and dizziness associated with motion sickness. In the past few years, nicotine patches have become common over-the-counter anti-smoking aids, and birth control patches have become common contraceptive alternatives for women. In addition, pain medication can be delivered by transdermal patch, which eliminates additional discomfort and abuse while keeping medication at a therapeutic level to control pain.

When you apply a transdermal patch, remember these tips:

- Apply the patch to a clean, dry, nonhairy area of intact skin.
- Remove the old patch when you put on a new one.
- Put the new patch in a different site so that it does not irritate the skin.
- Do not shave the new site, because the razor may also cause irritation.

## Intravenous Medications

The fastest way to get a drug into a patient's body is by injecting it directly into a vein. This route is called IV injection. Drug action occurs almost immediately.

As a medical assistant, you may not have contact with IV medications. IVs are usually administered in hospitals rather than in physician's offices. Furthermore, state law often allows only physicians, registered nurses, and other licensed health care professionals to insert an IV line into a vein. However, in a few states, medical practice laws do allow a medical assistant to establish peripheral IV lines. Also, you may see references to IV medications in a patient's medical record, so you should be familiar with them.

After an IV is started, the type of IV fluid and the drug added to the solution are documented in the patient's medical record. The rate of infusion, as it is called, should be checked every 15 to 30 minutes.

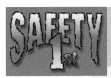

### WATCH FOR INFILTRATION AND EXTRAVASATION

For a patient receiving an IV infusion, the needle site should be inspected periodically for signs of redness, swelling, or other problems. Swelling around the needle may indicate infiltration or extravasation. **Extravasation** is the escape of fluid from a blood vessel into surrounding tissues while the needle is in the vein. If the needle or catheter slips out of the vein, fluid from the IV can leak out and build up inside the subcutaneous tissue. This problem is called **infiltration**. If either of these problems occurs, the IV infusion must be stopped. Then, the IV line must be taken out and inserted in another vein. Some drugs can cause severe tissue damage if extravasation or infiltration occurs. Because of this risk, the health care provider should be notified immediately.

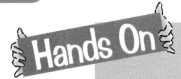

## HANDS ON PROCEDURE 8-1: ADMINISTERING ORAL MEDICATIONS

This procedure should take 5 minutes.

1. Wash your hands and gather your supplies, including the physician's order, the correct oral medication, a disposable calibrated cup, a glass of water, and the patient's medical record.

2. Check the medication label and compare it to the physician's order. Note the expiration date. Remember to check the medication label three times—when taking the medication from the shelf, when measuring, and when returning it to the shelf.

3. If necessary, calculate the correct dose.

4. For a multidose container, remove the cap from the container. Touch only the outside of the lid to avoid contaminating the inside. Single, or unit-dose, medications come individually wrapped. Packages may be opened by pushing the medication through the foil backing or by peeling back a tab on one corner.

5. Remove the correct dose of medication according to your calculations and the label.

   A. For solid medications:
      • Pour the correct dose into the bottle cap to prevent contamination.
      • Transfer the medication to a disposable cup.

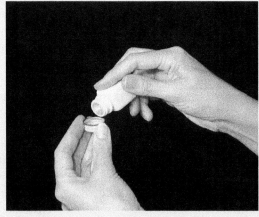

Pour the tablet into the bottle cap.

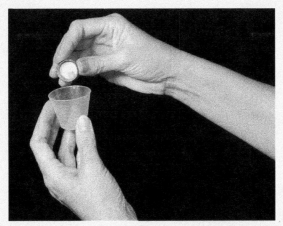

Transfer the medication to a disposable cup.

B. For liquid medications:
- Open the bottle and put the lid on a flat surface. The open end of the lid should face up to prevent contamination of the inside of the cap.
- Palm the label to prevent liquids from dripping onto the label. You do not want the label to become unreadable.
- With the opposite hand, place your thumbnail at the correct calibration on the cup. Holding the cup at eye level, pour the proper amount of medication into the cup. Use your thumbnail as a guide.

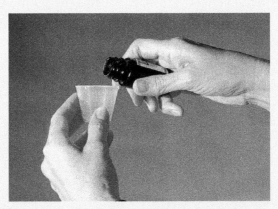

Palm the label of the container when pouring liquids.

6. Greet the patient and verify his name to avoid errors. Explain the procedure. Ask the patient about any medication allergies that may not be noted on the chart.

7. Give the patient a glass of water to wash down the medication, unless contraindicated (as in the case of lozenges or cough syrup). Hand the patient the disposable cup containing the medication.

8. Remain with the patient to be sure all the medication is swallowed. Observe any unusual reactions and report them to the physician.

9. Thank the patient and give any additional instructions as necessary.

10. Wash your hands and record the procedure in the patient's medical record.

**Charting Example:**

12/14/20XX 8:45 A.M. Ampicillin 125 mg PO given to patient—NKA. _____
_____ B. Rodriguez, CMA

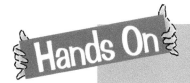

## HANDS ON PROCEDURE 8-2: PREPARING INJECTIONS

This procedure should take 5 minutes.

1. Wash your hands and gather your supplies, including the physician's order, medication for the injection in an ampule or vial, antiseptic wipes, a needle and syringe of appropriate size, a small gauze pad, a biohazard sharps container, and the patient's medical record. Choose the needle and syringe according to the route of administration, type of medication, and size of the patient.

2. Review the medication order and compare it to the label on the medication container. Check the expiration date. Remember to check the medication label three times— when taking the medication from the shelf, while drawing it up into the syringe, and when returning it to the shelf.

3. Calculate the correct dose, if necessary.

4. Open the needle and syringe package. Assemble if necessary. Make sure the needle is attached firmly to the syringe by grasping the needle at the hub and turning it clockwise on the syringe. A needle that isn't firmly attached may come off during the procedure.

5. Withdraw the correct amount of medication.

    A. From an ampule:
    - With the fingertips of one hand, tap the stem of the ampule lightly to remove any medication in or above the neck.
    - With an alcohol wipe, wipe the neck of the ampule where the break will occur. Wrap a piece of gauze around the neck to protect your fingers from broken glass. Snap the stem off the ampule with a quick downward movement of the gauze. Be sure to aim the break away from your face. Dispose of the ampule top in a biohazard sharps container.
    - After removing the needle guard, insert a filtered needle into the ampule. The needle lumen should be below the level of medication.
    - Withdraw the medication by pulling back on the plunger of the syringe. Take care not to touch the needle to the contaminated edge of the broken ampule. After you've withdrawn the correct amount, discard the ampule in the biohazard sharps container.

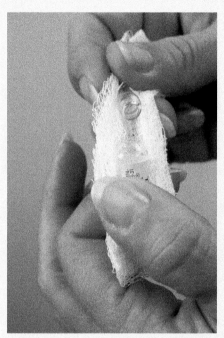

Grasp the gauze and ampule firmly when you
snap off the top of the ampule.

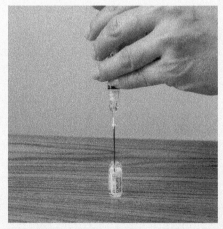

When withdrawing the medicine, be careful not
to touch the edge of the broken ampule.

- Hold the syringe with the needle up. Remove any air bubbles by gently tapping the barrel of the syringe until the bubbles rise to the top. Draw back on the plunger to add a small amount of air. Then, gently push the plunger forward to eject the air from the syringe. Be careful not to eject any medication.

B. From a vial:
  - Cleanse the stopper of the vial with an antiseptic wipe.
  - Remove the needle guard. Pull back on the plunger to fill the syringe with a small amount of air equal to the amount of medication to be removed from the vial.
  - Insert the needle into the vial through the center of the cleansed vial top. Inject the air from the syringe into the vial above the level of the medication so that you do not make bubbles or foam in the medication. Injecting air into the vial prevents a vacuum from forming in the vial, which would make it difficult to withdraw the medication.

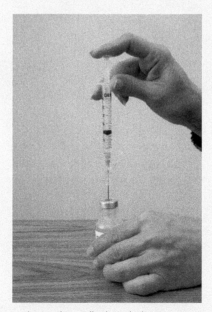

Insert the needle through the stopper
and inject the air into the vial.

- With the needle inside the vial, invert the vial, holding the syringe at eye level. Aspirate, or withdraw, the desired amount of medication into the syringe.

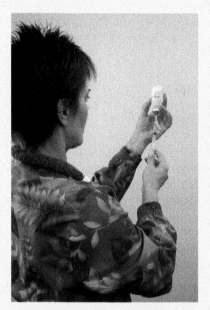

Invert the vial and withdraw
medicine at eye level.

- Gently tap the barrel of the syringe with your fingertips to displace any air bubbles. Remove the air by pushing the plunger slowly and forcing the air into the vial.

6. Place the needle guard on a hard, flat surface. Without contaminating the needle, insert the needle into the cap and scoop up the cap with one hand. It's best to place your other hand behind your back so you do not inadvertently puncture your finger with the needle. Recapping the needle protects the sterility of the needle until you administer the medication. You should use one hand to recap the needle to prevent needle sticks.

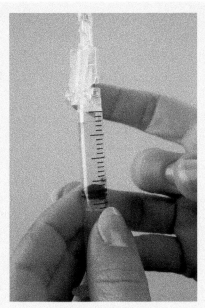

Tap the barrel gently to remove air
bubbles from the medication.

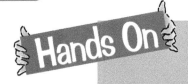

## HANDS ON PROCEDURE 8-3: ADMINISTERING A SUBCUTANEOUS INJECTION

This procedure should take 10 minutes.

1. Wash your hands and gather supplies, including the physician's order, medication for the injection in an ampule or vial, antiseptic wipes, a needle and syringe of appropriate size, a small gauze pad, a biohazard sharps container, clean examination gloves, an adhesive bandage, and the patient's medical record. Choose the needle and syringe according to the route of administration, type of medication, and size of the patient.

2. Review the medication order, select the correct medication, and compare it to the label on the medication container. Check the expiration date. Remember to check the medication label three times—when taking the medication from the shelf, while drawing it up into the syringe, and when returning it to the shelf.

3. Prepare the injection according to the steps in Hands On Procedure 8-2 on page 303.

4. Greet and identify the patient. Explain the procedure, and ask the patient about any known medication allergies.

5. Select the appropriate site for the injection. Recommended sites include the upper arm, thigh, back, and abdomen.

6. Prepare the site by cleansing with an antiseptic wipe. Use a circular motion starting at the intended injection site and working toward the outside. The circular motion will carry microorganisms away from the site. Do not touch the site after cleansing.

7. Put on gloves. You must follow standard precautions for your protection.

8. Remove the needle guard. Using your nondominant hand, hold the skin surrounding the injection site in a cushion fashion.

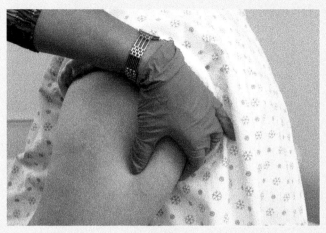

Holding the skin up and away from the underlying muscle will ensure
the needle's entrance into the subcutaneous tissues.

9. With a firm motion, insert the needle into the tissue
at a 45-degree angle to the skin surface. Make sure the
bevel of the needle is facing upward. Hold the barrel
between the thumb and index finger of the dominant
hand and insert the needle completely to the hub. A
quick, firm motion is less painful to the patient.

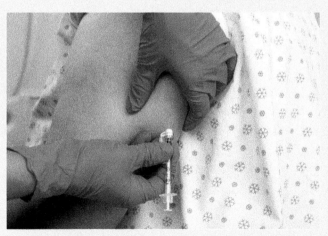

Insert the needle at a 45-degree angle. Full insertion of the needle
helps to make sure the medication goes into the proper tissue.

10. Inject the medication by slowly pressing down on the
plunger. If you press down on the plunger too quickly,
the pressure will cause discomfort and, possibly, tissue
damage to the patient.

11. Place a gauze pad over the injection site and remove the needle at the angle of insertion. With one hand, gently massage the injection site with the gauze pad and, with the other hand, discard the needle and syringe into the sharps container. Do not recap the used needle. Apply an adhesive bandage, if needed.

12. Remove your gloves and wash your hands.

13. An injection for allergy desensitization means the patient must stay in the office for at least 30 minutes so you can observe any reaction the patient might have. Note: If a patient has any unusual reaction after any injection, let the physician know immediately.

14. Document the procedure, site, and results, as well as any instructions to the patient.

**Charting Example:**

05/23/20XX 9:15 A.M. FBS 180. Regular insulin 5 units SubQ (R) anterior thigh. Manufacturer Eli Lilly Lot #114113-7 exp. 01/16/2007. Pt. tolerated injection well.

_____ C. L. Cho, RMA

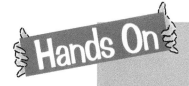

## HANDS ON PROCEDURE 8-4: ADMINISTERING AN INTRADERMAL INJECTION

This procedure should take 10 minutes.

1. Wash your hands and gather supplies, including the physician's order, medication for the injection in an ampule or vial, antiseptic wipes, a needle and syringe of appropriate size, a small gauze pad, a biohazard sharps container, clean examination gloves, and the patient's medical record. Choose the needle and syringe according to the route of administration and type of medication.

2. Review the physician's order and select the correct medication. Check the order carefully against the medication label. Make sure the expiration date hasn't passed. Remember to check the medication label three times—when taking the medication from the shelf, while drawing it up into the syringe, and when returning it to the shelf.

3. Prepare the injection according to the steps in Hands On Procedure 8-2 on page 303.

4. Greet and identify the patient. Explain the procedure and ask the patient about any known medication allergies.

5. Select the appropriate site for the injection. Recommended sites are the anterior forearm and the middle of the back.

6. Prepare the site by cleansing with an antiseptic wipe. Use a circular motion, starting at the injection site and working toward the outside. The circular motion will carry microorganisms away from the site. Do not touch the site after cleansing.

7. Put on gloves. You must follow standard precautions for your protection.

8. Remove the needle guard. Using your nondominant hand, pull the patient's skin taut. Stretching the patient's skin allows the needle to enter with little resistance and secures the patient against movement.

9. With the bevel of the needle facing upward, insert the needle at a 10- to 15-degree angle into the upper layer

of the skin. This angle ensures that penetration occurs within the dermal layer.

- The bevel of the needle must be facing up for a wheal to form.
- Stop inserting the needle when the bevel of the needle is under the skin. The needle should be slightly visible below the skin.

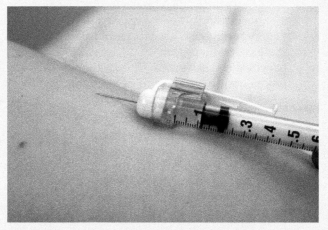

Insert the needle at a 10- to 15-degree angle.

10. Inject the medication slowly by depressing the plunger.
    - A wheal will form as the medication enters the dermal layer of the skin.
    - Hold the syringe steady! Moving the needle will be uncomfortable for the patient.

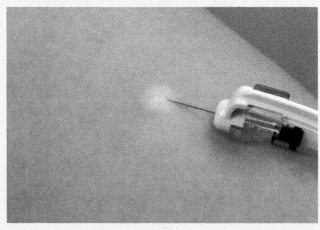

Observe for wheal while you're injecting the medication.

11. Remove the needle from the skin at the angle of insertion.
    - Do not use an antiseptic wipe or gauze pad when withdrawing the needle.
    - Do not press or massage the site. Pressure on the wheal may press the medication into the tissues or out of the injection site.
    - Do not apply a bandage—it may cause redness or swelling that could result in an inaccurate reading of the test.

12. To reduce the risk of an accidental needle stick, do not recap the needle. Dispose of the needle and syringe in a biohazard sharps container.

13. Remove your gloves and wash your hands.

14. Depending on the type of skin test administered, the length of time required for a reaction, and the policies of your medical office, perform one of the following:
    - Read the test results. Inspect and palpate the site for the presence and amount of induration.
    - Tell the patient when to return (date and time) to the office to have the results read.

15. Document the procedure, site, and results. Document any instructions to the patient.

**Charting Example:**

10/28/20XX 12:05 P.M. Mantoux test, 0.1 mL PPD ID to (L) anterior forearm. Manufacturer Sandoz Lot #3312666 exp. 02/15/2010. Pt. tolerated well. Pt. given verbal and written instructions to return to office in 48–72 hours for reading the results—verbalized understanding._____
_____ G. Ruiz, RMA

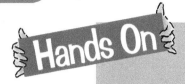

## HANDS ON PROCEDURE 8-5: ADMINISTERING AN INTRAMUSCULAR INJECTION

This procedure should take 10 minutes.

1. Wash your hands and gather supplies, including the physician's order, medication for the injection in an ampule or vial, antiseptic wipes, a needle and syringe of appropriate size, a small gauze pad, a biohazard sharps container, clean examination gloves, an adhesive bandage, and the patient's medical record. Choose the needle and syringe according to the route of administration, type of medication, and size of the patient.

2. Review the medication order and select the correct medication. Check the order carefully against the medication label. Make sure the expiration date hasn't passed. Remember to check the medication label three times—when taking the medication from the shelf, while drawing it up into the syringe, and when returning it to the shelf.

3. Prepare the injection according to the steps in Hands On Procedure 8-2 on page 303.

4. Greet and identify the patient. Explain the procedure and ask about any known medication allergies.

5. Select the appropriate site for the injection. Recommended sites include the deltoid, vastus lateralis, dorsogluteal, and ventrogluteal areas. Take into account the patient's age and size, as well as the medication, when choosing a site.

6. Prepare the site by cleansing with an antiseptic wipe. Use a circular motion starting at the injection site and working toward the outside. The circular motion will carry microorganisms away from the site. Do not touch the site after cleansing.

7. Put on gloves. You must follow standard precautions for your protection.

8. Remove the needle guard. Using your nondominant hand, hold the skin surrounding the injection site taut with the thumb and index or middle fingers. This makes the needle easier to insert in an average or overweight individual.

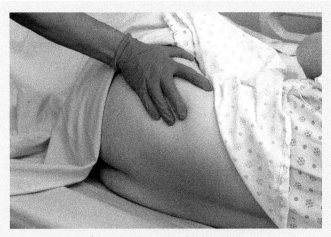

Hold the injection site taut with the fingers before administering
an intramuscular injection to ensure the needle's entrance into
the muscular tissue.

9. Hold the syringe like a dart. Use a quick, firm motion
to insert the needle into the tissue at a 90-degree angle
to the surface. Hold the barrel between the thumb and
index finger of your dominant hand and insert the
needle completely to the hub. This way, the medication will go into the muscle tissue.

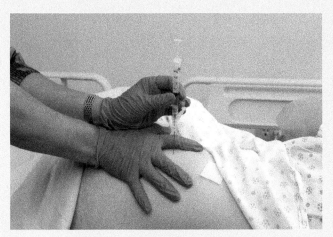

Insert the needle into the tissue at a 90-degree angle.

10. Remove your nondominant hand from the skin. Holding the syringe steady, pull back the syringe (aspirate).
    - If blood appears in the hub or the syringe, you've entered a blood vessel. Do not inject the medication! Injecting the medication into a blood vessel means the medication may be absorbed too quickly. Place a gauze pad over the injection site and remove the needle. Prepare a new injection.
    - If blood does not appear, you may continue with the procedure.

11. Inject the medication by slowly pressing down on the plunger. If you press down on the plunger too quickly, the pressure will cause discomfort and, possibly, tissue damage to the patient.

12. Place a gauze pad over the injection site. Remove the needle at the angle of insertion. With one hand, gently massage the injection site with the gauze pad. Massaging helps to distribute the medication. With your other hand, discard the needle and syringe into the biohazard sharps container. Do not recap the needle.

13. Apply an adhesive bandage to the site, if needed. Remove your gloves and wash your hands.

14. Observe the patient for any reactions. If the patient has any unusual reactions, let the physician know immediately.

15. Document the procedure, site, and results, as well as any instructions to the patient.

**Charting Example:**

04/13/20XX 9:35 A.M. Solu-Medrol 20 mg IM (L) DG.

_____ M. Santucci, CMA

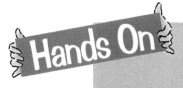

## HANDS ON PROCEDURE 8-6: ADMINISTERING AN INTRAMUSCULAR INJECTION USING THE Z-TRACK METHOD

This procedure should take 10 minutes.

1. Follow steps 1–7 as described in Hands On Procedure 8-5 on page 314. Note: The ventrogluteal, vastus lateralis, and dorsogluteal sites work well for the Z-track method, but the deltoid does not.

2. Remove the needle guard. Rather than pulling the skin taut or grasping the muscle tissue, pull the top layer of skin to the side and hold it with the nondominant hand throughout the injection.

3. Hold the syringe like a dart and use a quick, firm motion to insert the needle into the tissue at a 90-degree angle to the skin surface. Hold the barrel between the thumb and index finger and insert the needle completely to the hub.

4. Aspirate by withdrawing the plunger slightly. If no blood appears, push the plunger in slowly and steadily. Count to 10 before withdrawing the needle. This allows time for the tissues to begin absorbing the medication.

5. Place a gauze pad at the injection site. Remove the needle at the same angle at which it was inserted. Release displaced tissue after removing the needle. Do not massage the area. Discard the needle and syringe into the biohazard sharps container.

6. Apply an adhesive bandage to the site, if needed. Remove your gloves and wash your hands.

7. Observe the patient for any unusual reactions. Note: If a patient has any unusual reaction after an injection, let the physician know immediately.

8. Document the procedure, site, and results, as well as any instructions to the patient.

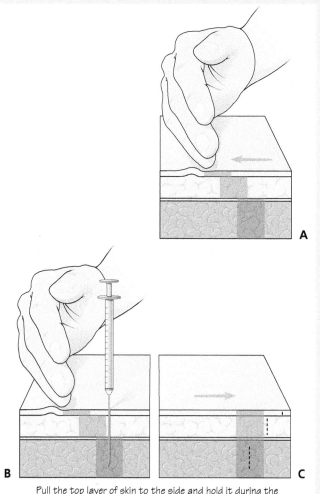

Pull the top layer of skin to the side and hold it during the injection (A). This way, when the needle is withdrawn (B) and the tissue returns to its normal position, the medication does not escape from the muscle tissue (C).

**Charting Example:**

01/19/20XX 4:15 P.M. Imferon 25 mg IM Z-track (R) dorsogluteal. Manufacturer Merck Lot# 339-095 exp. 01/31/2009.————————————————————
———————————————— B. Davis-Gumbs, CMA

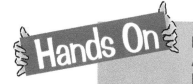

## HANDS ON PROCEDURE 8-7: APPLYING TRANSDERMAL MEDICATIONS

This procedure should take 5 minutes.

1. Wash your hands and gather supplies, including the physician's order, the medication, clean examination gloves, and the patient's medical record.

2. Review the medication order and select the correct medication. Check the order carefully against the medication label. Make sure the expiration date hasn't passed. Remember to check the medication label three times—when taking the medication from the shelf, when opening the medication package, and when returning it to the shelf.

3. Greet and identify the patient. Explain the procedure and ask about any known medication allergies.

4. Select the appropriate site for the medication. The usual sites are the upper arm, the chest or back, and behind the ear. Ideally, the best choice of site is a clean, dry, hairless patch of intact skin. These sites should be rotated with each new dose.

5. Perform any necessary skin preparation. Make sure the skin is clean, dry, and free from any irritation. Trim any hair close with scissors, but do not shave areas with hair. Shaving may wear away the skin and cause the medication to be absorbed too quickly.

6. Open the medication package by pulling the two sides apart. Do not touch the medicated side of the patch. The drug may be absorbed into your skin, causing an unwanted reaction.

7. Apply the medicated patch to the patient's skin following the manufacturer's directions. Starting at the center, press the adhesive edges down firmly all the way around. Starting at the center eliminates air spaces. If the edges do not stick, fasten with tape.

8. Wash your hands and document the procedure, including the site of the patch.

### Charting Example:

02/16/20XX 11:40 A.M. Transdermal nitroglycerin 0.2 mg/hr patch to left anterior chest._____

_____ J. Delgado, RMA

**Chapter Highlights**

- A medication label includes the name of the drug, the dose strength, and the expiration date.

- When you administer oral medications, check that you're giving the right drug at the right dose to the right patient. When preparing a dose, observe the necessary techniques and procedures to avoid contaminating the medication. Be sure that the patient swallows the full dose and watch for adverse reactions.

- For IM injections, the needle should be inserted directly into the muscle at a 90-degree angle to the skin. The appearance of blood in the syringe indicates that the needle has punctured a blood vessel instead of a muscle. If this occurs, a new injection must be prepared.

- The needle should be positioned at a 45-degree angle to the skin for SubQ injections. This places the drug into the tissues between the skin and the muscle. Drugs inserted this way include insulin and heparin.

- For intradermal injections, the needle should be inserted at a 15-degree angle between the upper layers of the skin. The intradermal route is usually used for sensitivity tests.

- Inhalant medications include bronchodilators, mucolytics, and some anti-inflammatory drugs. These drugs are administered through a face mask, nebulizer, or positive-pressure breathing machine.

- Topical medications such as creams and lotions act on the skin locally, but are usually not absorbed into the bloodstream. These medications are used to soften, disinfect, or lubricate the skin. They're also used to remove dead skin, cleanse skin ulcers, or treat minor skin infections.

- Transdermal medications are usually administered using a patch placed on the skin. The medication is absorbed into the body through the skin and produces systemic effects, delivering a slow, steady, stable level of medication.

- IV injection is the fastest way to get a drug into the bloodstream. Drug action occurs almost immediately.

- Infiltration occurs if the IV needle or catheter slips out of the vein, letting fluid from the IV leak into the subcutaneous tissue, causing swelling at the site. The IV line must be taken out and restarted in another vein.

# GLOSSARY

**acquired immunodeficiency syndrome (AIDS)**   A set of symptoms or infections resulting from a deficiency in the immune system caused by the human immunodeficiency virus (HIV) [Chapter 1]

**addiction**   A compulsive desire or craving to use a drug or chemical with a resultant physical dependence [Chapter 3]

**administer**   To give or apply medications in the health care provider's office; examples include flu shots, vaccinations for hepatitis or various childhood diseases, injections of penicillin or other antibiotics, and local anesthetics such as those given in a dentist's office before a procedure [Chapter 3]

**adverse reactions**   Undesirable effects caused by drugs [Chapter 1]

**akinesia**   Loss of muscle movement [Chapter 5]

**allergic reaction**   A drug reaction that occurs because the individual's immune system views the drug as a foreign substance [Chapter 4]

**alternative medicine or traditional medicine**   An option or substitute to the standard medical treatment plan; for example, herbal therapies, acupuncture, or hypnosis [Chapter 6]

**analgesic**   A drug that relieves pain [Chapter 5]

**anaphylactic shock**   A severe form of hypersensitivity reaction to a foreign substance [Chapter 4]

**antacids**   Over-the-counter medications that neutralize or reduce the acidity of stomach and duodenal contents [Chapter 5]

**antagonist**   A drug that joins with a receptor to prevent the action of an agonist at that receptor [Chapter 4]

**antianxiety drugs**   Drugs used to treat anxiety by depressing, or slowing down, the central nervous system [Chapter 5]

**antiarrhythmic drugs**   Drugs that treat arrhythmias, which occur when the heart beats too fast, too slow, or irregularly [Chapter 5]

**antibiotics**   Drugs that inhibit or destroy pathogenic microorganisms [Chapter 5]

**anticholinergics**   Drugs used to alleviate the symptoms associated with peptic ulcers; they work directly in the nervous system to inhibit the action of the neurotransmitter acetylcholine [Chapter 5]

**anticoagulants** Drugs that prevent or delay blood clotting [Chapter 5]

**anticonvulsants** Drugs used for the management of convulsive disorders; these drugs work to keep nerve cells from firing rapidly enough to cause a seizure [Chapter 5]

**antidepressants** Drugs used to treat depression [Chapter 5]

**antidiarrheals** Drugs used to treat diarrhea and constipation by slowing down peristalsis and decreasing the contractions throughout the colon that expel waste matter [Chapter 5]

**antiemetics** Drugs used to treat or prevent nausea [Chapter 5]

**antifungal drugs** or **antimycotic drugs** Drugs used to treat fungal infections such as diaper rash, oral thrush, and other infections of the skin and mucous membranes [Chapter 5]

**antigen** A substance that the immune system perceives as foreign and that causes the body to produce antibodies [Chapter 4]

**antihistamines** Drugs used to counteract the effects of histamine on body organs and structures [Chapter 5]

**antihypertensive drugs** Drugs that reduce blood pressure [Chapter 5]

**anti-inflammatory drugs** Drugs used to reduce inflammation or swelling and the discomfort of minor aches and pains [Chapter 5]

**antilipemic drugs** Drugs that lower the lipid levels in the blood [Chapter 5]

**antineoplastics** Drugs used for the cure, control, or palliative (relief of symptoms) treatment of neoplastic growth [Chapter 5]

**antiparkinsonian drugs** Drugs used to treat Parkinson disease by affecting the brain to decrease tremors and other parkinsonian symptoms [Chapter 5]

**antipsychotic drugs** Drugs used to treat psychotic disorders [Chapter 5]

**antipyretic** A drug that lowers an elevated body temperature [Chapter 5]

**antispasmodics** Drugs used to treat irritable bowel syndrome by slowing down or stopping smooth muscle contractions of the intestines [Chapter 5]

**antitubercular drugs** Drugs used to treat active cases of tuberculosis [Chapter 5]

**antitussives** Drugs used to relieve coughing [Chapter 5]

**antiviral drugs** Drugs used to treat infections caused by viruses [Chapter 5]

**autism** A developmental disorder characterized by impaired communication, extreme rigidity, and emotional detachment;

symptoms usually start to appear before a child is three years old [Chapter 6]

**anxiety**   A feeling of extreme worry or uneasiness that may or may not be based on reality [Chapter 5]

**bacteremia**   A serious infection of the blood [Chapter 6]

**barrel**   The part of the syringe and needle that holds the medication [Chapter 8]

**bioavailability**   The availability of a given amount of a drug after a portion of the drug has been absorbed into the bloodstream [Chapter 4]

**bipolar disorder**   A psychiatric disorder characterized by severe mood swings from extreme hyperactivity to depression (manic-depressive disease) [Chapter 5]

**bronchodilators**   Drugs used to relieve bronchospasm associated with respiratory disorders [Chapter 5]

**buffered caplets**   Medication specifically produced with a buffering ingredient, such as calcium carbonate, to prevent stomach irritation [Chapter 1]

**calcium**   A mineral found predominantly in dairy products that is necessary for many functions, such as the formation of strong bones and blood clotting [Chapter 6]

**calcium channel blockers**   Drugs that block calcium from reaching the muscle and prevent the smooth muscle walls of the arteries from contracting as much, thereby helping to keep coronary arteries open; may be prescribed for patients who suffer from hypertension or chronic stable angina [Chapter 5]

**capsule**   A gelatinous case enclosing a dose of medicine in powdered or granulated form [Chapter 1]

**chickenpox**   An infectious disease, caused by the varicella virus, typically affecting children under age 15; characterized by itching, fatigue, fever, and an uncomfortable blister-like rash usually appearing on the face, scalp, or upper body [Chapter 6]

**cholesterol synthesis inhibitors**   Antilipemic drugs that lower lipid levels by slowing the liver's production of cholesterol; sometimes called *statins* because their generic names end in the letters *-statin* [Chapter 5]

**common denominator**   The same denominator as another fraction's denominator; helpful in comparing the sizes of various fractions [Chapter 2]

**contraceptive drugs**   Drugs used to prevent pregnancy or to help manage certain menstrual disorders by preventing ovulation and by thickening the mucus produced in the cervix [Chapter 5]

**contraindications**   Situations or conditions that prohibit the prescribing or administering of a drug or medication [Chapter 4]

**controlled substances**    Drugs with high potential for abuse that are controlled by special regulations [Chapter 1]

**Controlled Substances Act of 1970**    The federal law that regulates the manufacture and distribution of dangerous drugs; requires that anyone who manufactures, prescribes, administers, or dispenses controlled substances register with the U.S. government [Chapter 1]

**convulsions**    The repeated contracting and relaxing of muscles that cause a person's body to shake in a rapid, out-of-control way [Chapter 5]

**corticosteroids**    Drugs that are often used to treat allergic reactions, skin conditions, rheumatic disorders, and other conditions [Chapter 5]

**cumulative drug effect**    A drug effect that occurs when the body has not fully metabolized a dose of a drug before the next dose is given [Chapter 4]

**cyanosis**    Blue, gray, or dark purple discoloration of the skin caused by abnormal amounts of reduced hemoglobin in the blood [Chapter 4]

**decimal fraction**    A proper fraction (meaning the numerator is less than the denominator) in which the denominator is a power of 10, indicated by a decimal point placed to the left of the numerator [Chapter 2]

**decimal numbers**    Numbers that have whole numbers to the left of the decimal point and parts of a whole number to the right of the decimal point [Chapter 2]

**decongestant**    A drug that reduces the swelling of nasal passages

**deficiency**    Occurs when the body has low levels of, or completely lacks, an essential vitamin [Chapter 6]

**denominator**    The bottom number of a fraction; shows the total number of equal parts in the whole [Chapter 2]

**depression**    A mood disorder in which feelings of sadness, loss, hopelessness, and helplessness get in the way of everyday life for periods of time [Chapter 5]

**diabetes**    A chronic disease of insulin deficiency or resistance; in type 1 diabetes, the body does not make enough insulin; in type 2 diabetes, the body makes enough insulin, but responds to it sluggishly [Chapter 5]

**dietary supplements**    Products containing ingredients that are meant to supplement, or add to, a person's regular diet; for example, vitamins, minerals, and herbs [Chapter 6]

**diuretics**    Drugs that decrease edema by increasing the secretion of urine (water, electrolytes, and waste products) by the kidneys [Chapter 5]

**diluent**  Diluting agent; used when preparing injections [Chapter 8]

**dispense**  To provide medications to patients either for current or future use [Chapter 3]

**dividend**  The number that is divided [Chapter 2]

**divisor**  The amount by which a number is divided [Chapter 2]

**dropper**  A tube with a rubber bulb attached to one end used to dispense medicine [Chapter 2]

**Drug Enforcement Administration (DEA)**  A federal service tasked with enforcing the Controlled Substances Act of 1970; monitors the use of controlled substances [Chapter 1]

**drug errors**  Mistakes including any occurrence that causes a patient to receive the wrong dose, the wrong drug, a drug by the wrong route, or a drug given at the incorrect time [Chapter 3]

**drug idiosyncrasy**  Any unusual or abnormal reaction to a drug [Chapter 4]

**drug tolerance**  A decreased response to a drug requiring an increase in dosage to achieve the desired effect [Chapter 4]

**DT vaccine**  A two-in-one vaccine that protects against diphtheria and tetanus [Chapter 6]

**DTaP vaccine**  A three-in-one vaccine that protects against diphtheria, tetanus, and pertussis [Chapter 6]

**dyspnea**  Labored or difficult breathing; shortness of breath [Chapter 4]

**elixir**  A form of medication dissolved in a solution that contains some percentage of ethyl alcohol, usually given to adults and taken orally [Chapter 1]

**emulsion**  A medication combined with water and oil; must be thoroughly shaken before it is taken so that the medication is evenly dispersed [Chapter 1]

**enteral medicines**  Drugs that enter the body through the gastrointestinal tract; most of these medications are administered orally in pill form [Chapter 1]

**enteric coated tablets**  Dry, compressed medication inside a coating that can resist stomach acids; the coating allows the medication to dissolve in the intestines instead of in the stomach [Chapter 1]

**excretion**  The elimination of drugs from the body [Chapter 4]

**expectorant**  A drug that aids in raising thick, tenacious mucus from the respiratory tract [Chapter 5]

**extract**  A highly concentrated form of medication administered as drops or in a liquid to hide its strong taste [Chapter 1]

**extravasation**  The escape of fluid from a blood vessel into surrounding tissues while the needle is in the vein [Chapter 8]

**fat-soluble vitamins**   Vitamins stored and then dissolved in the body's fatty tissues [Chapter 6]

**Federal Food, Drug, and Cosmetic Act of 1938**   A law that protects consumers from harmful health and beauty aids already on the market; an amendment of the Pure Food and Drug Act of 1906; also requires that a drug's safety be proved before it can be dispensed to the public [Chapter 1]

**fetal alcohol effects (FAE)**   A group of problems similar to but less severe than those of fetal alcohol syndrome [Chapter 7]

**fetal alcohol syndrome (FAS)**   A group of problems that includes low birth weight, developmental delays, behavior problems, and possible mental retardation [Chapter 7]

**fluoride**   A mineral that is essential for healthy teeth; found in some drinking water, but also prescribed as a supplement [Chapter 6]

**Food and Drug Administration (FDA)**   A federal agency responsible for approving and monitoring the sale of drugs and food products [Chapter 1]

**fractions**   Parts of a whole number [Chapter 2]

**gauge**   The diameter of the needle lumen [Chapter 8]

**gel**   A medication that is suspended in a thin gelatin or paste [Chapter 1]

**gelcap**   A soft gelatin capsule filled with an oil-based drug [Chapter 1]

**$H_2$-receptor antagonists**   Drugs used to heal gastric and duodenal ulcers by blocking histamine from getting into stomach cells [Chapter 5]

**half-life**   Time required for the activity of a substance to lose 50 percent of its primary efficacy [Chapter 4]

**hemoglobin**   A protein found in red blood cells [Chapter 6]

**hepatitis B**   An infection of the liver caused by the hepatitis B virus (HBV); spread by contact with blood, semen, or other body fluids from a person who has HBV [Chapter 6]

**hollow-handle spoon**   A spoon with markings to measure teaspoons and tablespoons of liquid medicine [Chapter 2]

**hormone**   A substance that is produced by an endocrine gland and travels through the blood to a distant organ or gland where it acts to modify the structure or function of the gland or organ [Chapter 5]

**hypersensitivity**   Condition of being allergic to a drug or other substance [Chapter 4]

**hypertension**   High blood pressure [Chapter 5]

**hypoglycemic drugs**   Drugs prescribed for patients with type 2 diabetes or those who cannot control their blood sugar levels with diet and exercise [Chapter 5]

**hypokalemia**  Low blood level of potassium

**immunization**  The act or process of rendering an individual immune to a specific disease [Chapter 6]

**infiltration**  The collection of fluid in a tissue [Chapter 8]

**inhalants**  Medications that are absorbed directly into the lungs by breathing, or inspiration [Chapter 1]

**insulin**  A hormone produced by the pancreas that helps maintain blood glucose levels within normal limits [Chapter 5]

**intramuscular injection**  Route of administration in which the drug is injected into the muscle tissue [Chapter 8]

**iron**  A mineral found in meat, liver, and egg yolks that is needed by the body to bring oxygen to cells [Chapter 6]

**laxatives**  Drugs that increase the urge to defecate [Chapter 5]

**lipids**  Fats or fat-like substances in the blood [Chapter 5]

**lowest common denominator**  The shared multiple of a denominator among a group of fractions [Chapter 2]

**lozenge or troche**  A small flavored tablet that is often used to release medication into the mouth or throat while dissolving slowly; the most common form is a cough drop [Chapter 1]

**lumen**  The inside diameter of a needle; measured by needle gauge [Chapter 8]

**monoamine oxidase inhibitors (MAOIs)**  Antidepressants which, because of their serious interactions with certain foods and other drugs, usually aren't considered unless all other antidepressants have proven to be ineffective; prescribed when the patient shows symptoms of atypical depression [Chapter 5]

**medication cup**  A liquid medicine container that often has markings for household, metric, or apothecary measurements [Chapter 2]

**meningitis**  An infection of the covering of the brain and the spinal cord characterized by vomiting, fever, headache, and stiff neck; frequently caused by a bacterial or viral infection [Chapter 6]

**meniscus**  The phenomenon in which the surface of a liquid may appear curved when observed from the side of a cup [Chapter 8]

**metered dose**  A measured amount of medicine [Chapter 8]

**mucolytics**  Drugs use to relieve coughing by acting directly on mucus; they break down sticky, thick secretions of mucus so that they may be eliminated more easily [Chapter 5]

**muscle relaxants**  Drugs that relax certain muscles in the body; used to treat a variety of conditions that range from stiffness to muscle spasms [Chapter 5]

**minerals**  Byproducts of the earth; found in food and needed by the body to stay healthy [Chapter 6]

**nebulizer**  A device that disperses a fine spray of medication to be inhaled directly into the lungs [Chapter 1]

**nicotine**  An addictive stimulant; nicotine from a cigarette enters the bloodstream and rapidly reaches the brain [Chapter 7]

**nitrofurantoin**  A drug used to treat acute and chronic urinary tract infections; once absorbed, the drug collects in the urine and works best when the urine is acidic [Chapter 5]

**nonprescription drugs**  Medications designated by the FDA to be obtainable without a prescription [Chapter 1]

**numerator**  The top number of a fraction; tells how many parts of the whole are being considered [Chapter 2]

**ophthalmic drugs**  Drugs used to treat bacterial infections of the eye [Chapter 5]

**otic drugs**  Antibiotics used specifically to treat middle ear infections and infections of the ear canal [Chapter 5]

**pharmaceutic phase**  The dissolution of a drug [Chapter 4]

**pharmacodynamics**  A drug's actions and effects within the body [Chapter 4]

**pharmacokinetics**  Activities occurring within the body after a drug is administered, including absorption, distribution, metabolism, and excretion [Chapter 4]

**phenazopyridine hydrochloride**  Drug used to relieve the symptoms of urinary tract infections [Chapter 5]

**physical dependence**  A compulsive need to use a substance repeatedly to avoid mild to severe withdrawal symptoms [Chapter 3]

**plunger**  The part of the syringe and needle that forces the medicine out of the barrel and into the patient's body [Chapter 8]

**pneumonia**  A serious infection of the lungs [Chapter 6]

**polypharmacy**  The use of multiple medications simultaneously [Chapter 4]

**potassium**  Mineral that aids with the functioning of the heart, kidneys, nerves, muscles, and digestive system; found in foods including bananas, oranges, and potatoes, and in supplements [Chapter 6]

**potentiation**  An effect that occurs when one drug increases or prolongs the effects of another drug [Chapter 4]

**powder**  A finely ground form of medication usually dissolved into liquid [Chapter 1]

**prescribe**  To order a medication or treatment plan [Chapter 3]

**prescription**  An order from a licensed health care provider to a pharmacist or a therapist for a treatment to be provided to the patient [Chapter 1]

**prescription drugs**  Drugs the federal government has designated as potentially harmful unless use is supervised by a licensed health care provider [Chapter 1]

**proton pump inhibitors**    Drugs with antisecretory properties [Chapter 5]

**psychological dependence**    A compulsion or strong desire to use a substance to obtain a pleasurable experience [Chapter 3]

**psychotic disorder**    A severe mental disorder that can have many causes [Chapter 5]

**Pure Food and Drug Act of 1906**    A law that regulates questionable practices within the food and drug industries [Chapter 1]

**reciprocal**    The fraction that results from switching the numerator and the denominator of another fraction [Chapter 2]

**quotient**    The number that results from the division of one number by another number [Chapter 2]

**Reye Syndrome (RS)**    An acute and potentially fatal disease of childhood that can occur after a viral infection; characterized by vomiting and lethargy, progressing to coma [Chapter 6]

**selective serotonin reuptake inhibitors (SSRIs)**    Antidepressants that cause fewer adverse reactions by allowing serotonin to build up in the neurosynapses [Chapter 5]

**seizure**    A periodic attack of disturbed cerebral function [Chapter 5]

**subcutaneous injection**    Route of administration in which the drug is injected just below the surface of the skin [Chapter 8]

**sublingual medications**    Drugs administered and absorbed under the tongue [Chapter 1]

**suppository**    Medication administered by insertion into a bodily passage or cavity; made partly of glycerin and cocoa butter, this melts at body temperature [Chapter 1]

**suspensions**    Particles of medication that are dissolved in liquid; must be shaken before they can be used effectively [Chapter 1]

**synergism**    An interaction that occurs when drugs produce an effect that is greater than the sum of their separate actions [Chapter 4]

**synthetics**    Drugs with foundations that are not organic; usually produced in a laboratory setting through chemical synthesis [Chapter 1]

**syringe**    A device used to inject or withdraw fluids; has ruler-like markings on the side of the barrel to show the amount of the drug inside [Chapter 8]

**syrup**    Very sweet, flavored form of medication that is high in sugar and usually administered to children [Chapter 1]

**tablets**    Medication that is colored and shaped for easy identification and easily cut to divide dosages; this form of medication usually dissolves in the gastrointestinal tract [Chapter 1]

**tar**    Cancer-causing particles from partly burned tobacco, marijuana, or other plant products; over time, these particles damage the smoker's lungs [Chapter 7]

**target place** The site within the body where a drug is intended to reach [Chapter 4]

**The Federal Food, Drug, and Cosmetic Act of 1938** A set of laws granting the FDA authority to oversee the safety of food, drugs, and cosmetics already on the market [Chapter 1]

**time-release capsule** Also called a spansule, a capsule that will release the medicine inside over time rather than all at once; the most common dosages are released over a period of either 12 or 24 hours [Chapter 1]

**topical** Applied as a cream or ointment for treatment of mild to severe itching [Chapter 5]

**toxic** Harmful [Chapter 1]

**transcutaneous medications** or **transdermal medications** Drugs administered in the form of a patch, topical cream, lotion, or ointment and absorbed through the skin [Chapter 1]

**urinary antiseptic, antibacterial,** and **analgesic drugs** Drugs used to treat urinary tract infections (UTIs), to relieve pain and other symptoms associated with UTIs, and to relieve the symptoms of an overactive bladder

**vaccine** Suspension of infectious agents or some part of them; administered to establish resistance to an infectious disease [Chapter 6]

**vasodilating drugs** Drugs that relax the muscles in veins and arteries, which allows them to open wider, or dilate; commonly prescribed to patients with hypertension [Chapter 5]

**vitamins** Organic substances needed by the body in small amounts for normal growth and nutrition [Chapter 6]

**water-soluble vitamins** Vitamins that pass through the bloodstream and leave the body through urination [Chapter 6]

**wheal** Transient elevation of the skin caused by edema of the dermis and surrounding capillary dilation [Chapter 8]

**whole numbers** The counting numbers 1, 2, 3, 4, 5, and so on [Chapter 2]

**zinc** A mineral that helps the body's immune system function properly; found naturally in seafood, meat, liver, eggs, peanuts, and in supplements [Chapter 6]

# INDEX

Page numbers in *italics* denote figures; page numbers followed by *t* indicate tables.